The evaluation and treatment of syncope

A handbook for clinical practice

EUROPEAN
SOCIETY OF
CARDIOLOGY®

The evaluation and treatment of syncope

A handbook for clinical practice

Second edition

A publication based on the Guidelines on Management (diagnosis and treatment) of Syncope by the European Society of Cardiology (www.escardio.org/knowledge/guidelines)

EDITED BY
David G. Benditt
Jean-Jacques Blanc
Michele Brignole
Richard Sutton

Blackwell
Publishing

Published by Blackwell Publishing
Blackwell Publishing, Inc., 350 Main Street, Malden, Massachusetts 02148-5020, USA
Blackwell Publishing Ltd, 9600 Garsington Road, Oxford OX4 2DQ, UK
Blackwell Science Asia Pty Ltd, 550 Swanston Street, Carlton, Victoria 3053, Australia

First published 2003
Second edition 2006

Library of Congress Cataloging-in-Publication Data

The evaluation and treatment of syncope: a handbook for clinical practice/edited by
    David G. Benditt ... [et al.]. – 2nd ed.
      p. XXX; cm.
Publication based on the Guidelines on management (diagnosis and treatment) of syncope
by the European Society of Cardiology.   Includes bibliographical references and index.
    ISBN-13: 978-1-4051-4030-0
    ISBN-10: 1-4051-4030-5
    1. Coronary heart disease–Handbooks, manuals, etc. I. Benditt, David G. II. European
Society of Cardiology.
    [DNLM: 1. Syncope–therapy. 2. Syncope–diagnosis. 3. Syncope–physiopathology.
WB 182 E92 2006]
RB150.L67E94 2006
616'.047–dc22
                                                                              2005021788

ISBN-13: 978-1-4051-4030-0
ISBN-10: 1-4051-4030-5

A catalogue record for this title is available from the British Library

Commissioning Editor: Gina Almond
Development Editor: Vicki Donald

Set in 9.5/12 points Meridien by Newgen Imaging Systems (P) Ltd, Chennai, India
Printed and bound in India by Replika Press PVT Ltd

For further information on Blackwell Publishing,
www.blackwellcardiology.com

Contents

List of contributors

*Member of the ESC Management of Syncope Task Force

Editors

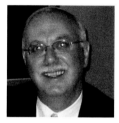

David G. Benditt, MD, FACC, FRCP(C), FHRS*, Professor,
Cardiac Arrhythmia Center, Department of Medicine,
Cardiovascular Division, University of Minnesota,
Minneapolis, USA

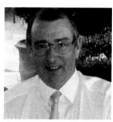

Jean-Jacques Blanc, MD, FESC*, Professor and Head,
Departement de Cardiologie, Universite de Brest, Hopital de la
Cavale Blanche, CHU de Brest, France

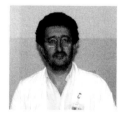

Michele Brignole, MD, FESC*, Chairman, European Society of
Cardiology Task Force on Syncope, Department of Cardiology
and Arrhythmologic Centre, Ospedali del Tigullio, Lavagna, Italy

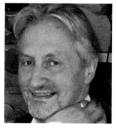

Richard Sutton, DScMed, FRCP, FESC, FACC*, Professor,
Imperial College of London, Royal Brompton Hospital,
London, UK

Contributors

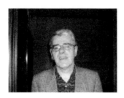

Paolo Alboni, MD*, Professor, Divisione di Cardiologia, Ospedale Civile, Cento, Italy

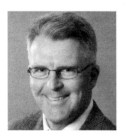

Lennart Bergfeldt, MD, PhD, FESC*, Professor of Cardiology, Sahlgrenska Academy, University of Gothenburg, Department of Cardiology, Sahlgrenska University Hospital Gothenburg, Sweden

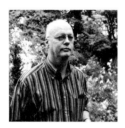

J. Gert van Dijk, MD, PhD*, Professor, Department of Neurology and Clinical Neurophysiology, Leiden University Medical Centre, Leiden, The Netherlands

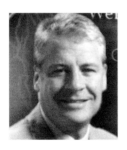

Adam P. Fitzpatrick, MD, FESC*, Manchester Heart Centre, Royal Infirmary, Manchester, UK

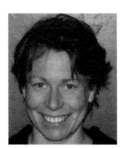

Karin S. Ganzeboom, MD, Department of Medicine, Academic Medical Centre, University of Amsterdam, Amsterdam, The Netherlands

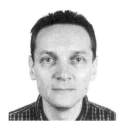

Jan Janousek, MD*, Klinik f. Kinderkardiologie, Herzzentrum, University of Leipzig, Leipzig, Germany

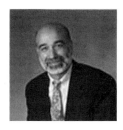

Wishwa N. Kapoor, MD MPH*, Professor, Department of Internal Medicine, University of Pittsburgh, Pittsburgh, PA, USA

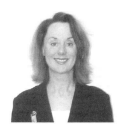

Rose Anne Kenny, MD, FESC*, Professor, Institute for the Health of the Elderly, University of Newcastle Upon Tyne, Royal Victoria Infirmary, Newcastle upon Tyne, UK, and Trinity College, Dublin, Ireland

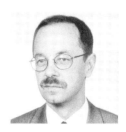

Piotr Kulakowski, MD, FESC*, Department of Cardiology, Med. Centre of Postgraduate Education, Grochowski Hospital, Warsaw, Poland

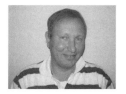

Johannes J. van Lieshout, MD, PhD, Department of Medicine, Academic Medical Centre, University of Amsterdam, Amsterdam, The Netherlands

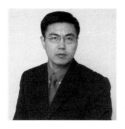

Fei Lü, MD, PhD, Assistant Professor, Director Cardiac Electrophysiology Laboratory, Cardiac Arrhythmia Center, Department of Medicine, Cardiovascular Division, University of Minnesota Medical School, Minneapolis, USA

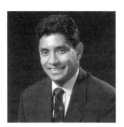

Christopher J. Mathias, DPhil DSc, FRCP, FMedSci, Professor of Neurovascular Medicine, Neurovascular Medicine Unit, Faculty of Medicine, Imperial College London at St Mary's Hospital, The Queen Elizabeth the Queen Mother Wing, London & Autonomic Unit, National Hospital for Neurology & Neurosurgery, Queen Square & Institute of Neurology, University College London, London, UK

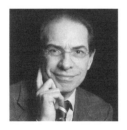

Angel Moya, MD, PhD, FESC*, Chief of Arrhythmia Unit, Department of Cardiology, Hospital General Vall d'Hebron, Barcelona, Spain

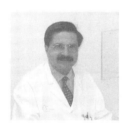

Antonio Raviele, MD, FESC*, Head, Divisione di Cardiologia, Ospedale Umberto I, Mestre-Venice, Italy

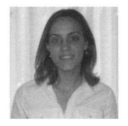

Anna Serletis, MD, Libin Cardiovascular Institute of Alberta, University of Calgary, Calgary, Alberta, Canada; Division of Cardiology, University of Calgary, Calgary, Alberta, Canada

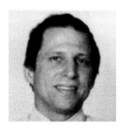

Robert S. Sheldon MD, PhD, FRCP(C), Head, Division of Cardiology, Libin Cardiovascular Institute of Alberta, University of Calgary, Calgary, Alberta, Canada; Division of Cardiology, University of Calgary, Calgary, Alberta, Canada

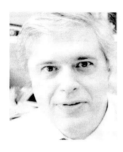

George Theodorakis, MD, FESC*, 2° Department of Cardiology, Onassis Cardiac Surgery Center, Athens, Greece

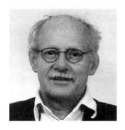

Wouter Wieling, MD, PhD*, Director, Syncope Unit, Academic Medical Centre, University of Amsterdam, Amsterdam, The Netherlands

Introduction

Michele Brignole

This handbook is based on *Guidelines on the Management (Diagnosis and Treatment) of Syncope* published by the European Society of Cardiology in 2001 and updated in 2004. The contributors are primarily comprised of Task Force members but other outstanding authorities in the field have also contributed to specific topics. The purpose was principally to provide a means for disseminating the *Guidelines* in a manner that was readily accessible to medical professionals and could be conveniently utilized in the office, clinic, and emergency department.

The Task Force was constituted in 1999 and the first edition of the *Guidelines* was published in 2001 (*Eur Heart J* 2001; **22**: 1256–1306). An updated edition of the *Guidelines* was published in 2004 (*Eur Heart J* 2004; **25**: 2054–2072 and *Europace* 2004; **6**: 467–537) and was the impetus for developing the second edition of this handbook.

The purpose of the ESC Syncope guidelines is to provide specific recommendations regarding the diagnostic evaluation and management of syncope. The creation of a panel of experts was justified by the fact that in this field, data from the literature are often not definitive, and there has been a lack of standardization regarding nomenclature, diagnostic procedures and their interpretation, and treatment strategies. There are several reasons for this. First, a major issue in the use of diagnostic tests is that syncope is a transient symptom and not a disease. Typically, patients are most often asymptomatic at the time of evaluation. The opportunity to capture a spontaneous event during diagnostic testing is rare. As a result, the diagnostic evaluation must focus on discerning susceptibility to physiological states that could cause loss of consciousness. This type of reasoning leads, of necessity, to uncertainty in establishing a cause. In other words, the causal relationship between a diagnostic abnormality and syncope in a given patient is often presumptive. Second, in the absence of documentation at the time of an event, the establishment of the cause of syncope depends critically on taking an accurate and detailed history. Currently, there is a great deal of variation in how physicians take the history and their knowledge base regarding the crucial information to be sought, and the interpretation of the findings. Third, since documentation of spontaneous syncope events is relatively rare, measurements of test sensitivity are not possible. Essentially there is lack of a 'gold standard' for most of the tests employed for this condition. Consequently, decisions have to be made based on the patient's history and abnormal findings usually obtained during asymptomatic periods. To overcome the lack of a gold standard, the diagnostic yield of many tests in syncope has been assessed indirectly by evaluation of the reduction of syncopal recurrences after administration of the specific therapy suggested by the results of the test(s) that were diagnostic. In the absence of randomized controlled treatment trials, inferences derived from follow-up observations are inherently suspect.

Given these issues the objectives of the Task Force were to provide:
• criteria for diagnosis of the cause(s) of syncope from history and physical examination;
• guidelines for choosing tests and determining test abnormalities in the further evaluation of syncope;
• advice regarding how to use the results of diagnostic procedures in defining the most probable cause of syncope; and
• recommendations regarding the most appropriate treatment strategy

The methodology for writing the basic Guideline document consisted of literature reviews and consensus development by the panel. The recommendations provided in this book are directly derived from that development process. However, since the goal of the handbook is to provide practicable specific recommendations for diagnosis and management for practicing care givers, recommendations are often provided even when the data from the literature is not definitive. In fact, as remains the case in much of medical practice, most of the recommendations are based on consensus expert opinion.

In order to facilitate reading, the handbook provides neither levels of evidence for every recommendation, nor literature citations for each statement. Key goals for each section are noted at the beginning of each section. Additional reading for each section will be found at the end of each segment of the text. Further, a relatively complete literature source, divided into major interest areas (e.g. pathophysiology, history taking, tilt-table testing) is provided separately at the end of the book. The interested reader is referred to the European Society of Cardiology Guidelines document for statements of levels of evidence and detailed literature citations (you can download this document from the guidelines section of the ESC website: www.escardio.org).

In this handbook the reader will find practical consideration of all the important clinical aspects of syncope:
• What are the diagnostic criteria for causes of syncope?
• What is the preferred approach to the diagnostic work up in various subgroups of patients with syncope?
• How should patients with syncope risk be stratified?
• When should patients with syncope be hospitalized?
• Which treatments are likely to be effective in preventing syncopal recurrences?

In respect to the initial document, the following sections of the *Guidelines* were widely revised in the updated 2004 document and, every effort has been made in this second edition to provide a parallel updated view of:

- classification of transient loss of consciousness;
- epidemiologic and prognostic considerations;
- initial evaluation and diagnostic flow;
- prolonged ECG monitoring;
- electrophysiological testing;
- ATP test;
- tools for risk stratification (e.g. signal averaged electrocardiogram, T-wave microvolt alternans);
- exercise testing;
- neurological and psychiatric evaluation;
- treatment of neurally mediated (reflex) syncope;
- syncope in the older adult;
- syncope in pediatric patients.

This book attempts to present the Guidelines information in a succinct form. It is directed toward practicing physicians who encounter syncope patients. Thus, we envision it being widely useful. It should be of particular value to practitioners in Emergency Medicine, Primary Care, Internal Medicine, Neurology, Pediatrics, and Cardiology.

Both the ESC Syncope Task Force Guidelines document and this handbook, owe their development to many individuals who planned the tasks, undertook the research, wrote the text, and provided the financial resources to bring these efforts to fruition. In particular, the authors very much appreciate the encouragement and support provided by the leadership and staff of the European Society of Cardiology and specifically the chairmen of the Committee for Practice Guidelines, Professor Jean Pierre Bassand (1998–2000), Professor Werner Klein (2000–2002), and Professor Silvia Priori (2002–2006), and their coordinating secretary, Ms Veronica Dean and her staff.

Section one:
Definition, pathophysiology, epidemiology

CHAPTER 1

Syncope: definition, classification, and multiple potential causes

Jean-Jacques Blanc and David G. Benditt

Introduction

The term 'syncope' is derived from an old Greek word meaning 'to cut short' or 'interrupt'. In modern usage, syncope refers to a transient and spontaneously reversible interruption of global cerebral activity resulting in loss of consciousness (and by inference, loss of postural tone). However, in the clinic, most English-speaking patients do not use the word 'syncope'. More commonly they will use terms that are more common in everyday language such as 'fainting', 'blacking out', 'collapse', or 'passing out'. In former days, the term 'swoon' was used, but this is rare today. Additionally, syncope must be considered as part of the differential diagnosis for patients who present with an apparent self-limited 'fall' or 'collapse' (Figure 1.1), even if it is unclear whether they suffered loss of consciousness.

The *'sine qua non'* of syncope (faint) is transient global diminution of blood flow to the brain, such that a disturbance of cerebral function occurs

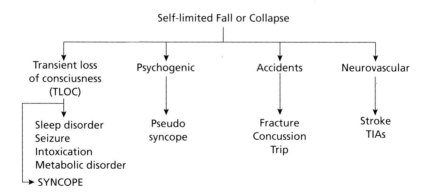

Figure 1.1 Scheme depicting differential diagnostic considerations for patients who present with a self-limited fall or collapse. Syncope is only one element of the differential, but is the primary focus of this book.

Table 1.1 Conditions often
mistakenly considered to be syncope.

Dizziness
Vertigo
Drop attacks
Falls
Psychogenic syncope
Transient ischemic attack (TIA)

(see Chapters 3 and 4). As discussed below and elsewhere in this book, this definition eliminates many other conditions that are often mistakenly (even in the literature) considered to be syncope (Table 1.1).

In terms of a practical approach to the clinical problem, physicians are most often first confronted with a patient who has apparently experienced an episode of transient loss of consciousness, or (as in the case of an unexplained 'fall' – suspicion of transient loss of consciousness). In this scenario, one should not immediately assume that the event was 'syncope', since it is not the only explanation for such symptoms. The broader term 'Transient Loss of Consciousness (TLOC)' is a better starting point, since it has a much more diverse set of etiologies and thereby requires the physician to consider a wider range of possibilities. Only if TLOC is due to transient inadequacy of global cerebral blood flow should the differential diagnosis begin to focus on those conditions typically responsible for 'syncope'.

Goals

This chapter provides an introduction to the concept of syncope as a symptom with many potential causes. Indeed, multiple possibilities frequently coexist in the same patient, thereby complicating the diagnostic dilemma. Specifically, the objectives of this section are to:
- define syncope;
- provide a classification of the principal causes of syncope in a manner consistent with the most recent ESC Syncope Task Force guidelines; and
- highlight the possibility that multiple potential contributing factors need to be considered when evaluating syncope patients.

Definition

Syncope is a symptom defined as a transient, self-limited loss of consciousness, and as a consequence the concomitant loss of voluntary muscle tone. The underlying mechanism is transient global cerebral hypoperfusion. The onset of syncope is relatively rapid and the subsequent recovery is by definition spontaneous, complete, and usually prompt. Residual symptoms (e.g. fatigue) may, however, persist for hours or longer in certain types of faints.

Elements of the definition of syncope

The definition of syncope incorporates five main components.

1 *Loss of consciousness.* This is a critical feature that has to be derived from the history taken from the patient or from those who witnessed the episode(s). If the history convincingly points to there not having been loss of consciousness associated with the patient's 'spell', the diagnosis of syncope is excluded – it is something else (for examples see Table 1.1). Beware, however, that the victim may deny (possibly due to memory deficit or embarrassment) having experienced loss of consciousness, and only careful interrogation of witnesses may determine the real state-of-affairs.

2 *Loss of voluntary muscle tone.* Loss of voluntary muscle control is inherent with loss of consciousness. Therefore, if standing, the fainter falls down; if seated he or she slumps over.

3 *Onset is relatively rapid.* As a rule, the onset of syncope is rapid, being no more than 10 to 20 s after onset of premonitory symptoms (if there are any such symptoms). Faints may be associated with any of a variety of warning symptoms (or none at all), and the nature of these (see Chapters 7 and 8 discussing the initial evaluation and medical history taking) may provide important clues as to the cause of the symptoms. On the other hand, many fainters either do not experience or are unaware of any premonitory symptoms. This lack of warning seems to be particularly prevalent in older individuals.

4 *Recovery is spontaneous, complete, and usually prompt.* This aspect of the definition excludes a number of conditions that may result in loss of consciousness, but which in fact do not reverse themselves to normal in the absence of medical intervention. Examples of such conditions are coma (e.g. hypoglycemia), intoxicated states (alcohol, narcotics, other drugs), stroke, or resuscitated 'sudden death' syndrome. Although states of intoxication usually reverse spontaneously, the relatively long time frame of the recovery distinguishes them from true syncope.

5 *Underlying mechanism is transient global cerebral hypoperfusion.* This element of pathophysiology differentiates 'true syncope' from loss of consciousness due to trauma (e.g. concussion) or seizures (epilepsy). Both trauma and epilepsy may lead to loss of consciousness with complete and spontaneous recovery, but their origins are not inadequacy of cerebral perfusion. With regard to epilepsy (see also Chapters 2, 17, and 23), perhaps the aspect that causes the most confusion is abnormal motor activity. In syncope, it is not uncommon for patients to exhibit jerky movements of the arms and legs for a brief period of time; nonexpert bystanders may incorrectly interpret these movements as a 'seizure' or a 'fit'. However, the jerky movements during a faint differ from those accompanying a grand mal epileptic seizure in several ways. They are of shorter duration, they tend to occur after the loss of consciousness has set in rather than before, and they are jerkier and do not have the 'tonic–clonic' features of a true grand mal epileptic seizure.

Causes of syncope: classification and single versus multiple etiologies

Later chapters in this book provide a comprehensive discussion of the most important causes of syncope and their appropriate investigation. Only a brief

Table 1.2 Syncope classification.

Neurally mediated reflex syncopal syndromes
Vasovagal (common) faint
Carotid sinus syndrome
Situational faint
  Acute hemorrhage
  Cough, sneeze
  Gastrointestinal stimulation (swallow, defecation, visceral pain)
  Micturition (postmicturition)
  Postexercise
Other (e.g. brass instrument playing, weightlifting, postprandial)
Glossopharyngeal and trigeminal neuralgia

Orthostatic
Primary autonomic failure syndromes (e.g. pure autonomic failure, multiple
 system atrophy, Parkinson's disease with autonomic failure)
Secondary autonomic failure syndromes (e.g. diabetic neuropathy, amyloid neuropathy)
  Volume depletion
  Hemorrhage, diarrhea, Addison's disease

Cardiac arrhythmias as primary cause
Sinus node dysfunction (including bradycardia/tachycardia syndrome)
AV conduction system disease
Paroxysmal supraventricular and ventricular tachycardias
Inherited syndromes (e.g. long QT syndrome, Brugada syndrome, short QT,
 arrhythmogenic dysplasia)
Implanted device (pacemaker, ICD) malfunction, drug-induced proarrhythmias

Structural cardiac or cardiopulmonary disease
Cardiac valvular disease
Acute myocardial infarction/ischemia
Obstructive cardiomyopathy
Atrial myxoma
Acute aortic dissection
Pericardial disease/tamponade
Pulmonary embolus/pulmonary hypertension

Cerebrovascular
Vascular steal syndromes

overview is provided here. Specifically, we provide a classification (Table 1.2) of the causes of syncope beginning with the most frequently encountered conditions, the neurally mediated reflex faints. However, it should be borne in mind that even after a thorough assessment, it may not be possible to assign a single cause for fainting. Often, patients have multiple comorbidities and as a consequence they may have several equally probable causes of fainting. Thus, individuals with severe heart disease may faint due to transient tachyarrhythmias, high-grade atrioventricular (AV) block, or even as a consequence of being excessively medicated. Thus, the physician must not be lured into the trap of accepting an observed abnormality as either the certain cause or the sole cause of fainting in a given individual.

Neurally mediated reflex faints are of several different types, but the best known is the common or vasovagal faint. This is the so-called swoon often seen in films (usually triggered in the movies by a painful or emotionally upsetting event). The vasovagal faint can occur in both healthy persons as well as those with health problems; it is not indicative of nervous system disease and should not typically initiate neurologic studies. The patient experiencing a vasovagal type of reflex faint is very likely to feel nauseated and sweaty before fainting, and often appears pale and feels clammy. After the faint, they often feel tired; this sensation may last for hours or days. Other reflex faints include carotid sinus syndrome, or faints triggered by micturition or defecation. Coughing, swallowing, laughing, or even forcibly blowing into a wind instrument may also trigger a faint, presumably on a reflex basis.

Orthostatic (postural) faints are also common, and most often are associated with movement from lying or sitting to a standing position. Many healthy individuals experience a minor form of this faint when they need to support themselves momentarily as they stand up. However, the most dramatic postural faints occur in older frail individuals, those who have underlying medical problems (e.g. diabetes, certain nervous system diseases), or persons who are dehydrated from hot environments or inadequate fluid intake. Certain commonly prescribed medications such as diuretics, beta-adrenergic blockers, antihypertensives, or vasodilators (e.g. nitroglycerin) predispose to postural faints.

Cardiac arrhythmias may cause faints if the heart rate is too slow or too fast. Occasionally, such faints occur in otherwise healthy people such as at the onset of a paroxysmal supraventricular tachycardia (SVT) episode. However, individuals with underlying heart disease (e.g. previous myocardial infarction, valvular heart disease) are at greater risk. In either case the faint tends to occur at the onset of the rhythm problem, before compensatory vasoconstriction has a chance to respond and support the central systemic pressure. Faints may also occur when a rapid abnormal rhythm stops suddenly, and a pause ensues before the normal heart rhythm takes over again. If this is for more than 5 s,

Table 1.3 Causes of 'spells' commonly misdiagnosed as syncope.

Disorders with impairment or loss of consciousness
Metabolic disorders, including hypoglycemia, hypoxia, hyperventilation with hypocapnia
Epilepsy
Intoxication (drugs, alcohol)
Vertebrobasilar transient ischemic attack

Disorders resembling syncope without loss of consciousness
Cataplexy
Drop attacks
Psychogenic syncope (somatization disorders)
Transient ischemic attacks of carotid artery origin

---

the patient can experience lightheadedness or a faint (especially if they are in an upright position at the time).

Structural cardiopulmonary diseases are relatively infrequent causes of faints. The most common cause in this category is fainting associated with an acute myocardial infarction or ischemic event. The faint in this case is primarily caused by an abnormal nervous system reaction similar to the reflex faints. In general, faints caused by structural disease of the heart or blood vessels are particularly important to recognize as they are warning of potentially life-threatening conditions.

Cerebrovascular disease is rarely the cause of a faint. Perhaps subclavian steal is the best example in this class, but it is extremely uncommon. In the absence of clear-cut fixed or transient localizing neurologic signs during physical examination, cerebrovascular disease as a cause of syncope is unlikely. As a rule, this category should be considered only after all other 'causes' have been eliminated.

As noted earlier, certain clinical presentations are unfortunately often mislabeled as 'syncope' (Table 1.1). In other situations, however, the medical history mimics that of a faint (see also Chapter 23), and the most important of these are worth noting here primarily because they are commonly confused with 'true' faints (Table 1.3). As a consequence of this confusion (often aggravated by the manner in which even well-known investigators present their findings in the literature), the process needed to arrive at the correct etiologic diagnosis is impeded. The most common conditions in this category include: seizures, sleep disturbances, accidental falls, and some psychiatric conditions (e.g. anxiety attacks, severe hyperventilation and hysterical reactions). Inner ear problems causing dizziness (vertigo) are also frequently mislabeled as faints. Neurologic and metabolic disturbances (such as diabetes) are rarely the cause of true fainting.

Summary

The methods recommended to determine the most probable cause of syncope and ascertain which treatment direction is most appropriate are reviewed in subsequent chapters of this book. Here, we have attempted to provide an introductory overview, so that the reader will better appreciate the value of understanding the pathophysiology, the differential diagnosis, and the need for a thoughtful evaluation strategy. In the end, however, it is important to bear in mind that neurally mediated reflex syncope, orthostatic syncope, and cardiac arrhythmias account for approximately 60 to 70% of the recognized causes of syncope. Further, in 20% of patients the cause of syncope may remain unknown in spite of an extensive and well-planned evaluation. In some of this latter 20% there may be multiple possible causes and distinguishing among them in an effort to find a 'sole' cause may be both impossible and incorrect.

Additional reading

Benditt DG, Goldstein MA. Fainting. *Circulation* 2002; **106**: 1048–1050.

Benditt DG, Sutton R. Tilt-Table testing in the evaluation of syncope. *J Cardiovasc Electrophysiol* 2005; **16**: 1–3.

Brignole M, Alboni P, Benditt DG *et al.* Guidelines on management (diagnosis and treatment) of syncope – Update 2004. *Europace* 2004; **6**: 467–537.

Kapoor W. Evaluation and outcome of patients with syncope. *Medicine* 1990; **69**: 160–175.

Sheldon R, Rose S, Ritchie D *et al.* Historical criteria that distinguish syncope from seizures. *J Am Coll Cardiol* 2002; **40**: 142–148.

Soteriades ES, Evans JC, Larson MG *et al.* Incidence and prognosis of syncope. *N Engl J Med* 2002; **347**(12): 878–885.

Thijs RD, Benditt DG, Mathias C, *et al.* Unconscious confusion. A literature search for definitions of syncope and related disorders. *Clin Auton Res* 2005; **15**: 35–39.

CHAPTER 2

What is syncope and what is not syncope: the importance of definitions

J. Gert van Dijk and Adam P. Fitzpatrick

Introduction

The literature surrounding syncope is extensive. However, its interpretation is undermined by the most basic of deficiencies, namely a consistent operational definition of the term syncope.

Goals
• Define syncope and review the rationale for the definition accepted by the European Society of Cardiology (ESC) Syncope Task Force.
• Illustrate that the use of imprecise definitions impairs understanding of the clinical problem.

The definition and its understanding

The European Society of Cardiology Task Force on Syncope defines syncope as:

> a transient, self-limited loss of consciousness, usually leading to falling. The onset of syncope is relatively rapid, and the subsequent recovery is spontaneous, complete, and usually prompt. The underlying mechanism is a transient global cerebral hypoperfusion.

The first part of the definition is wholly clinical in nature, while the last sentence describes an underlying cause. This distinction may be felt to be unwise because often neither the cause nor the mechanism of transient of loss of consciousness (TLOC) is clear. How useful is a definition of which an important part cannot always be assessed? Why was it necessary to include a nonclinical element?

The simple answer is that within the concept of syncope it was essential to include some disorders and also to exclude others that most clinicians would never label as syncope. A vasovagal faint should be included as should a temporary loss of consciousness due to cardiac arrhythmia, or to orthostatic hypotension, because all these phenomena have in common that TLOC is due to global lack of blood flow to the brain. However, TLOC due to a subarachnoid hemorrhage, an epilepsic seizure, or a brain concussion should clearly be excluded from this definition of syncope. These latter disorders may also present as TLOC, but often otherwise differ in many clinical features and in their underlying pathogenesis. For example, loss of consciousness in epilepsy is due to inappropriate firing of cortical neurons, whereas concussion is less well characterized but is not due to inadequate perfusion.

Various definitions of syncope
In the past, many researchers and textbooks used definitions along the following lines: syncope is 'a temporary self-limited loss of consciousness associated with loss of postural tone'. Such a definition is much broader than the one used in this book. Taken literally, such a broad definition encompasses both the disorders that were felt to be syncopal, but also the ones that most physicians would not now label as syncope. In fact, it is better used as a good definition of TLOC.

Readers may feel that these nomenclature distinctions are solely an academic question. Two examples are given in which a lack of precision was harmful:

1 A paper describing the prognosis associated with syncope was published in the *New England Journal of Medicine* in 2002. The report, part of the Framingham study, was retrospective in nature and spanned a period of 17 years. Syncope was defined as 'a sudden loss of consciousness associated with the inability to maintain postural tone, followed by spontaneous recovery'. One may wonder whether the physicians who diagnosed syncope over this period had done so according to this definition. If so, the study should result in a sizable number of epileptic seizures, concussion cases, etc. If, in contrast, physicians had applied a concept of syncope based on cerebral perfusion, such disorders (i.e. concussions, seizures) should not show up at all, meaning that the study was about something different than that which was implied by the definition provided in the manuscript itself.

Syncope was subclassified into various groups. For the present purpose only the group of 'neurological syncope' is relevant. In it, 47 cases of concussion are encountered, which seems a low number in view of the large number of person-years studied. These cases were not analyzed in the paper. The number of epileptic seizures also appears too low for the duration and size of the study. What is apparent from this paper is that some physicians had used a broad definition as stated in the paper, but most relied on another concept. The group of 'neurological syncope' also included cases of TIA's and stroke. This is most surprising, as TIA's almost never cause unconsciousness, and strokes are by definition not temporary. It is therefore apparent that many of the cases of syncope included in this study were cases of TLOC, and in this study syncope included TLOC with a wide variety of underlying causes, certainly not just cerebral hypoperfusion. The relative numbers of syncope due to an epileptic seizure, a concussion, a TIA, or a stroke must depend on the apparently rather individual concept of syncope used by individuals who entered patient data. What we can say with some confidence, is that different physicians used the term 'syncope' in different ways, and the clinical features, investigations and outcomes of syncope in this paper cannot be quoted with confidence.

2 A relatively recent manuscript published in the *British Medical Journal* defined syncope as 'a transient loss of consciousness, with loss of posture (that is, falling)'. This is also a broad definition, and again fits with a definition of TLOC, not of syncope. The authors divided syncope into cardiac, metabolic, psychiatric, and neurological groups. At first glance, this division appears to do justice to the definition, as consciousness may definitely be lost though a variety of means. But psychiatric mechanisms can only do so through circuitous mechanisms: some people can voluntarily evoke syncope through a Valsalva-like maneuver, but the cause of the unconsciousness is cerebral hypoperfusion, that is, it is true syncope. Somatization disorders and hyperventilation were stated as psychiatric causes of syncope. In the first, however, the brain keeps functioning so patients may look unconscious but are not. As for hyperventilation, it appears to be almost impossible to lose consciousness by hyperventilation (in subjects with autonomic failure it may worsen orthostatic hypotension, but if this contributes to unconsciousness, this too is true syncope). The group of 'neurological syncope' again includes epileptic seizures and TIA's, as well as normal pressure hydrocephalus (the latter two conditions would rarely be included even in the differential diagnosis of TLOC). 'Cardiac syncope' contained the four groups of syncope recognized by the ESC Syncope Task Force as true syncope. However, the ESC did not regard 'orthostatic syncope' and 'neurally mediated (i.e. reflex)' syncope as cardiac in origin.

These two examples, illustrate how an imprecise concept of syncope, that does not include a definition of the pathogenesis, leads to the inclusion of disorders in which consciousness merely appears to have been lost, but is not actually lost (i.e. it is not true TLOC), disorders where there is TLOC but it is not due to transient global cerebral hypoperfusion, or some conditions in which consciousness does not even look lost, (i.e., not even apparent TLOC). Imprecise usage such as exemplified here cannot help understanding, and runs the risk of complicating in the physicians' minds the most important distinction, that is the difference between syncope and epilepsy. Similar criticisms can be directed at many other published works, whose authors cannot be blamed for doing so in such a confused situation. However, henceforth it does mean that papers on syncope should be more precise in their nomenclature and should also be subjected to more critical reading. Readers must ask: was this really syncope?

Consequences of confusing TLOC and syncope

The inclusion of a pathogenesis in the definition of syncope has two important consequences. The first is that additional clinical features, not included in the definition, are needed to conclude syncope. An example is the presence of nausea and pallor in a young girl in whom TLOC was triggered by having her ears pierced; this points to neurally mediated reflex syncope; another example concerns a man fainting repeatedly after reaching the top of a flight of stairs, suggesting either autonomic failure or perhaps a cardiac origin, such as ischemia or rate-dependent block.

The second consequence is that the word syncope should not be used when there is insufficient evidence that TLOC was due to transient global cerebral hypoperfusion. In such cases, epilepsy cannot be discounted, and a term is needed to describe this situation. TLOC can be used to describe this condition. As said, its definition is akin to that of syncope, but with the cause removed and one addition. This important addition is that the term TLOC should not be used when the transient loss of consciousness is due to traumatic head injury; concussion should not cause much confusion with either syncope or epilepsy. Note that both the broad and narrow definitions referred to above are recognized in this view. Both are not just useful for clinical and scientific purposes, but also critically important for an accurate diagnosis and prescription of the correct treatment to prevent recurrences.

A word on epilepsy

Epilepsy is discussed elsewhere in this book (see Chapters 17 and 23). Nevertheless, a few remarks may be made regarding terms encountered when dealing with epilepsy. 'Seizures' are usually understood to mean 'epileptic attacks', but the International League against Epilepsy does not in fact firmly restrict the term to epilepsy. Every kind of attack associated with abnormal movement may be called a 'seizure', and sometimes is. 'Reflex anoxic seizures' is used to describe attacks in young children who are startled, often by a bump on the head, cry, lose consciousness, and who then exhibit jerking movements. The word seizures here does not refer to epileptic attacks, but to the movements that may accompany many types of TLOC. These attacks are examples of reflex syncope (equivalent to neurally mediated reflex syncope) of the emotionally induced or vasovagal type (in infants this often leads to asystole). The attacks are also described as pallid breath-holding spells, a term that also does not convey that this is syncope (in the cyanotic type prolonged expiratory apnea does appear to play a role, but neither term implies voluntary breath holding). The jerking movements that may accompany syncope, and that should be distinguished from epileptic clonic movements, are sometimes called convulsions giving rise to convulsive syncope. Again, this does not imply an epileptic nature, since 'syncope' with or without convulsions means that TLOC was due to transient cerebral hypoperfusion.

In the United States, the term 'seizure disorder' appears to be preferred over epilepsy. Apparently, the word seizure is restricted to epilepsy for some, while it can also include convulsive syncope for others. It would be preferable to restrict it to one sense, and the one that is preferable is the most widely used one: seizures mean an epileptic attack and nothing else.

Sometimes the term 'non-epileptic attack disorder (NEAD)' is used to indicate attacks that look like epilepsy but are not, and that are of a psychogenic nature. Syncope is obviously nonepileptic, but definitely not psychogenic. Moreover, there are also psychogenic attacks that resemble syncope (sometimes termed psychogenic pseudosyncope) more than they resemble epilepsy. Those working with syncope might choose to label this condition as 'non-syncopal attack disorder' but this would cause the same problems as NEAD. It might be better to label such attacks as psychogenic instead of emphasizing what they are not. Alternatives are pseudosyncope and pseudoseizures.

A wider framework

There is one further definition required, and that is for patients who have abrupt loss of postural tone, but in whom it is not certain whether consciousness was lost or not. Elderly patients may be completely unaware after the fact that they had temporarily lost consciousness. Such cases may present with falls of an undermined nature. Sometimes, the fall is clearly attributable to an external cause, such as a trip on an uneven floor and sometimes the cause appeared to reside in the patient, where the fall was actually precipitated by syncope. When consciousness was lost, one may conclude TLOC and then try to determine its cause. But when this is not the case, or the cause is uncertain, a term is needed that leaves all possibilities open, to stop physicians from jumping to conclusions, and forgetting the full range of possible causes. 'Collapse of unknown cause' may serve this purpose, but its use will depend on circumstances beyond those described in this book. This subject falls outside the scope of the ESC Task Force on syncope, and is discussed here only to broaden interest.

Summary

The syncope literature is extensive, but unfortunately it is characterized by substantial variability in the definition of what syncope really is. On first pass, this may seem to be an arcane academic concern, but as has been demonstrated in this chapter, nomenclature problems introduce real operational difficulties. The reader is encouraged to think of syncope in terms of the ESC Syncope Task Force definition provided above; specifically that subset of TLOC in which the pathophysiology is self-limited diminution of cerebral perfusion.

Additional reading

Benbadis SR. The problem of psychogenic symptoms: is the psychiatric community in denial? *Epilepsy Behav* 2005; **6**: 9–14.
Benditt DG, van Dijk JG, Sutton R, *et al.* Syncope. *Curr Probl Cardiol* 2004; **29**: 152–229.

Chen-Scarabelli C, Scarabelli TM. Neurocardiogenic syncope. *Brit Med J* 2004; **329**: 336–341.

Soteriades ES, Evans JC, Larson MG, Chen MH, Chen L, Benjamin EJ, Levy D. Incidence and prognosis of syncope. *N Engl J Med* 2002; **347**: 878–885.

Thijs RD, Wieling W, Kaufmann H, van Dijk JG. Defining and classifying syncope. *Clin Auton Res* 2004 **14**: 4–8.

Thijs RD, Benditt DG, Mathias CJ, *et al.* Unconscious confusion–a literature search for definitions of syncope and related disorders. *Clin Auton Res* 2005; **15**: 35–39.

Zaidi A, Clough P, Cooper P, Scheepers B, Fitzpatrick AP. Misdiagnosis of epilepsy: many seizure-like attacks have a cardiovascular cause. *J Am Coll Cardiol* 2000; **36**: 181–184.

CHAPTER 3

Pathophysiology and clinical presentation

Wouter Wieling, J. Gert van Dijk, Johannes J. van Lieshout, and David G. Benditt

Introduction

Syncope is a syndrome defined as a transient, self-limited loss of consciousness due to inadequate global cerebral blood flow. The underlying mechanism is in almost all instances due to a fall in systemic blood pressure resulting in transient global cerebral hypoperfusion (a few rare cases of cerebrovascular spasm have been reported but verification is uncertain). Loss of postural tone, often mentioned as an additional element, is in fact an inevitable consequence of loss of consciousness.

A sudden cessation of cerebral blood flow for only about 10 s has been shown to be sufficient to cause complete loss of consciousness. Experience with tilt-table testing has taught us that a decrease in systolic blood pressure to 60 mm Hg or less invariably leads to syncope. Furthermore, it has been estimated that a drop of as little as 20% in cerebral oxygen delivery is sufficient to cause unconsciousness.

In healthy young persons, cerebral blood flow lies in the range of 50–60 mL per 100 g of brain tissue per min, representing about 12–15% of resting cardiac output. A flow of this magnitude easily meets the minimum oxygen (O_2) requirement to sustain consciousness (approximately 3.0–3.5 mL O_2/100 g tissue/min). However, the safety factor for O_2 delivery may be markedly impaired in older individuals or in those with diseases like diabetes mellitus or hypertension.

The integrity of a number of control mechanisms is crucial for maintaining adequate cerebral O_2 delivery:

• Arterial baroreceptor-induced adjustments of systemic vascular resistance, cardiac contractility, and heart rate all act to modify systemic circulatory dynamics in order to protect cerebral blood flow.

• Intravascular volume regulation, incorporating renal and hormonal influences, helps to maintain central blood volume.

• Cerebrovascular autoregulation permits cerebral blood flow to be maintained over a relatively wide range of perfusion pressures.

Transient failure of protective mechanisms or the additional effects of other factors such as vasodilator drugs, diuretics, dehydration, or hemorrhage, any of which reduce systemic blood pressure below the autoregulatory range, may induce a syncope episode. Risk of failure of normal protective compensatory mechanisms is greatest in older patients or those who are ill.

This chapter discusses physiologic factors affecting the supply of blood to the brain, and discusses the clinical presentation of syncope, inasmuch as the clinical findings illuminate the pathophysiology of syncope. In addition, since failure of compensatory adjustments to orthostatic stress is thought to play an important role in the vast majority of patients with syncope (this concept forms the basis for the use of tilt testing in the evaluation of patients with syncope), a brief review of normal orthostatic blood pressure adjustment is provided first.

Goals

The goals of this chapter are to:
- review orthostatic blood pressure adjustment;
- discuss factors that may cause systemic hypotension and insufficient cerebral blood supply:
  - low cardiac output
  - low peripheral vascular resistance
  - increased cerebrovascular resistance to blood flow; and
- discuss clinical presentation patterns of syncope.

Orthostatic blood pressure adjustment

On moving from the supine to the erect posture there is a large gravitational shift of blood away from the chest to the distensible venous capacitance system below the diaphragm (Figure 3.1). This shift is estimated to total 0.5–1 L of thoracic blood, and largely occurs in the first 10 s of standing. In addition, with prolonged standing, the high capillary transmural pressure in dependent parts of the body causes a filtration of protein-free fluid into the interstitial spaces. It is estimated that this results in a decrease of about 15–20% (700 mL) in plasma volume in 10 min in healthy humans. As a consequence of this gravitationally induced blood pooling and the superimposed decline in plasma volume, the return of venous blood to the heart is reduced. This decline results in a rapid diminution of cardiac filling pressure and a decrease in SV.

Despite the decreased cardiac output associated with movement to the upright posture, a fall in mean arterial pressure is prevented by compensatory vasoconstriction of the resistance and the capacitance vessels in the splanchnic, musculocutaneous, and renal vascular beds and by an increase in heart rate. The vasoconstriction of systemic blood vessels is the key factor in the maintenance of arterial blood pressure in the upright posture. A pronounced heart rate increase on its own is insufficient to maintain cardiac output: the heart cannot pump blood that it does not receive.

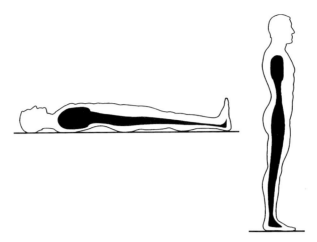

Figure 3.1 Schematic drawing illustrating the influence of posture on intravascular volume. Note that in the supine figure (left), central blood volume (intrathoracic) is greater than when the figure is upright (right). The shift in blood volume to the lower extremities reduces venous return and cardiac output.

Rapid short-term compensation for the hemodynamic instability associated with orthostatic stress is mediated exclusively by the autonomic nervous system. During prolonged orthostatic stress, further compensation is effected by the humoral limb of the neuroendocrine system (i.e. renin–angiotensin–aldosterone system and vasopressin).

The main sensory receptors involved in orthostatic neural reflex adjustments are the arterial mechanoreceptors (baroreceptors) located in the aortic arch and carotid sinuses (Figure 3.2). Mechanoreceptors located in the heart and the lungs (cardiopulmonary receptors) are thought to play a minor role. Reflex activation of central sympathetic outflow to the systemic blood vessels can be reinforced by local mechanisms such as the veno-arteriolar reflex and a myogenic response of the smooth muscle of the resistance vessels in the dependent parts. The skeletal muscle pump and the 'respiratory pump' play important adjunctive roles in maintenance of arterial pressure in the upright posture by promoting venous return. Static increase in skeletal muscle tone of the lower limbs opposes orthostatic pooling of blood in limb veins. This latter mechanism occurs even in the absence of physical movement by the patient. However, any such movement (e.g. walking) would be expected to be of additional benefit by enhancing muscle-pumping activity.

Factors that may cause insufficient cerebral blood supply
Pathophysiologic mechanisms
Cerebral perfusion pressure is largely dependent on systemic arterial pressure, which in turn depends on cardiac output and peripheral vascular resistance. Thus, anything that decreases either or both of these latter two factors

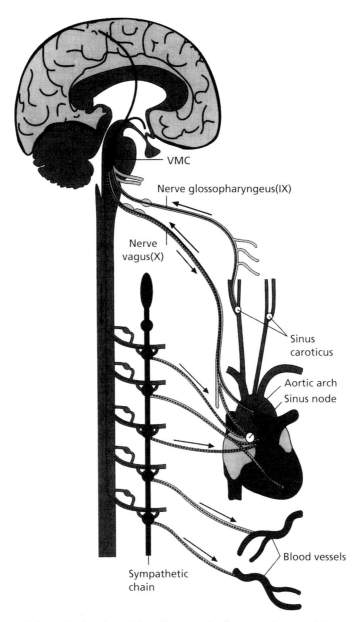

Figure 3.2 Schematic drawing of the afferent and efferent pathways of the arterial baroreceptor reflex arc. Nerve fibers from the lungs and the heart (not shown) join the vagus nerve as cardiopulmonary afferents. VMC indicates vasomotor centers in the brainstem. (Revised after Timmers HJ, Weiling W, Karemaker JM, Marres HA, Lenders JW. *Ned Tijdschr Geneeskd* 2001; **145**: 1413–1416.)

Table 3.1 A physiologic approach to the causes of syncope.

Syncope primarily due to low peripheral resistance
Neural reflex syncope disorders such as vasovagal faint
Widespread cutaneous vasodilatation such as occurs during thermal stress
Vasodilator drugs
Autonomic neuropathies

Syncope primarily due to low cardiac output
Inadequate venous return – due either to excessive venous pooling or to low blood volume
Cardiac causes such as bradyarrhythmias, tachyarrhythmias, valvular heart disease and
  diminished left ventricular function

Syncope primarily due to increased resistance to cerebral blood flow
Low PCO_2 due to hyperventilation (arguable)

---

will diminish systemic arterial pressure and cerebral perfusion pressure and may thereby predispose to syncope. In addition to these two factors, any impairment to blood flow in the cerebrovascular vessels themselves, such as vasoconstriction, will also increase the chances of syncope.

A physiologic classification of mechanisms leading to reduced cerebral perfusion and syncope can be derived from the basic principles outlined above. A simple classification is summarized in Table 3.1 and each category is discussed briefly here.

Low peripheral resistance
Widespread and excessive vasodilatation may play a critical role in decreasing arterial pressure and thereby diminishing cerebral blood flow. In fact, this is the most frequent cause of cerebral hypoperfusion leading to syncope. Excessive vasodilatation is the main cause of fainting in the neural reflex syncope disorders. These disorders refer to conditions in which neural reflexes that are normally useful in controlling the circulation (i.e. maintaining blood pressure) respond paradoxically. This results in a fall of systemic blood pressure due to vasodilatation and/or bradycardia (vasovagal reaction). In order to elicit this reflex a normal or functioning autonomic nervous system is necessary, in contrast to syncope due to orthostatic hypotension in patients with autonomic failure. Circumstances known to evoke neural reflex syncope are summarized in Table 1.2. It should be noted that the syncope induced by increased intrathoracic pressure is mainly due to a decrease in venous return and is only partially reflex mediated.

Impaired capacity to increase vascular resistance during standing is the principal cause of orthostatic hypotension and syncope in patients using vasoactive drugs, and in patients with various primary and secondary autonomic neuropathies. A similar problem may arise in some patients with paroxysmal tachycardias (supraventricular or ventricular). Apart from the potential adverse hemodynamic impact of the rapid heart rate alone, inadequate vasoconstriction (especially at the onset of an episode) may contribute to the severity of symptomatic hypotension.

Low cardiac output
With regard to maintenance of an adequate cardiac output, the most import-ant physiologic determinant is the adequacy of venous filling. Venous return may become inadequate if there is an improper distribution of the circulating volume. An example is when blood is pooled excessively in lower parts of the body such as occurs in some patients during movement to the upright posture. Obviously, a diminished total blood volume will also predispose to syncope, especially in conjunction with postural change. A reduction in the central blood volume raises the lower limit of cerebral autoregulation to approxim-ately 80 mm Hg compared to the commonly considered value of approximately 60 mm Hg. Cardiac output may also be impaired when the heart itself per-forms inadequately due to bradyarrhythmias, tachyarrhythmias, myocardial dysfunction, or valvular heart disease.

The physiologic significance of changes in heart rate in the context of ortho-static stress merits consideration in this context. The relationship between heart rate (HR) and cardiac output (CO) is well known, namely:

$$CO = HR \times stroke\ volume\ (SV)$$

Although this equation is mathematically straightforward, it may be some-what misleading in relation to understanding of physiologic control of blood pressure. This is because SV is not usually independent of HR. Unless cardiac inflow (i.e. venous return) and cardiac contractility are enhanced, as occurs during whole-body exercise by the action of the leg muscle pump and high catecholamine levels, an increase in HR is accompanied by a decrease in SV. At higher workloads the increase in SV reaches a limit or SV may even fall, and especially older endurance-trained subjects have an impaired ability to maintain SV at high levels of exercise. Consequently, the increase in CO is much less than expected. Conversely, if venous return is impaired (e.g. during venous pooling in the lower limbs), an increased HR may not compensate sufficiently.

Supraventricular tachycardia rarely causes syncope, except when rates are very high (usually >200 bpm), or there is significant concomitant intrinsic structural cardiac disease (e.g. coronary artery disease, valvular stenosis, obstructive cardiomyopathy), or there is concomitant inadequate neural reflex vasoconstriction as discussed earlier. Ventricular tachycardia, in contrast, is a frequent cause of syncope or near-syncope. However, in this case it is usually the presence of underlying heart disease (especially left ventricular dysfunction) that is responsible for the susceptibility to symptomatic hypo-tension. In the absence of structural heart disease, even relatively rapid ventricular tachycardias may not cause syncope.

As far as a low HR is concerned, the rate will have to decrease to well below 50 bpm (and more often below 30 bpm) for it to have a significant effect on CO (in the absence of concomitant significant structural heart disease).

Increased resistance to cerebral blood flow
Cerebral hypoperfusion may also result from an abnormally high cerebral vascular resistance. Studies both in healthy subjects and in patients with cardiac insufficiency support the view that cerebral perfusion may be affected by sympathetically mediated cerebral vasoconstriction as a consequence of a reduction in CO. Vasoconstriction induced by low carbon dioxide tension due to hyperventilation is probably the main cause but sometimes the cause remains unknown. It has been suggested that this mechanism may contribute to the vasovagal faint in some patients, but the concept is controversial.

Clinical presentation patterns
Documented records of the hemodynamic and clinical events that precede syncope during daily life are difficult to obtain. Consequently, voluntarily induced syncopal episodes under laboratory conditions have been studied. Two main approaches have been used. First, syncope may be induced instantaneously by using the combination of hyperventilation and straining. Second, the sequence of events during more gradually induced arterial hypotension can be studied by inducing vasovagal reactions in volunteers and patients using passive head-up tilt or subatmospheric pressure applied to the lower part of the body. In addition, observations in patients with cardiac syncope and patients with autonomic failure have contributed to the understanding of the events that are of importance for developing pre (near)-syncope or frank syncope symptoms.

The 'fainting lark': voluntary self-induced instantaneous syncope
The 'fainting lark' (see also Chapter 21) is a maneuver that combines the effects of acute arterial hypotension due to the effect of gravity and raised intrathoracic pressure with cerebral vasoconstriction due to hypocapnia. The maneuver can be applied to induce almost instantaneous syncope in volunteers and may be used as a research tool. It consists of squatting in a full knee bend position and overbreathing. The subject then stands up suddenly and performs a forced expiration against a closed glottis. This maneuver provokes a precipitous and deep fall in arterial pressure, and hyperventilation further reduces cerebral blood flow and the subject loses consciousness (Figure 3.3).

Lempert and coworkers applied the 'fainting lark' to study the sequence of events during syncope. Fifty-nine students aged 20–39 years volunteered for self-induction of syncope. Out of 59, complete syncope was induced in 42. Prodromal symptoms were short lasting (<5 s), which is not surprising given the precipitous and deep fall in arterial pressure and cerebral blood flow induced by the 'fainting lark' maneuver (Figure 3.3). The loss of consciousness

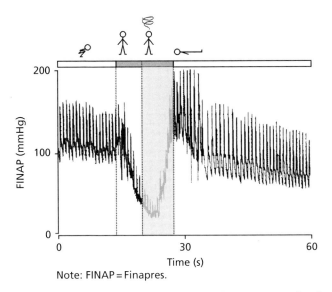

Note: FINAP = Finapres.

Figure 3.3 Effect of the 'fainting lark' on finger arterial pressure. For details about the procedure see text. Tracing obtained in a 54-year-old subject. Note instantaneous, deep fall in arterial pressure. At the nadir of blood pressure, the subject experienced a 'blackout'. Lying down, blood pressure recovers almost immediately and did overshoot. (Unpublished; by N. van Dijk and W. Wieling.)

lasted for 5–22 s. Myoclonic jerks were observed in almost all of the 42 syncope episodes. They occurred always after falling down and lasted for 1–16 s. During syncope, the EEG first shows large slow waves, signifying a profound disturbance of cortical function. When blood supply is not restored, these slow waves quite abruptly make way for a 'flat' EEG, pointing to a complete cessation of function of cortical neurons. Unless blood flow is restored quickly, neurons will start dying, which is not reflected in any further EEG change. Provided that blood flow is restored before irretrievable damage has occurred, the EEG changes back to the normal state in reverse order. Myoclonic jerks occurring during the slow and flat stages apparently originate on a subcortical level.

Vasovagal syncope
Vasovagal syncope, also known as the common faint, is the most common of the neural reflex disorders (Table 3.2). The key circulatory alterations responsible for a vasovagal faint are vasodilatation (the vaso component) and bradycardia (the vagal component).

   Prodromal symptoms and signs are usually present in individuals experiencing spontaneous vasovagal syncope in daily life or induced vasovagal syncope under laboratory conditions. There are two types of symptoms. The first, such as diminished vision and inability to think clearly, is due to a disturbance of retinal and cortical perfusion. Patients only become aware of such sensations

Table 3.2 Circumstances known to evoke neural reflex syncope.

Vasovagal syncope
Emotionally induced
Orthostatic induced

Spontaneous carotid sinus syncope

Eyeball pressure

Gastrointestinal
Swallow syncope
Glossopharyngeal neuralgia
Esophageal stimulation
Gastrointestinal tract instrumentation
Rectal examination
Defecation syncope

Urogenital
(Post)micturition syncope
Urogenital tract instrumentation
Prostatic massage

Pulmonary
Airway instrumentation

Increased intrathoracic pressure
Cough and sneeze syncope
Wind instrument player's syncope
Weightlifter's syncope
Mess trick and fainting lark
Stretch syncope

Special situations
High altitude
Exercise induced, diving

---

when there is sufficient time for symptons to develop (i.e. when the fall in arterial pressure and cerebral perfusion pressure is gradual). A gradual fall in pressure is common in vasovagal syncope but not in the fainting lark (compare Figures 3.3 and 3.4). However, about one out of three individuals with vasovagal syncope (especially older patients) have little or no prodromal symptoms and the syncope essentially occurs instantaneously without any warning (usually because of a severe sudden-onset period of asystole). A second type of prodromal symptoms is presumed to be the result of 'autonomic activation' with symptoms and signs of sympathetic overactivity such as tachycardia, sweating and pallor, and later of parasympathetic overactivity such as bradycardia and nausea.

Prodromal symptoms sometimes occur minutes prior to the actual faint, but a period of only about 30 s is probably more common. The patient begins to feel uncomfortable in an ill-defined way. This may be manifested by symptoms of epigastric discomfort and vague nausea, sweating, and a desire to sit down or to leave the room. If these early warning symptoms are ignored, the disturbances increase and symptoms like lightheadedness, fatigue, blurred and fading vision, palpitations, and tingling of the ears occur. The visual prodromal sensations are due to a reduction in blood supply to the retina. The eye, unlike the brain and brainstem, is not protected by the pressure-equalizing effects of the cerebrospinal fluid. Consequently, the retina is exposed to the intraocular pressure and visual symptoms that result from collapse of retinal perfusion become manifest before consciousness is lost. This relationship has been studied in detail by exposure of subjects to large G-forces in whole-body centrifuges. Sensations begin with diminution of vision, gray-out (loss of color vision), which can then lead to 'blackout'. The moment of 'blackout' occurs when the ischemic retina essentially ceases to function.

Objective signs of an impending vasovagal faint are facial pallor, sweating, restlessness, yawning, sighing and hyperventilation, and pupillary dilatation. The prodromal phase is most often associated with a relatively rapid heart rate (HR) (patient may note 'palpitation' during this phase). With continuing hypotension the individual has difficulty in concentrating and becomes unaware of his or her surroundings. Some patients at this stage can still hear the conversation, but cannot move. When blood pressure falls further, the patient loses consciousness, and if standing falls to the floor. Severe bradycardia usually occurs late, immediately prior to the actual faint (Figure 3.4).

The clinical picture during the actual faint resembles that of voluntarily induced syncope by the fainting lark. Myoclonic jerks, however, appear to be less common in spontaneous vasovagal syncope than in voluntarily induced syncope using the fainting lark. The duration of unconsciousness is almost always brief, usually lasting less than 5 min. Of additional importance in the overall clinical picture of vasovagal syncope are the postsyncopal findings, characterized by a persistence of pallor, nausea, weakness, sweating and oliguria, and a tendency toward recurrence of the reaction if the individual is returned to the upright posture too early. Fatigue, often lasting for several hours after the event, is also common (the latter observation led to the as yet controversial association of vasovagal physiology with certain forms of chronic fatigue syndrome).

Cardiac syncope
Syncope associated with heart block or with cardiac arrhythmias is usually characterized by sudden onset and absence of premonitory warning symptoms. However, in some patients with arrhythmias or heart block the onset is less abrupt, loss of consciousness need not be complete, and sweating along with a sense of palpitation may occur. Nausea is rare in cardiac syncope. The syncope episode may occur in either the erect or the prone posture. With cardiac arrest the patient is pulseless. Loss of consciousness usually ensues

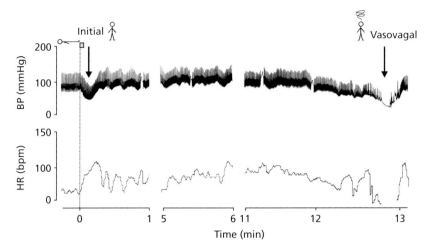

Figure 3.4 Vasovagal fainting in a healthy 22-year-old male subject. Note normal initial HR and blood pressure response and marked increase in HR after 6 min standing. After 11–12 min standing, BP and HR start to decrease to very low values during the faint; the HR tracing during the faint is interrupted by a period of asystole of 7 s. On lying down, HR and BP recover quickly, but BP does not overshoot (with permission from Van Lieshout JJ, Weiling W, Karemaker JM, Eckberg D. *Clin Sci* 1991; **81**: 575–586).

within 10 s. It is reported that the loss of consciousness occurs more rapidly when the individual is standing than when he or she is recumbent. Recovery after termination of the arrhythmia is rapid with a sudden return of the pulse, flushing of the face, and usually full orientation of the patient. The flush occurs during an overshoot in arterial pressure following the hypotensive arrhythmia.

Syncope due to orthostatic hypotension in patients with autonomic failure
Symptomatic orthostatic hypotension is the main problem in patients with autonomic failure (see also Chapter 18). With a significant and persistent decrease in arterial pressure characteristic symptoms include:
• lightheadedness and blurring of vision;
• neck ache radiating to the occipital region of the skull and to the shoulders (coat-hanger distribution) often precedes actual loss of consciousness. The postulated mechanism of this virtually unique symptom of postural hypotension is ischemia in continuously contracting postural muscles;
• symptoms suggesting impaired perfusion of muscle tissue such as lower back and buttock ache or angina pectoris.

Typically symptoms develop within minutes on standing or walking and resolve on lying down. In many patients symptoms start during standing still after physical exercise such as climbing stairs. Postexercise hypotension should always raise the possibility of autonomic failure. This also holds for the shoulder and neck pain associated with orthostatic hypotension.

The symptoms described above can be considered as a prodrome and patients with autonomic failure quickly learn to use them as a warning sign that they must lie down to restore an adequate perfusion pressure. If the patient remains upright, a gradual fading of consciousness occurs and the patient falls slowly to his or her knees. Sudden postural attacks may, however, also occur. Symptoms and signs of autonomic activation like sweating or a vagally induced bradycardia are absent in patients with autonomic failure.

Summary

The most important underlying mechanism of syncope is a transient pronounced fall in systemic blood pressure with cerebral hypoperfusion and loss of postural tone as its inevitable consequence. The most frequent causes are the neural reflex syncope disorders (such as a vasovagal faint). A low cardiac output, for example, due to heart block, can also cause syncope. Cardiac syncope is characterized by the suddenness of its onset and the lack of premonitory warning symptoms, thereby distinguishing it from the more slow onset of cerebral hypoxia and enhanced autonomic discharge in vasovagal syncope. Clinical presentation patterns of syncope often reveal the underlying pathophysiology.

Additional reading

Calkins H, Shyr Y, Frumin H, Schork A, Morady F. The value of clinical history in the differentiation of syncope due to ventricular tachycardia, atrioventricular block and neurocardiogenic syncope. *Am J Med* 1995; **98**: 365–373.

Giese AE, Li V, McKnite S, *et al.* Impact of age and blood pressure on the lower arterial pressure limit for maintenance of consciousness during passive upright posture in healthy vasovagal fainters: preliminary observations. *Europace* 2004; **6**: 457–462.

Gisolf J, van Lieshout JJ, van Heusden K, Pott F, Stok WJ and Karemaker JM. Human cerebral venous outflow pathway depends on posture and central venous pressure. *J Physiol* 2004; **560**, 317–327.

Gisolf J, Westerhof BE, Van Dijk N, Wesseling KH, Wieling W, Karemaker JM. Sublingual nitroglycerin used in routine tilt testing provokes a cardiac output-mediated vasovagal response. *J Am Coll Cardiol* 2004; **44**: 588–593.

Gisolf J, Wilders R, Immink RV, van Lieshout JJ and Karemaker JM. Tidal volume, cardiac output and functional residual capacity determine end-tidal CO(2) transient during standing up in humans. *J Physiol* 2004; **554**: 579–590.

Grubb BP. Neurocardiogenic syncope and related disorders of orthostatic intolerance. *Circulation* 2005; **111**: 2997–3006.

Hainsworth R. Syncope and fainting. In: Mathias CJ & Bannister R. *Autonomic failure. A Textbook of Clinical Disorders of the Autonomic Nervous System*. Oxford University Press, Oxford, 1999: 429–436.

Lempert T, Bauer M, Schmidt D. Syncope: a videometric analysis of 56 episodes of transient cerebral hypoxia. *Ann Neurol* 1994; **36**: 233–237.

Smit AAJ, Halliwill JR, Low PA, Wieling W. Topical review. Pathophysiological basis of orthostatic hypotension in autonomic failure. *J Physiol* 1999; **519**: 1–10.

Sutton R. Vasovagal syncope: prevalence and presentation. An algorithm of management in the aviation environment. *Eur Heart J* 1999; **1**: 109–113.

Van Lieshout JJ, Wieling W, Karemaker JM, Secher NH. Syncope, cerebral blood velocity and oxygenation. *J Appl Physiol* 2003; **94**: 833–848.

Van Lieshout JJ, Wieling W, Karemaker JM, Eckberg D. The vasovagal response. *Clin Sci* 1991; **81**: 575–586.

CHAPTER 4

Maintaining blood pressure while upright – physiology and potential for disturbances to cause syncope

Christopher J. Mathias

Introduction

A suitable level of blood pressure is essential to ensure an adequate supply of oxygen and nutrients to different organs, to enable them to function appropriately in a variety of circumstances. In humans, amongst the many factors (cardiac, vascular, endocrine, and neural) that contribute to blood pressure control, the autonomic nervous system plays a key role through the baroreceptor reflex.

This chapter covers various aspects concerned with physiological blood pressure control, with an emphasis on function of the autonomic nervous system and its disturbances, which result in syncope.

Goals

• To provide an outline of physiological aspects of blood pressure control, both nonneurogenic and neurogenic.
• To indicate the potential sites where failure of the system can result in syncope.
• To classify nonneurogenic and neurogenic disorders of blood pressure control that result in syncope.

Physiological aspects of blood pressure control

The maintenance of blood pressure is dependent on a combination of factors that include the heart and vasculature, endocrine and paracrine systems, intravascular volume, and the autonomic nervous system. The heart functions as a pump, with arterial vessels providing appropriate resistance and the venous vasculature contributing to capacitance. This is especially important when subjects are upright, because of gravitational strains affecting arterial

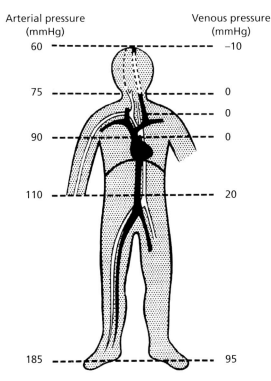

Arterial pressure (mmHg)
60
75
90
110
185

Venous pressure (mmHg)
−10
0
0
0
20
95

Figure 4.1 Effects of gravity on arterial and venous blood pressures in an erect, motionless man. Arterial and venous pressures in the lower part of the body are increased and in the upper part of the body decreased. Note that cerebral arterial pressure is about 15 mm Hg lower than aortic root pressure. Because the brain is enclosed by the rigid skull, the venous pressures may be below atmospheric pressure. This results in a relatively constant arterial–venous pressure difference in different parts of the brain. (From: Hainsworth R. Arterial blood pressure. In: GEH Henderby, ed, *Hypotensive Anaesthesia*, Churchill Livingstone, Edinburgh, 1985: 3–29).

and venous pressure (Figure 4.1). The vasculature is affected by circulating hormones, such as angiotensin II and adrenaline, and by locally active hormones, which include endothelin and nitric oxide. Intravascular and extravascular fluid volumes are maintained by various factors including hormones such as the renin–angiotensin–aldosterone system and atrial natriuretic peptide. However, these different mechanisms do not have the sensitivity of the baroreceptor reflex, which controls blood pressure on a beat-by-beat basis (Figure 4.2). Afferents from the carotid sinus, heart, and major cardiopulmonary vessels relay information to the brain through the vagus and glossopharyngeal nerves. There are numerous cerebral connections that influence efferent pathways, which consist of the sympathetic outflow to blood vessels and heart, and parasympathetic (vagus) nerves to the heart.

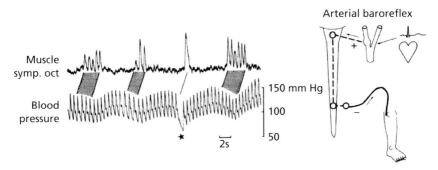

Figure 4.2 Relationship between spontaneous fluctuations of blood pressure and muscle nerve sympathetic activity (left panel) recorded in right peroneal nerve (right panel). The baroreceptor reflex accounts for the pulse synchrony of nerve activity and the inverse relationship to blood pressure fluctuations. ★ indicates diastolic blood pressure fall due to sudden AV block. Stippling indicated corresponding sequences of bursts and heart beats. (From: Wallin BG, Linblad L-E. Baroreflex mechanisms controlling sympathetic outflow to the muscles. In: P Sleight, ed, *Arterial Baroreceptors and Hypertension*, Oxford University Press, Oxford 1988: 101).

Levels of blood pressure need to be adequately maintained during activities, ranging from food ingestion to exercise, that imposes various constraints and necessitates changes in organ blood flow, which need to be rapidly adjusted. The latter is especially so when subjects are upright, because gravity imposes further strains on hemodynamic stability. The flexibility and responsiveness of the autonomic nervous system enables appropriate activation of autonomic nerves to different regions, thus maintaining the 'milieu interieur'.

Failure to maintain blood pressure – potential sites, situations, and sequelae

The inability to maintain blood pressure, especially when upright, leads to reduced perfusion of organs and in particular those vital organs above the level of the heart, such as the brain. A critical reduction in cerebral perfusion results in loss of consciousness or syncope. This failure of cerebral perfusion may be due to nonneurogenic or neurogenic causes, as described below; the former are more common. Some, such as cardiac malfunction through arrhythmias, result in syncope even while lying flat. The additional effects of gravity often contribute, particularly when neurogenic failure results in an inability to activate sympathetic nerves and cause vasoconstriction. Keeping upright a subject who has fainted, does not allow blood pressure and thus cerebral perfusion to recover, and may lead to hypoxia-induced convulsions, that may be mistaken for epilepsy.

Multiple factors may impair ability to maintain blood pressure (Tables 4.1–4.4). Essential activities in daily life, such as food ingestion and

Table 4.1 Examples of nonneurogenic causes of inability to maintain blood pressure especially when upright, that cause syncope.

Cardiac	
Arrhythmia	Stoke–Adams attacks, bradydysrhythmias, tachydysrhythmias
Myocardial	Myocarditis
Impaired ventricular filling	Atrial myxoma, constrictive pericarditis
Impaired output	Aortic stenosis
Low intravascular volume	
Blood/plasma loss	Hemorrhage, burns, hemodialysis
Fluid/electrolyte deficiency	Anorexia nervosa
Fluid intake	
loss from gut	Vomiting, ileostomy losses, diarrhea
loss from kidney	Salt losing nephropathy, diuretics
endocrine deficiency	Adrenal insufficiency (Addison's disease)
Vasodilatation	
Endogenous	Hyperpyrexia
	Hyperbradykininism
	Systemic mastocytosis
	Varicose veins
Exogenous	Exercise
	Heat
	Drugs such as glyceryl trinitrates (GTN)
	Alcohol

(Adapted from Mathias CJ. Autonomic diseases: clinical features and laboratory evaluation. *J Neurol Neurosurg Psychiatry* 2003; **74**: iii31–iii41).

exertion, can lower blood pressure, especially when neurogenic factors impair autonomic compensatory mechanisms (Figures 4.3 and 4.4). Thus, splanchnic vasodilatation during food ingestion and increased skeletal muscle blood flow during exercise can contribute to syncope, especially when upright. Recognition of these factors is important as they often warrant further consideration and investigation, with appropriate management based on knowledge of the pathophysiological processes.

Inability to maintain blood pressure – nonneurogenic causes
An inability to maintain blood pressure, particularly when upright, may result from impairment of nonneurogenic factors (Table 4.1):
• Cardiac causes include impairment of cardiac output, by diseases affecting the musculature, or by tachyarrhythmias or bradyarrhythmias.
• Intravascular volume may be inadequate for reasons that include blood loss, diminished intake, or endocrine deficiency.
• Vasodilatation may be compounded by disease and commonly by the actions of drugs.

Table 4.2 Examples of neurogenic causes of inability to maintain blood pressure, especially while upright, that can cause syncope.

Neurally mediated syncope
Vasovagal syncope
Carotid sinus hypersensitivity
Situational syncope

Drugs (see Table 4.3)
by their direct effects
by causing a neuropathy
Primary autonomic failure
Acute/subacute dysautonomias
Pure pandysautonomia
Pandysautonomia with neurological features

Chronic autonomic failure syndromes
Pure autonomic failure
Multiple system atrophy (Shy-Drager syndrome)
Autonomic failure with Parkinson's disease
Secondary autonomic failure
Congenital
Nerve growth factor deficiency

Hereditary
Autosomal dominant trait
   Familial amyloid neuropathy
Autosomal recessive trait
   Dopamine beta-hydroxylase deficiency

Metabolic diseases
Diabetes mellitus
Alcohol induced

Inflammatory
Guillain-Barre syndrome
Transverse myelitis

Infections
Viral
human immuno-deficiency virus infection
Neoplasia
Paraneoplastic, to include adenocarcinomas of lung and pancreas
Trauma
Cervical and high thoracic spinal cord transection

(Adapted from Mathias CJ. Role of autonomic evaluation in the diagnosis and management of syncope. *Clin Auton Res* 2004; **14**: S1, 45–54.)

Table 4.3 Examples of mechanisms by which drugs, chemicals, poisons and toxins may cause syncope.

By decreasing sympathetic activity
Centrally acting
  Clonidine, reserpine, anaesthetics
Peripherally acting via
  Sympathetic nerve endings (guanethidine, bethanidine)
  α-Adrenoceptor blockade (phenoxybenzamine)
  β-Adrenoceptor blockade (propranolol)

By increasing cardiac parasympathetic activity
Organophosphates
Ciguatera (reef fish) poisoning
By vasodilatation
Jellyfish and marine animal venoms

By a first dose effect
Prazosin, Captopril

By causing an autonomic neuropathy
Alcohol, thiamine (vitamin B_1) deficiency
Vincristine, perhexiline maleate

(Adapted from Mathias CJ. Role of autonomic evaluation in the diagnosis and management of syncope. *Clin Auton Res* 2004; **14**: S1, 45–54.)

Table 4.4 Factors in addition to head-up posture that further influence the inability to maintain blood pressure and contribute to syncope while upright.

Speed of positional change
Time of day (worse in the morning)
Prolonged recumbency
Warm environment (hot weather, hot bath)
Raising intrathoracic pressure – micturition, defecation, or coughing
Food and alcohol ingestion
Physical exertion
Drugs with vasoactive properties

(Adapted from Mathias CJ. Autonomic diseases: clinical features and laboratory evaluation. *J Neurol Neurosurg Psychiatry* 2003; **74**: iii31–iii41.)

Inability to maintain blood pressure – neurogenic factors

Neurogenic causes are listed in Table 4.2. Common causes of intermittent autonomic dysfunction include the three major forms of neurally mediated syncope.

1 Vasovagal syncope is the most common (Figure 4.5).

2 Carotid sinus hypersensitivity occurs predominantly in older patients (Figure 4.6).

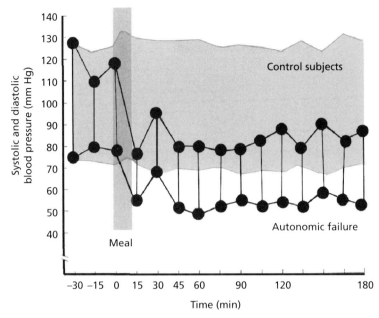

Figure 4.3 Supine systolic and diastolic blood pressure before and after a standard meal in a group of normal subjects (stippled area) and in a patient with autonomic failure (filled dots). Blood pressure does not change in the normal subjects after a meal taken while lying flat. In the patient there is a rapid fall in blood pressure to levels around 80/50 mm Hg, which remains low while in the supine position over the 3-h observational period. (Adapted from: Mathias CJ, Bannister R. Postprandial hypotension in autonomic disorders. In: Mathias CJ, Bannister R, eds, *Autonomic Failure: A Textbook of Clinical Disorders of the Autonomic Nervous System*, 4th edn. Oxford University Press, Oxford, 2002: 283–295.)

3 Miscellaneous (situational) syncope may occur in a variety of situations. The key provocative stimulus is either physiological or emotional; it may be specific to the individual and not necessarily reproducible in the laboratory, which accounts for why people do not always faint even in an identical situation.

Another increasingly recognized cause of intermittent neurogenic dysfunction is the postural tachycardia syndrome (PoTS) (Figure 4.7). Orthostatic and exercise-induced intolerance is common, and syncope may occur.

There are less common, but increasingly recognized, disorders that damage autonomic centers and pathways in the brain, spinal cord, or peripheral nerves. They include primary and secondary autonomic failure, and drugs that damage autonomic nerves, sometimes irreparably (Table 4.3). These disorders often result in orthostatic hypotension (Figure 4.8), which is arbitrarily defined as a fall in systolic blood pressure of 20 mm Hg or more and in diastolic blood pressure of 10 mm Hg or more, on either standing or head-up tilt to 60° for 3 min.

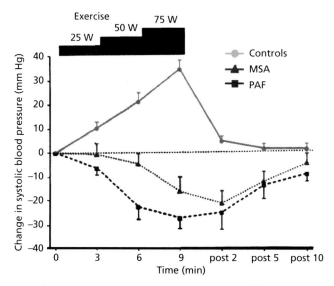

Figure 4.4 Changes in systolic blood pressure during supine bicycle exercise at three incremental levels (25, 50, and 75 W) in normal subjects (controls) and patients with multiple system atrophy (MSA) and pure autonomic failure (PAF). The bars indicate standard error of the mean. Unlike controls in whom there is a rise, there is a fall in blood pressure in both MSA and PAF. Blood pressure returns rapidly to the baseline in controls, unlike in the two patient groups in whom it takes almost 10 min. All subjects remained horizontal during and for 10 min postexercise. (From: Smith GDP, Watson LP, Pavitt DV, Mathias CJ. Abnormal cardiovascular and catecholamine responses to supine exercise in human subjects with sympathetic dysfunction. *J Physiol* (London) 1995; **485**: 255–265.)

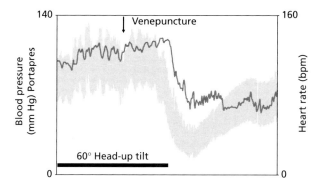

Figure 4.5 Blood pressure and heart rate with continuous recordings from the Portapres II noninvasive recording system during head-up tilt testing in a patient with the mixed (cardioinhibitory and vasodepressor) form of vasovagal syncope. (From Mathias CJ. Orthostatic hypotension and orthostatic intolerance. In: JL Jameson, LJ DeGroot, eds, *Endocrinology*, 5th edn. Elsevier, Philadelphia. (In press))

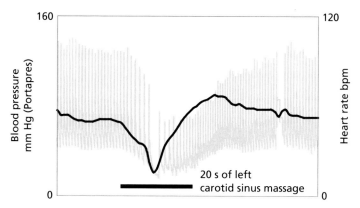

Figure 4.6 Continuous blood pressure and heart rate measured noninvasively (by Finapres) in a subject with falls of unknown cause. Left carotid sinus massage (LCSM) caused a fall in both heart rate and blood pressure. The findings indicate the mixed (cardioinhibitory and vasodepressor) form of carotid sinus hypersensitivity. (Adapted from Mathias CJ, Armstrong E, Browse N *et al.* Value of non-invasive continuous blood pressure monitoring in the detection of carotid sinus hypersensitivity. *Clin Auton Res* 1991; **2**: 157–159.)

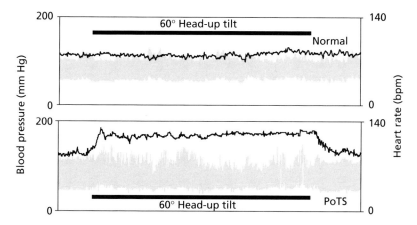

Figure 4.7 Blood pressure and heart rate measured continuously by the Portapres II before, during and after 60° head-up tilt in a normal subject (upper panel) and in subject with the postural tachycardia syndrome (PoTS) (lower panel). Note the marked increase in heart rate characteristic of PoTS. (Adapted from Mathias CJ. To stand on ones' own legs. *Clin Med* 2002; **2**: 237–245.)

Summary

The preservation of blood flow to the brain through maintenance of blood pressure is essential in preventing syncope. This especially is so in bipedal

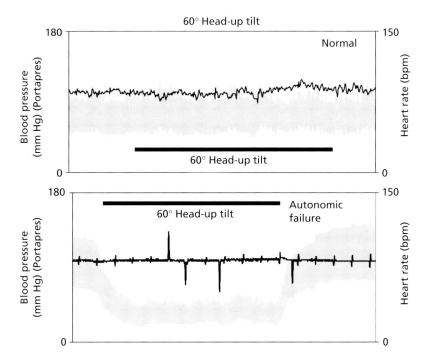

Figure 4.8 Blood pressure and heart rate before, during, and after head-up tilt in a normal subject (upper panel), and in a patient with autonomic failure due to multiple system atrophy (MSA; lower panel). In the normal subject there is no fall in blood pressure during head-up tilt, unlike the patient with MSA in whom blood pressure falls promptly and remains low with a blood pressure overshoot on return to the horizontal. In the patient with MSA there is only a minimal change in heart rate despite the marked blood pressure fall. In each subject, continuous blood pressure and heart rate was recorded with the Portapres II. (From Mathias CJ. Cardiovascular Autonomic Dysfunction in Parkinson's Disease and Parkinsonian Syndromes. In: Ebadi M & Pfeiffer RF, eds, *Parkinson's Disease*. CRC Press LLC, New York, 2005: 295–317.)

humans when upright. The autonomic nervous system, through the barore-flex pathways, and in combination with various other mechanisms, is essential in these processes. There are many nonneurogenic and neurogenic disorders that impair control of blood pressure and heart rate and thus cause syncope. Determining the precise cause of the underlying dysfunction and its pathophysiological basis is essential for appropriate targeting of therapy.

Additional reading

Mathias CJ. Role of autonomic evaluation in the diagnosis and management of syncope. *Clin Auton Res* 2004, **14**: S1, 45–54.

Mathias CJ. Disorders of the autonomic nervous system. In: WG Bradley, RB Daroff, GM Fenichel, J Jancovich, eds, *Neurology in Clinical Practice*. 3rd edn. Butterworth-Heinemann, United States, 2004; 2403–2240.

Mathias CJ. Autonomic diseases – clinical features and laboratory evaluation. *J Neurol Neurosurg Psychiatry* 2003; **74**: 31–41.

Mathias CJ. Autonomic diseases – Management. *J Neurol Neurosurg Psychiatry* 2003; **74**: 42–47.

Mathias CJ, Bannister R. (eds) *Autonomic Failure: A Textbook of Clinical Disorders of the Autonomic Nervous System*. 4th edn. Oxford University Press, Oxford, 2002.

Mathias CJ, Deguchi K, Schatz I. Observations on recurrent syncope and presyncope in 641 patients. *Lancet* 2001; **357**: 348–353.

CHAPTER 5
Epidemiology and social costs of syncope

Rose Anne Kenny and Wishwa N. Kapoor

Introduction

Syncope is a common problem. Forty percent of us will experience syncope at least once in our lifetime. The majority of events are simple faints not requiring detailed investigation. Recurrent syncope, injurious events, or syncope in patients with structural heart disease or neurologic disorders require further attention.

Goals

The goals of this chapter are to provide an overview of:
• epidemiology of syncope including estimates of incidence and prevalence;
• prognosis;
• quality of life issues; and
• economic impact.
Certain of these issues are revisited in other chapters addressing specific causes of syncope.

Epidemiology

The reported prevalence of syncope in the population varies depending on the group being studied. Thus, reports range widely: 15% of children before the age of 18; 25% of a military population aged 17–26; 16% and 19% in men and women aged 40–59 years; and up to 23% in a nursing home population of people greater than 70 years.

The highest frequency of syncope occurs in patients with cardiovascular comorbidity and older patients in institutional care settings. However, it should be noted that the quoted syncope prevalence figures for older people are undoubtedly an underestimate given that up to 20% have amnesia for loss of consciousness and present with a 'fall' rather than 'syncope'.

Prognosis

The 1-year mortality of patients with cardiac syncope is consistently higher (ranging between 18 and 33%) than for patients with noncardiac cause

(0 to 12%), or unexplained syncope (6%). One-year incidence of sudden death is 24% in patients with a cardiac cause compared with 3% in the other two groups. Although patients with cardiac syncope have higher mortality rates compared with those of noncardiac or unknown causes, patients with cardiac causes do not appear to exhibit a higher mortality when compared with matched controls who have similar degrees of heart disease. The presence and severity of structural heart disease are the most important predictors of mortality. It may reasonably be expected that syncope patients with multiple comorbidities, and thereby multiple potential causes for syncope, will have an even higher mortality.

Excess mortality rates in syncope patients with ventricular tachyarrhythmias are highest in those with severe ventricular dysfunction (Table 5.1). One-year mortality in patients with syncope due to cardiac arrhythmias increases exponentially from 4% (no other risk factor) to 80% in patients with three or more risk factors – this algorithm incorporating risk factors is useful for risk stratification.

Structural heart disease is a major risk factor for sudden death and overall mortality in patients with syncope (Table 5.1). The association of syncope with aortic stenosis has been long recognized as having an average survival without valve replacement of 2 years. Similarly, in hypertrophic cardiomyopathy, the combination of young age, syncope at diagnosis, severe dyspnea, and a family history of sudden death best predict sudden death. In arrhythmogenic right ventricular dysplasia (arrhythmogenic right ventricular cardiomyopathy), patients with syncope or symptomatic ventricular tachycardia have a similarly poor prognosis. Syncope patients with ventricular tachyarrhythmias have high rates of total mortality and sudden death, but the excess mortality rates seem to depend primarily on the severity of underlying heart disease; patients with severe ventricular dysfunction have the worst prognosis. Some of the cardiac causes of syncope do not appear to be associated with increased mortality. These include most types of supraventricular tachycardias and sinus node dysfunction.

A number of subgroups of patients can be identified who have an excellent prognosis (Table 5.1). These include young healthy individuals without heart disease and normal electrocardiogram (ECG), neurally mediated reflex syndromes, orthostatic hypotension (the mortality rates of patients with orthostatic hypotension depend on the causes of this disorder), and syncope of unknown cause (5% first-year mortality in patients with unexplained syncope).

Recurrences

One-third of patients have recurrences of syncope at 3 years of follow-up. The majority of these recurrences occur within the first 2 years (but presumably continue into the future in untreated individuals). Predictors of recurrence of syncope include having had recurrent syncope at the time of presentation, age <45 years or a psychiatric diagnosis. After positive tilt-table testing, patients

Table 5.1 Syncope: prognostic stratification.

Cardiac disease – general
Age ≥45 years, history of congestive heart failure, history of ventricular arrhythmias, and abnormal ECG (other than nonspecific ST changes)
Cardiac arrhythmias are a cause of syncope or death (or cardiac death) within 1 year of follow-up in 4% without any of these risk factors, increasing to 80% in patients with three or more factors

Structural heart disease – specific conditions with poor prognosis
Aortic stenosis
  In syncopal patients without valve replacement, the average survival is 2 years
Hypertrophic cardiomyopathy
  The combination of young age, syncope at diagnosis, severe dyspnea, and a family history of sudden death best predict sudden death
Arrhythmogenic right ventricular dysplasia (cardiomyopathy)
  Patients with syncope or symptomatic ventricular tachycardia have poor prognosis
Ventricular tachyarrhythmias
  Patients have higher rates of mortality and sudden death but the excess mortality rates depend on underlying heart disease; patients with severe ventricular dysfunction have the worst prognosis

Structural heart disease – specific conditions with better prognosis
Young healthy individuals (less than 45 years of age) without heart disease and normal ECG
  There is no evidence that these patients have an increased mortality risk. Most have neurally mediated or unexplained syncope
Neurally mediated reflex syncope
  The mortality at follow-up is near 0%. Most of these patients have normal hearts
Orthostatic hypotension
  The mortality rates of patients with orthostatic hypotension depend on the causes of this disorder and comorbid illnesses
Supraventricular tachycardias and sick sinus syndrome
  These cardiac causes of syncope are not associated with increased mortality
Syncope of unknown cause (after thorough evaluation)
  First-year mortality is 5%. Although the mortality is largely due to underlying comorbidity, such patients continue to be at risk for physical injury, and may encounter employment and lifestyle restrictions

---

with more than six syncope spells have a risk of recurrence of more than 50% over 2 years.

Recurrences are not proven to be associated with increased mortality or sudden death rates, but patients with recurrent syncope have a poor functional status similar to patients with other chronic diseases.

Physical injury
Syncope may result in injury to the patient or to others. This may occur when a patient is driving or working in an environment where injury might result

from loss of postural control. Major morbidity such as fractures and motor vehicle accidents are reported in 6% of patients, and minor injury such as laceration and bruises in 29%. There is no data on the risk of injury to others. Recurrent syncope is associated with fractures and soft tissue injury in at least 12% of patients.

Quality of life

Functional impairment in syncope patients is similar to chronic illnesses such as rheumatoid arthritis, low back pain, and psychiatric disorders. Impairment is evident in domains such as mobility, usual activities, self-care, pain and discomfort, and anxiety and depression. There is a marked negative relationship between the frequency of spells and overall perception of health.

Economic implications

Patients with syncope are often admitted to hospital and undergo expensive and repeated investigations, many of which do not provide a definite diagnosis. Despite the advent of multiple diagnostic tests (e.g. tilt testing, wider use of electrophysiologic testing, ambulatory ECG 'loop' monitoring) the management of syncope remains disparate and unstructured in most centers (see Chapters 7 and 11). Patients often undergo a great number of tests at considerable cost.

Estimated hospital costs are in excess of 10 billion US dollars per year. This is undoubtedly an underestimate because many patients with syncope are not admitted to hospital, and the costs of their care may not be adequately captured. In the United Kingdom, syncope and collapse are the sixth most common cause of emergency admission, and 80% of cost incurred by those diagnostic categories is accrued via emergency activity.

An extant conservative estimate of total annual costs for syncope-related hospitalizations is $2.4 billion, with an average cost of $5400 per hospitalization. Efforts to decrease syncope-related admissions and increase rapid access elective activity can reduce hospital costs by half (see Chapter 10).

Summary

Syncope occurs frequently in the population and recurrences are common. The evaluation of syncope remains largely unstructured in most centers. The result is frequent use of ineffective testing strategies at considerable cost to the health care system.

Additional reading

Kapoor WN, Peterson J, Wieand HS, Karpf M. Diagnostic and prognostic implications of recurrences in patients with syncope. *Am J Med* 1987; **83**: 700–708.
Kenny RA, O'Shea D, Walker HF. Impact of a dedicated syncope and falls facility for older adults on emergency beds. *Age Ageing* 2002; **31**: 272–275.

Lewis DA, Dhala A. Syncope in the pediatric patient. The cardiologist's perspective. *Pediatr Clin North Am* 1999; **46**: 205–219.

Lipsitz LA, Wei JY, Rowe JW. Syncope in an elderly, institutionalized population: prevalence, incidence, and associated risk. *Q J Med* 1985; **55**: 45–54.

Martin TP, Hanusa BH, Kapoor WN. Risk stratification of patients with syncope. *Ann Emerg Med* 1997; **29**: 459–466.

Oh JH, Hanusa BH, Kapoor WN. Do symptoms predict cardiac arrhythmias and mortality in patients with syncope? *Arch Intern Med* 1999; **159**: 375–380.

Rose MS, Koshman ML, Spreng S, Sheldon R. The relationship between health-related quality of life and frequency of spells in patients with syncope. *J Clin Epidemiol* 2000; **53**: 1209–1216.

Shen WK, Decker WW, Smars PA *et al.* Syncope Evaluation in the Emergency Department Study (SEEDS): a multidisciplinary approach to syncope management. *Circulation* 2004; **110**: 3636–3645.

Soteriades ES, Evans JC, Larson MG *et al.* Incidence and prognosis of syncope. *N Engl J Med* 2002; **347**: 878–885.

Sun BC, Emond JA, Camargo CA Jr. Direct medical costs of syncope-related hospitalizations in the United States. *Am J Cardiol* 2005; **95**: 668–671.

The Multicentre Post Infarction Group. Risk stratification and survival after myocardial infarction. *N Engl J Med* 1983; **309**: 331–336.

Section two:
Syncope evaluation strategy

CHAPTER 6
Overview of recommended diagnostic strategies

Richard Sutton and Michele Brignole

Introduction

Many conditions may present as transient loss of consciousness (TLOC). Syncope is one of the most common and clinically important of these. However, apart from determining whether TLOC was due to true syncope (see Chapters 1 and 2), it is crucial to determine, as precisely as possible, the cause of syncope in each patient. In this regard, it is important to keep in mind that multiple causative factors may interact and thereby trigger syncope (e.g. abrupt movement to upright posture in a patient with diabetic neuropathy, overdiuresis in a patient with heart failure and paroxysmal atrial fibrillation).

The starting point for the evaluation of syncope is a careful history and physical examination including orthostatic blood pressure measurements. These aspects of the initial evaluation are discussed in more detail in subsequent chapters. Techniques for appropriate and complete medical history taking in syncope patients (reviewed in Chapters 7 and 8) merit particular attention given the importance of the history in providing a presumptive diagnosis, and directing subsequent diagnostic testing (Table 6.1).

Goals

The aim of this chapter is to provide a succinct overview of a reasonable strategy for assessment of patients with suspected syncope. Three issues will be addressed:

1 approach to the patient in whom the basis for syncope seems 'certain' after 'initial evaluation';

2 approach when the etiology is suspected but nonetheless remains 'uncertain'; and

3 approach when the diagnosis remains 'unknown' after the initial evaluation.

Table 6.1 Clinical features suggestive of specific causes of syncope and certain syncope – mimicks

Symptom or finding	Possible cause
After sudden unexpected, unpleasant sight, sound, or smell	Vasovagal
Prolonged standing at attention or crowded, warm places	Vasovagal or autonomic failure
Nausea, vomiting associated with syncope	Vasovagal
Within 1 h of a meal	Postprandial (autonomic failure)
After exertion	Vasovagal or autonomic failure
Syncope with throat or facial pain	Neuralgia (glossopharyngeal or trigeminal neuralgia)
With head rotation, pressure on carotid sinus	Spontaneous carotid sinus syncope (as in tumors, shaving, tight collars)
Within seconds to minutes upon active standing	Orthostatic hypotension
Temporal relationship with start of medication or changes of dosage	Drug induced
During exertion or supine	Cardiac syncope
Preceded by palpitation	Tachyarrhythmia
Family history of sudden death	Long QT syndrome, Brugada syndrome, right ventricular dysplasia, hypertrophic cardiomyopathy
In course of a migraine attack	Migraine
Associated with vertigo, dysarthria, diplopia	Brainstem transient ischemic attack (TIA)
With arm exercise	Subclavian steal
Differences in blood pressure or pulse in the two arms	Subclavian steal or aortic dissection
Syncope mimicks	
Confusion after attack for more than 5 min	Seizure (see Chapter 17)
Tonic–clonic movements, automatism, tongue biting, blue face, epileptic aura	Seizure (see Chapter 17)
Frequent attack with somatic complaints, no organic heart disease	Psychiatric illness (see Chapter 18)

The initial evaluation

The 'Initial Evaluation' (see also Chapter 7) of a patient presenting with TLOC, in whom syncope is suspected, consists of undertaking:
• careful medical history with detailed assessment of symptom events;
• complete physical examination with orthostatic (supine and upright) blood pressure measurements;

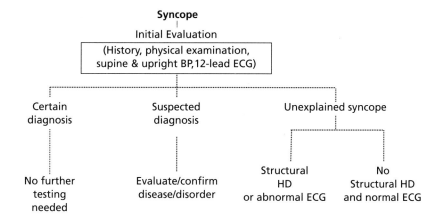

Abbreviations; BP, blood pressure.

Figure 6.1 Schematic illustrating a recommended strategy for the diagnostic evaluation of syncope patients. The first step is the initial evaluation (see Chapter 7). Thereafter, patients can be categorized as having a certain diagnosis, or a suspected but uncertain diagnosis (i.e. likely but not absolutely sure in the eyes of the physician), or unexplained.

- standard 12-lead electrocardiogram (ECG); and
- in some cases an echocardiogram may be considered reasonable at this stage, given the need to determine whether there is evidence of underlying structural heart disease.

Three key questions need to be considered during the initial evaluation.

1 Is TLOC attributable to syncope or not? In other words, the physician must differentiate true syncope from nonsyncope TLOC (e.g. seizures, concussion, etc.).

2 Are there features in the medical history that suggest the etiologic diagnosis? Accurate and detailed history taking is essential.

3 Is heart disease present or absent? The absence of signs or symptoms of heart disease virtually exclude a cardiac etiology (with the exception of paroxysmal supraventricular tachycardias). On the other hand, the presence of heart disease at the initial evaluation is a strong predictor of a cardiac cause and necessitates evaluation of a potential cardiac etiology early in the subsequent assessment. Ultimately, however, about one-half of cardiac patients with syncope have a noncardiac cause.

The diagnostic outcome from the initial evaluation may be a certain etiologic diagnosis, a suspected but uncertain diagnosis, or unexplained syncope (i.e. no known or suspected cause) (Figure 6.1). In each instance, the experience of the physician plays a major role in determining the most likely diagnosis, and in judging whether further testing is desirable. In those cases in which the cause of syncope is seemingly certain after the 'initial evaluation', further testing may be unnecessary depending on the physician's confidence in the certainty of the assessment. In the case of a suspected but as yet uncertain diagnosis, the subsequent direction for confirmatory testing is established by having come to at least a presumption of the cause. The latter paves the way for an efficient and cost-effective evaluation. When the initial evaluation is unable to provide any clue as to the diagnosis (here termed as unexplained syncope) the strategy for subsequent diagnostic steps depends on the frequency and severity of the episodes and the nature of any underlying heart disease.

Certain diagnosis
On occasion, the initial evaluation may lead to a relatively certain diagnosis based on symptoms, signs, or ECG findings (Table 6.1). Under such circumstances, no further evaluation is needed and treatment, if any, can be planned. The following are examples of such situations.
• Vasovagal syncope (the most frequent of the neurally mediated reflex faints) is diagnosed if precipitating events such as fear, severe pain, emotional distress, instrumentation, or prolonged standing are associated with typical prodromal symptoms in patients without evidence of underlying heart disease.
• Situational syncope (i.e. a subset of neurally mediated reflex faints) is diagnosed if syncope occurs during or immediately after certain circumstances, such as urination, defecation, coughing, or swallowing.
• Orthostatic syncope is diagnosed when there is documentation of orthostatic hypotension associated with syncope or presyncope. Orthostatic blood pressure measurements are recommended after 5 min of lying supine, followed by each minute, or more often, after standing for 3 min. Measurements may be continued longer if blood pressure is still falling at 3 min. If the patient does not tolerate standing for this period, the lowest systolic blood pressure during the upright posture should be recorded. A decrease in systolic blood pressure of $\geq$20 mm Hg or a decrease of systolic blood pressure to <90 mm Hg is defined as orthostatic hypotension regardless of whether or not symptoms occur.
• Cardiac ischemia-related syncope is diagnosed when symptoms are present with ECG evidence of acute ischemia with or without myocardial infarction. However, whether the syncope was due to a neurally mediated reflex (i.e. bradycardia and vasodilatation) or the result of an ischemia-induced cardiac arrhythmia may require further assessment.

Suspected but uncertain diagnosis
More commonly, the initial evaluation leads to a 'suspected' diagnosis, which needs to be confirmed by directed testing. Thus, in the case of suspected vasovagal faint, a head-up tilt-table test would be the next step. Thereafter, depending on how convincing the result is (i.e. did it reproduce

patient symptoms?), further steps might be needed. The reader is referred to Chapters 12 through 18 for details regarding appropriate diagnostic procedures.

Arrhythmias are often responsible for syncope, but are rarely diagnosed with certainty by 12-lead ECG alone during the initial evaluation. More often, an ambulatory long-term ECG (AECG, see Chapter 12) recording or electro-physiological evaluation is needed. However, the 12-lead ECG may provide evidence suggesting an arrhythmic cause if one of the following is recorded:
• sustained sinus bradycardia <40 bpm (other than during sleep) or repetitive asystolic pauses (i.e. sinoatrial block, sinus pauses) >3 s in duration in the absence of negative chronotropic medications;
• Mobitz II second or third degree atrioventricular block;
• alternating left and right bundle branch block;
• rapid paroxysmal supraventricular tachycardia or ventricular tachycardia; or
• pacemaker malfunction with cardiac pauses.

Unexplained syncope
The strategy for subsequent assessment of patients in whom the initial evaluation fails to provide a plausible diagnosis varies according to the severity and frequency of the episodes and the presence or absence of structural heart disease (Figure 6.2). Apart from the prognostic importance of the presence of heart disease, its absence excludes a cardiac cause of syncope with

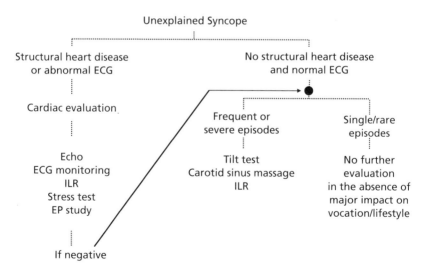

Abbreviations: ILR = insertable loop recorder.

Figure 6.2 Schematic illustrating the basic evaluation strategy for patients in whom the diagnosis remains unexplained after the steps in Figure 6.1 have been completed.

very few exceptions. In a recent study, heart disease was an independent predictor of cardiac cause of syncope, with a sensitivity of 95% and a specificity of 45%; by contrast, the absence of heart disease allowed exclusion of a cardiac cause of syncope in 97% of patients.

For patients without structural heart disease and who have a normal ECG, evaluation for neurally mediated reflex syncope is recommended for those with recurrent episodes or syncope that has caused injury, accidents, or impairs job safety or performance. The tests for neurally mediated syncope primarily consist of tilt testing and carotid massage.

The majority of patients with single or infrequent syncope episodes in this category probably have neurally mediated syncope. Since treatment is generally not recommended for most patients with infrequent events, close follow-up without additional evaluation is reasonable. For patients with signs of autonomic failure or neurologic disease, a specific diagnosis should be made. An additional consideration in patients without structural heart disease, with a normal ECG, and with many faints, is psychiatric illness. Psychiatric assessment is especially recommended for patients with very frequent syncope (actually pseudosyncope, see Chapter 18) recurrences. The latter is particularly warranted if, in addition to complaints of syncope, the affected individual appears to be exhibiting other somatic complaints, anxiety, and possibly other psychiatric disorders. Video-EEG monitoring may be helpful for assessing these individuals, inasmuch as documentation of a faint without supportive evidence of cerebral dysfunction could solidify the suspected diagnosis.

In patients with structural heart disease or who have an abnormal ECG (Table 6.2), cardiac evaluation consisting of echocardiography, stress testing, and tests for arrhythmia detection such as prolonged AECG monitoring (including use of implantable loop recorders, ILRs) and/or electrophysiologic study are recommended. If cardiac evaluation does not show evidence of arrhythmia as a cause of syncope, evaluation for neurally mediated reflex syndromes is recommended.

Table 6.2 ECG abnormalities suggesting an arrhythmic syncope.

Bifascicular block (defined as either left bundle branch block or right bundle branch block combined with left anterior or left posterior fascicular block)
Other intraventricular conduction abnormalities (QRS duration $\geq$0.12 s)
Mobitz I second degree atrioventricular block
Sinus bradycardia (<50 bpm) or sinoatrial block
Preexcited QRS complexes
Prolonged QT interval
Right bundle branch block pattern with ST elevation in leads V1–V3 (Brugada syndrome)
Negative T waves in right precordial leads, epsilon waves, and ventricular late potentials suggestive of arrhythmogenic right ventricular dysplasia (cardiomyopathy)
Q waves suggesting myocardial infarction

For patients with palpitations associated with syncope, AECG monitoring and echocardiography are recommended. Internet-based mobile cardiac outpatient telemetry (MCOT) and ILR monitoring are valuable tools and should be used in patients with recurrent unexplained syncope whose symptoms are suggestive of arrhythmic syncope. In patients with chest pain suggestive of ischemia before or after loss of consciousness, stress testing and echocardiography are recommended. AECG monitoring may have additional value in certain cases. Similarly, for patients with syncope during or after effort, echocardiography and stress testing are recommended as first evaluation steps.

Summary

The medical history provides the cornerstone for diagnosing the cause of syncope. A detailed history must be obtained in each case and whenever possible should incorporate observations of witnesses. Thereafter, the experienced physician can judge whether additional diagnostic testing is needed. The European Society of Cardiology Syncope Task Force statement provides useful guidance for appropriate diagnostic testing for syncope patients. The subsequent chapters of this handbook provide practical clinical advice.

Additional reading

Alboni P, Brignole M, Menozzi C *et al*. The diagnostic value of history in patients with syncope with or without heart disease. *J Am Coll Cardiol* 2001; **37**: 1921–1928.

Benditt DG, Brignole M. Syncope: is a diagnosis a diagnosis? *J Am Coll Cardiol* 2003; **41**: 791–794.

Brignole M, Alboni P, Benditt D *et al*. Guidelines on·management (diagnosis and treatment) of syncope. Guidelines on Management (Diagnosis and Treatment) of Syncope – Update 2004. Executive Summary. *Europace* 2004; **6**: 467–537.

Brignole M, Menozzi C, Moya A *et al*. The mechanism of syncope in patients with bundle branch block and negative electrophysiologic test. *Circulation* 2001; **104**: 2045–2050.

Menozzi C, Brignole M, Garcia-Civera R *et al*. Mechanism of syncope in patients with heart disease and negative electrophysiologic test. *Circulation* 2002; **105**: 2741–2745.

Moya A, Brignole M, Menozzi C *et al*. Mechanism of syncope in patients with isolated syncope and in patients with tilt-positive syncope. *Circulation* 2001; **104**: 1261–1267.

CHAPTER 7
Initial evaluation of the syncope patient

Antonio Raviele and Paolo Alboni

Introduction

Syncope is a subset of a broad range of conditions causing transient loss of consciousness (TLOC, see Chapter 2). In this chapter, we summarize the appropriate steps to be taken as part of the initial examination of the TLOC patient in terms of discerning the basis of syncope. However, the prudent examiner will always keep in mind the possibility that other causes of TLOC may be pertinent considerations at this stage in patients who are thought to have experienced syncope. Furthermore, it is equally prudent to be alert to the possibility that loss of consciousness may have caused physical injury that needs attention. Some of these injuries may be readily apparent, but others (e.g. intracranial bleeds, subtle fractures) may be less obvious, but nevertheless important to the patient's immediate care.

The initial diagnostic approach to patients with presumed syncope comprises a detailed medical history (incorporating documentation of eyewitness accounts), a thorough physical examination (including supine and standing blood pressure measurements, and often carotid sinus massage), and 12-lead electrocardiogram (ECG).

Other commonly ordered tests may be relevant to assessing concomitant injuries or illness, but are not recommended for the usual diagnostic evaluation of syncope itself. Thus, basic laboratory tests such as measurement of electrolytes, blood counts, and tests of renal function and glucose level are usually not indicated in the initial evaluation of patients with syncope. As a rule, such tests have a low diagnostic yield (2–3%) and are recommended only if a loss of circulating volume, severe anemia, marked dehydration, or a syncope-like disorder with a metabolic cause is suspected. Similarly, neurological studies (e.g. head CT or MRI, EEG) are of little value in the syncope assessment and should be reserved for evaluation of trauma if head injury is part of the clinical picture.

The history and physical examination are the core of the workup for patients with syncope. Alone, they permit the cause of loss of consciousness to be established in approximately 45% of cases, as a metanalysis of data from six population-based studies has shown (Table 7.1).

Table 7.1 Causes of syncope found by history and physical examination or electrocardiography.

Study	Patients (*n*)	Diagnosis by history and physical examination [*n* (%)]	Diagnosis by ECG [*n* (%)]
Kapoor	433	140 (32)	30 (7)
Ben-Chetrit	101	33 (33)	11 (11)
Martin	170	90 (53)	2 (1)
Eagle and Black		100	52 (52)
Silverstein	108	42 (38)	
Day	198	147 (74)	4 (2)
All studies	1110	504 (45)	47 (5)

Source: Adapted from Linzer M, Yang EH, Estes NA 3rd et al. *Ann Intern Med* 1997; **126**: 989–996.

Goals

The goals of this chapter are to provide:
• a review of the elements essential to the initial diagnostic evaluation of syncope patients; and
• a technique for obtaining a detailed medical history for evaluation of syncope.

Taking the medical history in syncope patients: a method

The first important issue in the medical evaluation is to determine whether the patient has suffered a significant injury that requires immediate medical attention. In its absence, the next step is differentiating true syncope from other conditions that resemble or mimic syncope (i.e. those that may produce or appear to produce TLOC but are not due to cerebral hypoperfusion). Examples of such conditions include seizures, drop attacks, and somatization disorders (see also Chapters 2, 18, and 19).

Obtaining a detailed medical history is the first step in the assessment of the cause or causes of TLOC, and for our purposes syncope in particular. If the history taking is careful and thorough, the story provided by the patient (and witnesses) will often reveal the most likely cause and will provide a means of guiding an efficient and cost-effective subsequent evaluation to confirm the clinical suspicion. On average, the history alone provides a sufficiently precise basis for syncope in about 40% of cases.

A classification of the principal causes of syncopal episodes has been provided earlier in this book (see Chapter 1). This classification provides a means of organizing one's thoughts when initiating the medical history-taking in a new patient, and it should be kept in mind throughout the process. In this section we highlight some of the most important clinical features often associated with various causes of syncope. In order to take advantage of this information, the details surrounding syncope events must be documented in considerable detail by the careful history-taker. Thereafter, we provide a basis upon which the historical features may be used to suggest a specific cause for the faint. However, history-taking is very user experience-dependent, and even in the best circumstances the sensitivity of the process is not established. False positives and false negatives are bound to occur. Consequently, confirmatory testing (albeit focused by virtue of having considered the historical findings) is often essential in order to establish a confident diagnosis.

Important components of the medical history in syncope

Before beginning the history-taking it is important to determine whether the patient can give an accurate account of events. This limitation particularly applies to older patients who commonly (as high as 20%) exhibit sufficient cognitive deterioration that impairs their relating the story accurately. In such cases, it is crucial that an informant in regular contact with the patient should attend the consultation and be interviewed as part of the history-taking process. Indeed, whenever possible, try to secure an eye-witness account of the loss of consciousness events.

General features

In order to characterize the patient's symptoms, it is helpful to have the patient focus on the most recent event. After a thorough description is obtained, turn the patient's attention to the next most recent episode. Be demanding of details. Witnesses can be very valuable in filling in items that the patient may not recall. Obtain details regarding as many events as you feel is necessary to assess whether there are features common to all or at least some of the episodes.

In many patients multiple causes may be responsible for symptoms. These may be identified or at least suggested by the medical history. Pay attention to the presence of comorbidities. Comorbidities may act synergistically (e.g. diabetic neuropathy and drug-induced orthostasis), or they may act independently thereby resulting in more than one 'cause' for the faint.

Among other general factors that are of importance in characterizing the nature and severity of the reported symptoms, and determining strategy for subsequent studies are:
- Frequency of episodes?
- Over what period of time?
- Duration of loss of consciousness (this is often inaccurately reported or at least is hard to substantiate)?
- Associated prodromal symptoms?
- History of falls or unexplained accidents/injuries?

Table 7.2 Important historical features.

Questions about circumstances just prior to attack
Position (supine, sitting, or standing)
Activity (rest, change in posture, during or after exercise, during or immediately after
  urination, defecation, cough or swallowing)
Predisposing factors (e.g. crowded or warm places, prolonged standing, postprandial
  period) and precipitating events (e.g. fear, intense pain, neck movements)

Questions about onset of attack
Nausea, vomiting, abdominal discomfort, feeling of cold, sweating, aura, pain in neck or
  shoulders, blurred vision, chest pain, palpitations

Questions about attack (eyewitness)
Way of falling (slumping or kneeling over), skin color (pallor, cyanosis, flushing), duration
  of loss of consciousness, breathing pattern (snoring), movements (tonic, clonic,
  tonic–clonic, or minimal myoclonus, automatism) and their duration, onset of
  movement in relation to fall, tongue biting

Questions about end of attack
Nausea, vomiting, feeling of cold, sweating, confusion, muscle aches, skin color, injury,
  chest pain, palpitations, urinary or fecal incontinence

Questions about background
Family history of sudden death, congenital arrhythmogenic heart disease
Previous cardiac disease
Neurologic history (Parkinsonism, epilepsy, narcolepsy)
Metabolic disorders (diabetes etc.)
Medication (antihypertensive, antianginal, antidepressant agent, antiarrhythmic,
  diuretics, and QT prolonging agents)
(In the case of recurrent syncope) Information on recurrences such as the time from the
  first syncopal episode and the number of spells

- Nature of physical injuries sustained if any?
- Any common thread with regard to time of onset?

Characterizing situations in which syncope tends to occur: is there a pattern?
Document position activity and circumstances in detail (Table 7.2).

Identifying prodromal symptoms
Is Syncope associated with nausea, vomiting, feeling of cold, sweating, visual
aura, pain in neck or shoulders, blurred vision, palpitations (Table 7.2)?

Documenting eyewitness observations during the faint
Obtain detailed description of the manner in which the loss of consciousness or
fall occurred (e.g. abrupt fall with possibility of injury, purposeful avoidance
of injury) (Table 7.2). Additionally, inquire if the patient was told by witnesses of any skin color changes associated with the faint; the duration of the
event; alterations in breathing pattern; physical movements (e.g. tonic–clonic

or myoclonic movements); incontinence; tongue biting. Not infrequently, only eyewitnesses can provide sufficient detail to be of value.

Symptoms noticed after the event
Confusion, palpitations, fatigue, headache, nausea, vomiting, sweating, feeling of cold, muscle aches, skin color, injury, chest pain (Table 7.2).

Characterizing patient risk for syncope recurrence and/or life-threatening consequences
Family history
Is there a family history of sudden death or known genetically transmitted arrhythmogenic states (e.g. long/short QT syndromes, Brugada syndrome, arrhythmogenic ventricular cardiomyopathy) (Table 7.2)? Characterize any familial predisposition to syncope (fainting, 'blackouts', 'spells', etc.)? Migraine history?

Fainter's medical history
Is there any evidence of structural cardiac disease (e.g. prior myocardial infarction, valvular heart disease, congenital conditions, previous cardiac surgery, etc.)? Neurologic conditions (e.g. Parkinsonism, epilepsy, migraine)? Metabolic/intoxication disorders (e.g. diabetes, alcoholism)? Drug abuse (e.g. cocaine, diuretics)?

Prescribed medication predisposing to syncope
Is the patient taking drugs known to predispose to syncope? Most important among these are:
• antihypertensives;
• beta-adrenergic blockers;
• antianginal drugs;
• antidepressant agents;
• antiarrhythmics;
• diuretics; and
• QT prolonging agents (including commonly used antibiotics, and psychoactive agents)?
Has there been any recent dosing change of prescribed medications? Have any new drugs been added that might produce an undesirable interaction?

Indicators from the history suggestive of specific causes of syncope
Perhaps the most frequent, important, and troublesome problem confronted by physicians during the initial evaluation of a patient with TLOC spells is the elimination of a seizure disorder as the cause of TLOC. Distinguishing syncope from a generalized seizure (epilepsy) may be difficult using medical history and bystander observations alone (see also Chapter 17).

In brief, features that are more supportive of epilepsy include:
• tonic–clonic movements that are usually prolonged and coincident with or precede onset of loss of consciousness;
• hemilateral clonic movements;
• automatisms such as chewing, lip smacking, or frothing at the mouth (partial seizure);
• tongue biting, blue face;
• aura such as unusual or distinctive smell before the event; and
• prolonged confusion and aching muscles after the event.

The development of jerky muscular movements in association with a loss of consciousness episode often raises the spectre of seizure or fit in the eyes of witnesses. However, jerky muscular movements often occur in syncope patients. Consequently, it is crucial to obtain a detailed account of the events in order to distinguish between a true seizure and a syncope event. In this regard, it should be kept in mind that jerky movements during syncope differ from epileptic-type movements by being of relatively short duration (<15 s), always starting after the loss of consciousness, and typically being asynchronous and limited in scope (so-called 'myoclonic').

Table 7.3 provides a short list of historical findings that suggest specific causes of syncope. The reader is referred to chapters dealing with each of these diagnoses for greater detail.

Additional elements of the initial evaluation

Physical findings that are useful for suggesting a basis for loss of consciousness are orthostatic hypotension, cardiovascular signs, and response to carotid sinus massage. Orthostatic hypotension has been found in 8% of patients with syncope. Carotid sinus massage is a recommended diagnostic step in all older (>55 years) syncope patients, and has until recently been underestimated in terms of diagnostic utility. A carotid massage-induced pause >3 s duration may be very valuable in suggesting a basis for syncope (see Chapter 14 for more detail). Important cardiovascular findings include differences in blood pressure/pulse in each arm (suggests subclavian steal or aortic dissection), pathologic cardiac and vascular murmurs, signs of pulmonary embolism, and peripheral pulse findings suggestive of severe aortic stenosis or idiopathic hypertrophic obstructive cardiomopathy. Signs of focal neurologic lesions, such as hemiparesis, dysarthria or diplopia and vertigo, or signs of Parkinsonism suggest but are not diagnostic of a neurologic cause for impairment of consciousness. Such patients warrant a neurologic evaluation. In general, however, neurologic disease is almost never a cause of true syncope.

The 12-lead ECG identifies with certainty a specific (arrhythmic) cause of syncope in only a small percentage of cases (about 5%). However, from time-to-time, 12-lead ECG findings such as a Q wave, left ventricular hypertrophy, a prolonged QT interval, or ventricular preexcitation may suggest the presence of organic heart disease and thereby provide a basis for proceeding with further directed testing. Echocardiography is increasingly considered to be

Table 7.3 Clinical elements considered diagnostic of a specific cause of syncope.

Vasovagal syncope
Association of precipitating events (fear, severe pain, emotional distress,
  instrumentation, prolonged standing) with typical prodromal symptoms (nausea,
  vomiting, sweating, feeling of cold, tiredness)

Situational syncope
Occurrence of syncope during or immediately after urination, defecation, cough, or
  swallowing

Orthostatic syncope
Documentation of orthostatic hypotension (decrease in systolic blood pressure (20 mm Hg
  or to <90 mm Hg) associated with reproduction of symptoms (syncope or presyncope)

Ischemia-related syncope
Simultaneous presence of symptoms and ECG signs of acute ischemia with or without
  myocardial infarction

Arrhythmia-related syncope
Sinus bradycardia <40 bpm or repetitive sinoatrial blocks or sinus pauses >3 s; Mobitz II
  second or third degree atrioventricular block; alternating left and right bundle branch
  block; rapid paroxysmal supraventricular tachycardia or ventricular tachycardia;
  pacemaker malfunction with cardiac pauses

an element of the initial evaluation, although its use may be best reserved
for instances when the status of underlying cardiac disease is unclear based
on history or prior studies. For the most part, the value of the echocardiogram is in assessing left ventricular function and occasionally identifying subtle
structural abnormalities such as severe aortic stenosis, intracardiac tumors, or
pulmonary hypertension.

When the initial evaluation (history, physical examination, 12-lead ECG,
and occasionally the echocardiogram) is diagnostic (Table 7.3), the workup
can be stopped, and if indicated, treatment may be planned and started. On
the other hand, in most cases the initial evaluation is at best suggestive of a
basis for loss of consciousness or is nondiagnostic for a specific cause. In such
cases, the investigation must be continued. Other investigations beyond the
initial evaluation are discussed elsewhere in this book.

Even when inconclusive (Table 7.4), the carefully performed initial evaluation is often useful because it may reveal abnormalities that suggest the
possible cause of syncope. The latter leads to a cost-effective subsequent evaluation strategy. For patients with a suggested but not definitive diagnosis
after the initial evaluation, specific confirmatory testing is often warranted in order to solidify the suspected diagnosis, or rule out the diagnosis.
Such testing may also aid in the planning of treatment. Tilt-table testing
is an example of a confirmatory test that is often used when the diagnosis
of a vasovagal faint is suspected, but the presentation was not classical.
Tilt testing is most valuable in individuals without evident structural heart

Table 7.4 ECG findings supporting a cardiac arrhythmia basis for syncope*.

Sinus bradycardia <40 bpm
Sinoatrial blocks or sinus pauses >3 s
Mobitz II or third degree atrioventricular block
Alternating left and right bundle branch block
Rapid paroxysmal supraventricular tachycardia or ventricular tachycardia
Pacemaker malfunction with cardiac pauses
Long QT syndrome, Brugada syndrome
Preexcitation (Wolff–Parkinson–White) syndrome

*The nature of the causal arrhythmia requires further evaluation, which may encompass ambulatory ECG monitoring (see Chapter 12), and electrophysiologic testing (see Chapter 5).

disease. Invasive electrophysiologic (EPS) testing is another example. EPS study (see Chapter 15) is most effective in terms of suggesting a basis for syncope when carried out in patients with evidence of structural cardiac disease or ECG evidence of a paroxysmal tachycardia. The use of long-term ECG monitoring strategies, such as insertable loop recorders (ILRs) or mobile outpatient telemetry (MCOT), is also to be reconsidered at this stage (see Chapter 12).

When the results of the initial evaluation are completely nondiagnostic, the patient may be considered to have unexplained syncope. Decisions about further testing should be based on an assessment of the patient's risk factors. In patients with structural heart disease and/or abnormal ECG, additional cardiac evaluation is indicated to exclude a mechanical or arrhythmic cause of syncope. In patients without structural heart disease and having a normal ECG, an evaluation for a neurally mediated reflex origin of syncope will need to be revisited because the majority of these patients ultimately are shown to have had vasovagal or related form of reflex syncope (i.e. high pretest probability). However, patients with single or rare spells and without clinical evidence of organic heart disease may not need an especially invasive evaluation because they have a low risk of syncope recurrences and a good overall prognosis.

Summary

This chapter focuses on the initial evaluation of the syncope patient. The medical history is the key in every case. Reports from witnesses should also be sought and recorded. The 12-lead ECG and perhaps an echocardiogram are reasonably included in the initial evaluation. In many cases, no further evaluation is needed after the initial evaluation. However, even when inconclusive, this stage of the syncope assessment sets the stage for efficient and cost-effective selection of subsequent confirmatory studies.

Additional reading

Hoefnagels WAJ, Padberg GW, Overweg J *et al*. Transient loss of consciousness: the value of the history for distinguishing seizure from syncope. *J Neurol* 1991; **238**: 39–43.

Martin GJ, Adams SL, Martin HG *et al*. Prospective evaluation of syncope. *Ann Emerg Med* 1984; **13**: 499–504.

Alboni P, Brignole M, Menozzi C *et al*. The diagnostic value of history in patients with syncope with or without heart disease. *J Am Coll Cardiol* 2001; **37**: 1921–1928.

Calkins H, Shyr Y, Frumin H, Schork A, Morady F. The value of clinical history in the differentiation of syncope due to ventricular tachycardia, atrioventricular block and neurocardiogenic syncope. *Am J Med* 1995; **98**: 365–373.

Oh JH, Hanusa BH, Kapoor WN. Do symptoms predict cardiac arrhythmias and mortality in patients with syncope? *Arch Intern Med* 1999; **159**: 375–380.

Linzer M, Yang EH, Estes III M *et al*. Diagnosing syncope. Part 1: Value of history, physical examination, and electrocardiography. *Ann Intern Med* 1997; **126**: 989–996.

Kapoor WH. Syncope. *N Engl J Med* 2000; **343**: 1856–1862.

Brignole M, Alboni P, Benditt D *et al*. Guidelines on management (diagnosis and treatment) of syncope-Update 2004. *Europace J* 2004; **6**: 467–537.

Colman N, Nahm K, van Dijk JG, Reitsma JB, Wieling W, Kaufmann H. Diagnostic value of history taking in reflex syncope. *Clin Auton Res* 2004 Oct; **14** Suppl 1: 37–44.

CHAPTER 8

The role of the prepared questionnaire in initial evaluation of transient losses of consciousness

Anna Serletis and Robert S. Sheldon

Introduction

There are numerous causes of transient loss of consciousness (TLOC). Although some of the less common causes of TLOC such as ventricular tachycardia are potentially life threatening and some such as epilepsy have substantial implications for lifestyle issues such as driving, in most patients TLOC is benign and does not pose an immediate threat to life. All the dangerous causes of TLOC and many of the benign causes merit treatment, and treating patients successfully begins with an accurate diagnosis.

The accurate and efficient diagnostic workup of TLOC can be difficult. Although many patients pose no diagnostic problems, not infrequently, clinicians must consider a number of possible etiologies. One of the problems in diagnosing the cause of loss of consciousness has been a reluctance to trust the history of unconsciousness, and the situations and symptoms that surround it, as an important source of information. This has led to reliance on investigative tools that measure structural and functional aspects of the central nervous system; ischemic, electrical, and structural aspects of the cardiovascular system; and various endocrinologic disorders. Most of these tools have a very limited diagnostic yield for unselected patients with a history of TLOC, most are expensive or invasive or both, and most continue to be used early in the diagnostic cascade. Are there other tools that might have a higher diagnostic yield?

Goals

- Identify limitations of current diagnostic strategies for evaluating TLOC;
- introduce the concept of a predefined questionnaire as a means of enhancing diagnostic assessment of TLOC.

Two popular diagnostic tools in the syncope evaluation are tilt-table tests and implantable loop recorders (ILRs). Tilt tests are thought to reproduce some aspect of the disturbed physiology that underlies the syndrome of neurally mediated reflex syncope and have been enormously useful in its study. They have provided a diagnosis in many patients with otherwise unexplained syncope, have been useful tools in the study of its physiology, and have provided uniformly diagnosed populations for natural history studies and clinical trials. ILRs record the ECG during syncope, and are therefore a screen for arrhythmic causes of syncope and for neurally mediated syncope syndromes associated with transient, autonomically mediated bradycardias. They have established the diagnostic outcomes of patients at higher risk for arrhythmic syncope and have provided valuable information about the heart rate of patients with probable neurally mediated syncope during their spells.

Tilt tests, although seemingly simple, are precariously balanced on a number of important variables. Not surprisingly, protocols that use a longer observation period, a steeper tilt angle, and drug interventions, have higher diagnostic accuracy but lower specificity. If two tilt test protocols come to divergent conclusions about any one patient, which one are we to accept? And can the approach in general be useful with this type of discrepancy? Patients with otherwise idiopathic syncope have the same baseline symptoms and symptom burden, the same clinical outcome, and the same statistical relationships between baseline symptoms and clinical outcome regardless of whether they have a positive or negative tilt test. Finally, there appears to be an intractable trade-off between diagnostic accuracy and specificity.

The ILR also has potential problems. It is a passive tool that relies on the patient having another syncopal spell. While this may be tolerable to some, it is not optimal for evaluation of patients with potentially fatal or harmful causes of syncope. Therefore, its use may be best restricted to patients with benign causes of syncope (although the benign nature of the cause cannot be readily predicted ahead of time). Further, ILRs are invasive and cost-effectiveness depends upon its sensitivity and the consequences of a diagnosis. Finally, TLOC due to causes such as epilepsy may have sinus tachycardia during the event, the same rhythm as is seen in many episodes of vasovagal syncope.

Can we take a better history?

Limitations of diagnostic tools highlight the potential importance of the medical history in assessing patients with TLOC. Compared to diagnostic techniques such as tilt testing, a careful medical history is not only cost- and time-effective, but may also reduce patient anxiety and morbidity.

Specific symptoms have traditionally been used to differentiate among various causes of TLOC. For example, generalized convulsions, tongue biting, and physical trauma have often been linked to seizure disorders. The presence of nausea, vomiting, and diaphoresis historically suggests vasovagal syncope, as do precipitating events such as severe pain, fear, and prolonged standing. Such associations are based on anecdotal accretion rather than evidence and have been further complicated by the recognition of syncope with apparently convulsive-like activity. They have been the subject of several reports of symptoms associated with TLOC in patients with vasovagal syncope in the older literature and have been reviewed recently (see Additional Reading). The problem with using these early reports for diagnosis is that the studies were usually not controlled by the inclusion of patients with other causes of TLOC and the results were reported as prevalences. Although prevalence data contribute to the overall sense of the diagnosis they are not definitively applicable.

Quantitative histories and diagnostic scores have increased diagnostic accuracy in other fields of medicine. Members of the American Rheumatology Association released a series of quantitative analyses of the diagnostic utility of various symptoms and signs in several chronic inflammatory disorders. Using both logistic regression and recursive partitioning, they developed and validated criteria with diagnostic accuracies around 90%. Further, we know that the use of a structured history improves the ability of clinicians to discriminate among some causes of seizures. These studies suggested the potential usefulness of similar tools for the assessment of TLOC patients.

Quantitative Histories

Several groups have reported progress in developing historical criteria for the diagnosis of causes of TLOC. In a study of 80 syncopal patients with neurally mediated syncope, atrioventricular block, or ventricular tachycardia, Calkins *et al.* compared clinical histories to determine features predictive of each cause of syncope. Some of the patients had a variety of causes of heart disease, while others had no apparent heart disease. A standard questionnaire was administered to each patient and they were also asked to describe their two most recent syncopal episodes in detail. The historical features of syncope due to ventricular tachycardia and atrioventricular block were quite similar, differing largely from those of neurally mediated syncope. Loss of consciousness due to ventricular tachycardia was associated with male sex, age >54 years, ≤2 episodes of syncope, and a duration of warning ≤5 s. In contrast, palpitations, blurred vision, nausea, warmth, diaphoresis, or lightheadedness prior to syncope, and nausea, warmth, diaphoresis, or fatigue following syncope were more predictive of neurally mediated syncope. The combination of four factors could predict the cause of syncope with 98% sensitivity and 100% specificity: age, sex, duration of the recovery period, and presence of mild or severe fatigue following syncope. However these may have been useful to some degree because they simply discriminated between patients with and without structural heart disease. How they would perform within specific subgroups of patients, for example those without structural heart disease, is unknown.

Alboni *et al.* evaluated 341 patients with causes of syncope established by standardized diagnostic criteria, including cardiac, and neurally mediated syncope. A standard questionnaire was administered to each patient, focusing on the historical findings surrounding their syncopal event. Not surprisingly, heart disease independently predicted a cardiac cause of syncope with 95% sensitivity and 45% specificity. Absence of heart disease excluded cardiac syncope in 97% of patients. In the presence of known or suspected heart disease, the most specific predictors of cardiac syncope were loss of consciousness while supine or during effort, blurred vision, and convulsive syncope. The most important predictors of neurally mediated syncope were time between the first and last episode >4 years, abdominal discomfort before syncope, and nausea and diaphoresis during recovery. In patients without heart disease, the only significant finding suggestive of a cardiac cause was palpitations prior to syncope.

While such features are helpful in generally classifying causes of syncope, they do not provide physicians with a simple, useful diagnostic tool. Diagnostic reliability of the first loss of consciousness is surprisingly low but this can be improved with a point score. A structured questionnaire based on firm quantitative evidence may prove very helpful in managing patients with TLOC.

The syncope symptom study

We hypothesized that evidence-based diagnostic criteria could distinguish between syncope and seizures as causes of TLOC. The Syncope Symptom Study was performed to test this hypothesis. A uniform questionnaire was completed by 671 patients who were referred to three academic centers in Canada and Wales for assessment of TLOC. Patients with securely defined diagnoses, based upon conventionally accepted objective tests, were tested first. Their responses were analyzed to identify the historical features that most accurately correlated with their diagnoses. We planned to develop three diagnostic questionnaires based upon a conventional and clinically relevant diagnostic approach. We addressed three questions in sequence. First, can we discriminate accurately between syncope and epilepsy? Second, can we discriminate accurately between vasovagal syncope and ventricular tachycardia in patients with structural heart disease? Third, can we discriminate between vasovagal syncope and other causes of syncope in patients without apparent structural heart disease?

The first study addressed the symptoms that discriminate between epileptic seizures and syncope. The causes of TLOC were known satisfactorily in 539 patients and included complex partial epilepsy, primary generalized epilepsy, tilt-positive vasovagal syncope, ventricular tachycardia, and other diagnoses such as complete heart block and supraventricular tachycardias. The point score based on symptoms alone correctly classified 94% of patients, diagnosing seizures with 94% sensitivity and 94% specificity. Therefore, a simple point score of historical features distinguished syncope from seizures with very high sensitivity and specificity.

Recently, we developed two similar questionnaires. The first of these was designed to assess patients with syncope in the setting of structural heart disease. An important diagnostic dilemma is that 20–40% of this patient population has ventricular tachycardia as a cause of syncope. A recurrence of this arrhythmia may be fatal, thus emphasizing the need for an accurate initial diagnosis. Other patients in this group have complete heart block and many have vasovagal syncope. Current investigations such as electrophysiologic testing have variable sensitivities and specificities, and may be inadequate. For example, invasive electrophysiologic testing is only 50% and 70% sensitive for ventricular tachycardia in the settings of idiopathic dilated cardiomyopathy and old inferior myocardial infarction. A brief quantitative questionnaire has been developed, which can distinguish between ventricular tachycardia and vasovagal syncope with 90% sensitivity and 90% specificity. The second brief questionnaire has similar accuracy in the population of patients with syncope and apparently structurally normal hearts. This too distinguishes between vasovagal syncope and other causes of syncope such as complete heart block and supraventricular tachycardia with about 90% accuracy.

Summary

Quantitative diagnostic criteria have specific uses, but cannot replace the richness of the classic history elicited by a skilled clinician. We have found that only about a dozen criteria are necessary to discriminate between major diagnostic groups, which means that numerous other descriptors are not captured. Some of these may help with patient counselling and treatment, and some may point to important diagnostic subgroups not discerned by the questionnaires. Importantly, the questionnaires reflect the patient groups used to develop them. For example, only patients with primary generalized convulsions and partial complex epilepsy with loss of consciousness were included in the development of the first questionnaire; therefore other less common causes of epileptic seizures may not be accurately detected. Rather, the questionnaires may prove to be useful diagnostic adjunctive tools rather than relying on more expensive or invasive tools such as tilt tests and ILRs. Although not meant to be the sole factor in diagnostic decisions, questionnaires may prove helpful to the clinician in the initial diagnostic assessment. They will provide inclusion criteria for population-based studies and clinical trials, permit a quantitative link among the various causes of vasovagal syncope, and allow us to examine the physiology of syncope in subgroups of patients who share common diagnostic criteria. If accepted by clinicians, they may significantly reduce the time, expense, and inaccuracy of the assessment of patients with TLOC.

Acknowledgment

From the Libin Cardiovascular Institute of Alberta, University of Calgary, Calgary, Alberta, Canada. This study was supported in part by grant 73-1976 from the Canadian Institutes for Health Research, Ottawa, Ontario, Canada.

References

1. Alboni P, Brignole M, Menozzi C *et al*. Diagnostic value of history in patients with syncope with or without heart disease. *J Am Coll Cardiol* 2001; **37**: 1921–1928.
2. Arnett FC, Edworthy SM, Bloch DA *et al*. The American Rheumatism Association 1987 revised criteria for the classification of rheumatoid arthritis. *Arthritis Rheum* 1988; **31**: 315–324.
3. Calkins H, Shyr Y, Frumin H, Schork A, Morady. The value of the clinical history in the differentiation of syncope due to ventricular tachycardia, atrioventricular block, and neurocardiogenic syncope. *Am J Med* 1995; **98**: 365–373.
4. Colman N, Nahm K, van Dijk JG, Reitsma JB, Wieling W, Kaufmann H. Diagnostic value of history taking in reflex syncope. *Clin Auton Res* 2004; **14**: 37–44.
5. Sheldon R. Tilt testing for syncope: a reappraisal. *Curr Opin Cardiol* 2005; **20**: 38–41.
6. Sheldon R, Rose S, Ritchie D et al. Historical criteria that distinguish syncope from seizures. *J Am Coll Cardiol* 2002; **40**: 142–148.
7. Van Donselaar CA, Geerts AT, Meulstee J, Habbema JDF, Staal A. Reliability of the diagnosis of a first seizure. *Neurology* 1989; **39**: 267–271.

CHAPTER 9

Who should be evaluated and treated in hospital, and who can be managed as an outpatient?

David G. Benditt

Introduction

When confronted with the dilemma of evaluating an individual who may have suffered a faint or syncope, it is prudent to first consider within the differential diagnosis the much broader category of conditions that cause periods of transient loss of consciousness (TLOC, see Chapter 2). Only after this first step leads to the conclusion that the TLOC was indeed true syncope should the physician focus on the more limited number of conditions that cause faints.

For purposes of this chapter, the assumption is made that we are dealing with true syncope. In this circumstance, it must be presumed from the outset that the patient had lost the capability to maintain postural tone for at least a short period of time on one, or often more than one, occasion. In this setting, the outcome may have been anything from serious injury to simple embarrassment. Nevertheless, whether physical injury was sustained or not, by virtue of the apparent susceptibility to loss of consciousness, there remains the need to assess future risk of personal injury as well potential for accidents and even harm to others, should syncope recur.

In terms of whether the patient with suspected syncope should be hospitalized in order for the physician to be able to undertake the diagnostic evaluation and if necessary initiate treatment safely, the driving force is most often concern regarding the patient's immediate mortality risk. Secondary issues of importance include potential for physical injury and to a lesser extent the issue of whether certain treatments inherently require hospital monitoring for safe initiation.

Goals

The goals of this chapter are to:
• identify those risk factors that favor hospitalizing a patient for the syncope evaluation;

- classify conditions in which hospitalization is not needed; and
- summarize treatment choices that may necessitate hospitalization for their safe initiation.

Overview of need for hospitalization

Admission to hospital may be appropriate for undertaking diagnostic studies in a safe environment or for initiating therapy, or both. For patients with syncope in whom the etiology remains unknown after the initial clinic or emergency department evaluation, a form of risk stratification can be used to determine if hospitalization is prudent.

In instances when the etiology of syncope has been diagnosed after the initial clinical evaluation, the need for hospitalization depends in part on the immediate risk posed to the patient by the underlying problem and in addition on the treatment proposed. Thus, for example, patients with syncope accompanying an acute myocardial infarction, or pulmonary embolism, or *torsade de pointes* ventricular tachycardia should be admitted to hospital and preferably to a monitored unit. Patients with dehydration due to excess diuretic therapy usually do not need admission, and more often than not can be treated sufficiently well in the emergency department or clinic and released after a few hours. Similarly, in terms of therapy considerations, patients needing pacemakers or implantable cardioverter defibrillators (ICDs) will usually need to be admitted possibly along with those in whom initiation of certain types of antiarrhythmic drugs is contemplated. On the other hand, for patients being treated with advice to increase salt and volume or in whom education regarding physical maneuvers like tilt-training or leg-crossing is to be provided, an outpatient visit is usually adequate.

When is hospitalization advised or out-of-hospital management safe?

The following provides an overview of common circumstances for which hospitalization is or is not recommended.

Strongly recommended

Several prognostic markers identify syncope patients who should be considered for inhospital evaluation. Syncope associated with an acute myocardial ischemia or infarction, and/or structural heart disease severe enough to cause hemodynamic impairment is associated with the highest immediate mortality risk. At similar high risk are syncope patients with certain ECG abnormalities, including high-grade AV block, preexcitation syndromes (e.g. Wolff–Parkinson–White syndrome), arrhythmogenic RV cardiomyopathy (ARVD), long QT syndrome (LQTS), Brugada syndrome, and the recently recognized short QT syndrome. Patients with syncope during exercise may also need to be evaluated in hospital. Some of these latter patients may have unrecognized myocardial ischemia, or exercise-induced AV block, while others may be susceptible to catecholamine-triggered tachyarrhythmias (e.g. idiopathic ventricular tachycardia, hypertrophic cardiomyopathy).

An additional troublesome prognostic marker is a family history of premature sudden death. This history may be indicative of ischemic heart disease but also of any of a variety of familial conditions, which may first present as syncope (e.g. LQTS, Brugada syndrome, familial cardiomyopathies, arrhythmogenic RV cardiomyopathy, etc). A number of these conditions are also discussed in more detail in later chapters (see Chapter 20).

Table 9.1 summarizes those conditions in which hospitalization for syncope assessment is strongly recommended. Tables 9.2 and 9.3 provide details of ECG findings and specific clinical scenarios that favor hospitalization.

Hospitalization desirable on case-by-case basis
These situations generally involve patients in whom the immediate risk of death is thought to be low and there is low likelihood of a near-term recurrence

Table 9.1 When to hospitalize a patient with syncope for diagnosis.

Strongly recommended for diagnosis
Suspected or known significant heart disease
ECG abnormalities suggestive of arrhythmic syncope (Table 9.2)
Syncope occurring during exercise (Table 9.3)
Syncope causing severe injury
Strong family history of sudden death
Occasionally may need to be admitted
Patients with or without heart disease but with:
• sudden onset of palpitations shortly before syncope;
• syncope in supine position;
• worrisome family history;
• significant physical injury.
Patients with minimal or mild heart disease when there is high suspicion for cardiac syncope
Suspected pacemaker or ICD problem

Table 9.2 ECG findings supporting hospital admission for diagnosis.

Acute myocardial infarction
Acute pulmonary embolism
Complete or high-grade atrioventricular block
Long QT syndrome
Brugada syndrome
Preexcitation (e.g. Wolff–Parkinson–White) syndrome, especially if documented atrial fibrillation and rapid ventricular response

Table 9.3 Causes of syncope during exercise or exertion.

Critical coronary artery disease
Congenital coronary artery anomaly
Severe valvular/subvalvular disease
• aortic stenosis
• hypertrophic cardiomyopathy (HCM)
Cardiomyopathies
High-grade atrioventricular block
Cathecholamine-triggered ventricular tachyarrhythmias
• Long QT (LQTS, KvLQT1)
• Idiopathic ventricular tachycardias
• Certain primary autonomic diseases
(Rare) Exercise/postexercise variant of neurally mediated reflex faint

Table 9.4 When to hospitalize a patient with syncope for treatment.

Cardiac arrhythmias as cause:
• drug initiation (particularly QT prolonging agents);
• proposed radiofrequency ablation (RFA);
• pacemaker/ICD implantation.

Ischemic cause:
• revascularization;
• drug initiation;
• exercise testing.

Neurally mediated:
• when pacemaker proposed;
• after significant injury/accident.

Severe orthostatic hypotension associated with:
• focal neurologic abnormality;
• injury/fracture;
• motor vehicle accident.

Social constraints:
• absence of adequate/safe home care

precipitating injury or harm to the public health (Table 9.4). Clearly, this is a judgment call and one ought to err on the side of caution. Some of the genetically transmitted disorders noted above may fall into this group, if the symptom events have been infrequent and the family history is not excessively worrisome. Additionally, some patients may not have sufficiently adequate or safe home environments to be assured that they will remain safe during outpatient evaluation.

Table 9.5 Low-risk scenarios favoring outpatient evaluation.

Isolated or rare syncope without:
• cardiac disease or significant ECG abnormality
• pacemaker or ICD present
• worrisome physical injury
• public health hazard in compliant patient
History typical of vasovagal or situational faint
History suggestive of syncope mimic (see Chapter 23)

Hospitalization can be avoided

For patients with isolated or rare syncope episodes, in whom there is no evidence of structural heart disease and who have a normal baseline ECG, the probability is high that the event was of neurally mediated reflex origin (see also Chapter 20, Part 1). In this setting, the risk of a life-threatening cardiac syncope is low. These patients have a good prognosis in terms of survival and generally their evaluation can be completed entirely on an outpatient basis. Nevertheless, for individuals with multiple faints over a lengthy period of time (years), recurrences may be expected and cautionary advice regarding driving, occupation, and avocation should be provided until such time as one is confident that the susceptibility to fainting has been suppressed. Further, it is important to be certain that the individual's home environment is safe and that there is sufficient home-care support to permit the subsequent evaluation to be carried out in an outpatient environment. Individuals with solitary faints have a much lower recurrence risk. These latter individuals should be provided insight into their condition in the clinic, but may not need to be hospitalized if the diagnosis is clear.

Most often, patients with neurally mediated reflex faints (especially vasovagal faints) do not need specific treatment apart from counseling and the general measures discussed in Chapter 20, Part 1. If treatment is needed because of recurrences, it can usually be initiated on an ambulatory basis in even the most frequent fainter.

Table 9.5 summarizes clinical findings associated with low risk of severe injury and/or death in a syncope patient. These individuals usually represent good candidates for outpatient evaluation and treatment.

Summary

The decision to hospitalize a patient with syncope for diagnostic evaluation and/or initiation of therapy depends primarily on the short-term mortality risk to the patient. In older individuals, the short-term morbidity risk also plays a role (i.e. fracture risk if syncope recurs in the elderly). Additional concerns relate to public well-being. These concerns may become relevant, should a noncompliant fainter resume driving an automobile or commercial vehicle, piloting an aircraft, or resuming an occupation or avocation the performance of which might cause risk to others if loss of consciousness were to recur.

There are no convincing data regarding risk of death or injury during the out-of-hospital evaluation of syncope patients. However, if the risk stratification provided here is used, the chances of an adverse outcome during the evaluation and treatment initiation phase should be remote.

Additional reading

Blanc JJ, L'Her C, Touiza A, *et al.* Prospective evaluation and outcome of patients admitted for syncope over 1 year period. *Eur Heart J* 2002; **23**: 815–20

Brignole M, Alboni P, Benditt DG *et al.* Guidelines on management (diagnosis and treatment) of syncope. *Europace* 2004; **6**: 467–537.

CHAPTER 10

Organizing management of syncope in the hospital and clinic (the syncope unit)

Rose Anne Kenny and Michele Brignole

Introduction

Inasmuch as syncope is a common symptom – experienced by 15% of persons under 18 years and up to 23% of older nursing home residents – it is important to consider optimizing strategies for the management of these patients. The strategy selected will inevitably differ from place-to-place depending on patient volume, available resources, and the expertise of medical personnel. However, ultimately an organized structure will offer more cost-effective care.

Goals

The goals of this chapter are to:
• outline possible health care delivery models for syncope management;
• review current status of the organization of syncope care; and
• summarize the Newcastle experience to illustrate the value of a multidisciplinary approach to the organized management of syncope patients.

General features of the syncope care delivery organization

There is no single syncope care delivery model suitable for all environments. The following offers a list of some of the more important features to consider when establishing such an organization.
• The model of care delivery should be the one that it is most appropriate to existing practice and will maximize resources and local expertise while ensuring implementation of published practice guidelines.
• Models of care delivery will vary from a single 'one site–one stop' syncope facility to a wider-based multifaceted practice where a number of specialists are involved in syncope management. The management strategy should be agreed upon and practiced by all practitioners (encompassing a range of specialties) involved in syncope management.

• The age range and symptom characteristics of patients appropriate for syncope investigation should be determined in advance. Some facilities are prepared to evaluate both pediatric and adult syncope patients while others limit practice to adult or pediatric cases.

• Potential referral sources should be taken into consideration. Referral can be directly from family practitioners, from the accident and emergency department, from hospital admissions, and from patients in institutional settings. The scope of referral source has implications for resources and skill mix.

• In a single dedicated facility, the skill mix will depend on the specialty designated to take a lead in the development of the facility. There are existing models where cardiologists (commonly with an interest in cardiac pacing and electrophysiology), neurologists (commonly with an interest in autonomic disorders and/or epilepsy), general physicians, and geriatricians (with an interest in age-related cardiology or falls) have each led syncope facilities. There is no evidence for superiority of any model.

• One factor, which will determine the skill mix (i.e. the types of professionals/expertise required to staff the facility), is the extent to which screening of referrals occurs prior to presentation at the facility. If referrals hail directly from the community and/or from the accident and emergency department, a broader skill mix is required. Under these circumstances, other differential diagnoses such as epilepsy, neurodegenerative disorders, metabolic disorders, and falls are more likely to be referred.

• It is essential to establish a mechanism through which regular communication can be established with all stakeholders (i.e. patients, referring physicians, hospital/clinic management, consultant physicians, nurses, and other allied medical professionals) in order to ensure an ongoing consensus for and understanding of proposed management strategies. This includes the implications of, and implementation of published guidelines. Among the medical profession stakeholders it is important to consider staff members in cardiology, the accident and emergency department, neurology department, general medicine service, orthopedic surgery, geriatric medicine, psychiatry and ear, nose and throat (ENT) department.

Need for coordinating the syncope evaluation

Emerging data suggests that up to 20% of cardiovascular syncope in older patients (over 70 years) presents as nonaccidental falls. There is also evidence from the 'falls' literature that multifactorial intervention that includes cardiovascular interventions (treatment of orthostatic hypotension, carotid sinus hypersensitivity, arrhythmias, and vasovagal susceptibility) significantly reduces subsequent falls in fallers with recurrent episodes – even if these are accidental falls. This has enormous implications for the volume of patients seen. It requires access to, or incorporation of, assessments and interventions for other common comorbid risk factors such as gait and balance instability, cerebrovascular disease, home hazard modifications, etc. An example of the scope of this issue is illustrated in a study from Newcastle. Forty-four percent of all accident and emergency attendees over 65 years came because of a fall or syncopal event. Of these patients, 35% had accidental falls, 25% were patients who had cognitive impairment or dementia (therefore a clear distinction between falls/syncope was often not possible), 22% had a medical explanation for the event (stroke, epilepsy, arrhythmia, etc), and 18% had unexplained falls or syncope.

Present syncope management (diagnosis and treatment) situation

Syncope is a common symptom in the community and in emergency medicine. For example, in the United Kingdom, syncope and collapse (International Classification of Diagnoses code 10) are the sixth most common reason for admission of adults aged >65 years to acute medical hospital beds. Given that half of all emergency admissions are >65 years of age, this constitutes a large volume of activity. The average length of stay for these admissions is 5 to 17 days – emphasizing the diversity of syncope management strategies and availability of existing investigations.

Currently, strategies for assessment of syncope vary widely among physicians and among hospitals and clinics. More often than not, the evaluation and treatment of syncope is haphazard and unstratified. The result is a broad and largely inexplicable variance from center to center in the frequency with which various diagnostic tests are applied, in the distribution of apparent attributable causes of syncope arrived at by attending clinicians, and in the proportion of syncope patients in which the diagnosis remains unexplained. One example of this is pacing rates for carotid sinus syndrome that vary even within countries from 1 to 25% of implants, depending on whether carotid sinus hypersensitivity is systematically assessed in the investigation profile. Another example is the prevalence of syncope that remains unexplained. This varies from 10 to 70%.

Assuming the status quo of the syncope evaluation is maintained, diagnostic and treatment effectiveness is unlikely to improve substantially. Even implementation of the published syncope management guidelines is likely to be diverse, uneven in application, and of uncertain benefit. It is the ESC Syncope Task Force's view that a cohesive, structured care pathway – delivered either within a single syncope facility or as a more multifaceted service – is now timely. In this manner, considerable improvement in diagnostic yield and cost effectiveness (i.e. cost per reliable diagnosis) can be achieved by focusing skills and following well-defined up-to-date diagnostic guidelines.

Newcastle syncope management unit model

The service model adopted by the Newcastle group is a multidisciplinary approach to referrals with syncope or falls. All patients attend the same facility (with access to cardiovascular equipment, investigations, and trained staff) but are investigated by a geriatrician or cardiovascular physician according to the dominant symptom cited in referral correspondence – falls or syncope. Recently, this group showed that activity at the acute hospital at which the day case falls and syncope evaluation unit was based, experienced 6116 fewer bed-days during the course of 1 year for the ICD code 10 categories comprising syncope and collapse compared to peer teaching hospitals in the United Kingdom. This reduction translated into a significant saving in emergency hospital costs (about four million euros or US dollars). The savings were attributed to a combination of factors – reduced readmission rates, rapid access to day case facility for accident and emergency and community patients, and implementation of effective targeted treatment strategies for syncope and falls. A similar US model (from workers at the Mayo Clinic), which randomized syncopal patients at the time of ER attendance to 'syncope unit' evaluation or 'standard care', demonstrated a four times higher diagnostic yield and a halving of hospital admission

Professional skill mix for the syncope evaluation facility

It is probably not appropriate to be dogmatic regarding the training needs of personnel responsible for a dedicated syncope facility. These skills will depend on the predetermined requirements of local professional bodies, the level of screening evaluation provided prior to referral, and the nature of the patient population typically encountered in a given setting. In general, experience and training in key components of cardiology, neurology, and geriatric medicine that are pertinent to the assessment and diagnosis of syncope, in addition to access to other specialties such as psychiatry, physiotherapy, occupational therapy, ENT, and clinical psychology are recommended.

Staff responsible for the clinical management of the facility should be conversant with the various appropriate diagnostic and treatment guidelines. The principal guidelines are as follows: 'Guidelines on management (diagnosis and treatment) of syncope', 'Guidelines for the prevention of falls in older persons', and 'Clinical guidelines for treatment and practical tools for aiding epilepsy management' (see Additional Reading for citations). A structured approach to the management of syncope also expedites clinical audit, patient information systems, service developments, and continuous professional training.

Equipment

Core equipment for the syncope evaluation facility includes surface electrocardiogram (ECG) recording, phasic blood pressure (BP) monitoring, tilt table testing equipment, external and implantable ECG, loop recorder systems, and 24-hour ambulatory BP, 24-hour ambulatory ECG, and autonomic function testing. The facility should also have access to intracardiac electrophysiologic testing, stress testing, cardiac imaging, CT, and MRI head scans and electroencephalography.

Setting

The majority of syncope patients can be investigated as outpatients or day cases.

Indications for hospital admission (see also Chapter 9) and investigation are those cases in which syncope occurs in association with one or more of the following:
• significant heart disease (particularly critical valvular or subvalvular aortic stenosis, severe coronary artery disease);
• suspected potentially serious cardiac arrhythmias (e.g. long QT syndromes, Brugada syndrome, preexcitation syndromes);
• physical exercise;
• severe injury; or
• family history of sudden death.

Summary

In summary, the role of a local integrated syncope service is to set standards for, and optimize the effectiveness of, the evaluation and treatment of syncope patients at a given center. This is best accomplished by a multidisciplinary approach and should be in keeping with appropriate guidelines such as those established by the objectives of the European Society of Cardiology Syncope Task Force Guidelines. The standards should consider, at a minimum, the following issues.
• The diagnostic criteria for causes of syncope.
• The preferred approach to the diagnostic workup in subgroups of patients with syncope.
• Risk stratification of the patient with syncope.
• Treatments to prevent syncope recurrences.
When establishing a newly structured service, current experience suggests that careful audit of the syncope unit activity and performance will rapidly justify the initial resource allocation and requests for additional funding, fuel further service development, and provide a legitimate magnet for increasing patient referrals.

Additional reading

Brignole M, Alboni P, Benditt D *et al*. Guidelines on management (diagnosis and treatment) of syncope. *Europace* 2004; **6**: 467–537.

Brignole M, Disertori M, Menozzi C *et al*. Evaluation of Guidelines in Syncope Study group. Management of syncope referred urgently to general hospitals with and without syncope units. *Europace* 2003; **5**: 293–298.

Department of Health. Improving services for people with epilepsy. Department of Health Action Plan in response to the National Clinical Audit of Epilepsy-related Death. London: Department of Health, 2003. Available from: URL: http://www.dh.gov.uk

Guideline for the prevention of falls in older persons. American Geriatrics Society, British Geriatrics Society, and American Academy of Orthopaedic Surgeons Panel on Falls Prevention. *J Am Geriatr Soc* 2001; **49**: 664–672.

Kenny RA, Richardson DA, Steen N *et al.* Carotid sinus syndrome: a modifiable risk factor for nonaccidental falls in older adults (SAFE PACE). *J Am Coll Cardiol* 2001; **38**: 1491–1496.

Kenny RA, O'Shea D, Walker HF. Impact of a dedicated syncope and falls facility for older adults on emergency beds. *Age Ageing* 2002; **31**: 272–275.

Shaw FE, Bond J, Richardson DA *et al.* Multifactorial intervention after a fall in older people with cognitive impairment and dementia presenting to the accident and emergency department. *Br Med J* 2003; **326**: 73–77.

Shen WK, Decker WW, Smars PA *et al.* Syncope Evaluation in the Emergency Department Study (SEEDS): a multidisciplinary approach to syncope management. *Circulation* 2004; **110**: 3636–3645.

CHAPTER 11

Impact of syncope guidelines on clinical care

Michele Brignole

Introduction

Despite the publication of clinical guidelines detailing the preferred approach to the diagnosis and treatment of syncope, strategies for the assessment of syncope continue to vary widely among physicians and among hospitals. Consequently, the evaluation and treatment of syncope often remains haphazard and unorganized. The outcome is often:
- use of inappropriate diagnostic tests,
- a large residual of misdiagnosed and still unexplained syncope, and
- excessive, cost-inefficient utilization of medical resources.

Goals

The goal of this chapter is to highlight the as yet inadequate acceptance of professional management guidelines for care of syncope patients.

A picture from the real world

Assuming the status quo of the syncope evaluation unchanged, diagnostic and treatment effectiveness is unlikely to improve substantially. Even implementation of published syncope management guidelines is likely to be diverse, uneven in application, and of uncertain benefit.

Guidelines from scientific societies should provide the standard of care but guidelines are often poorly publicized even among specialists, and are sometimes difficult to apply in clinical practice. Furthermore, physicians of specialties different from those that established the guidelines or who practice outside the geographical boundaries of the guideline-sponsoring agency are often reluctant to apply the guidelines to their patients. Thus, guidelines alone cannot change customary practice.

A prospective observational registry from a sample of 28 general hospitals was performed in Italy in order to evaluate the impact of the 2001 syncope guidelines of the European Society of Cardiology (ESC) on usual practice of management of syncope patients admitted via the emergency department.

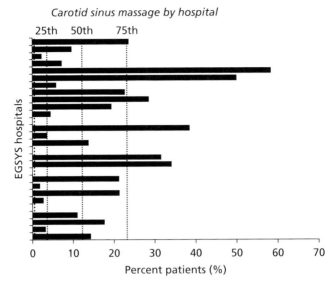

Figure 11.1 Incidence with which carotid sinus massage was undertaken at each of the 28 hospitals participating in the EGSYS-1 study expressed as percentage of total patients admitted. Each bar represents one hospital. The vertical dotted lines are those corresponding to the twenty-fifth, fifty and seventy-fifth percentiles of distribution.

The Evaluation of Guidelines in Syncope Study 1 (EGSYS-1) enrolled all consecutive patients referred to their emergency rooms from 5 November 2001 to 7 December 2001 for evaluation of transient loss of consciousness as the principal symptom. Data gathering began approximately 3 months after initial publication of the ESC Syncope guidelines. Observations obtained at each of the 28 participating hospitals were evaluated separately. The authors observed marked inter-hospital and inter-department heterogeneity with regard to the incidence of emergency admission, inhospital evaluation and treatment pathways, most of the tests performed, and the final assigned diagnosis. For example, the performance of carotid sinus massage as part of the diagnostic assessment ranged from 0% in one hospital to 58% in another (median 12.5%) (Figure 11.1); tilt testing ranged from 0% to 50% (median 5.8%); the final diagnosis of neurally mediated syncope ranged from 10% to 78.6% (median 43.3%). This heterogeneity may be partially explained by differences in the clinical characteristics of the population referred to the hospitals participating in the study. However, this proportion of the overall variability was calculated <10% of total variance. Thus, we can assume that the main determinant of inter-institution differences of behavior lies in the attitudes of the staff. As consequence of the great inter-hospital variability, the authors were unable to identify any uniformity of strategy for the management of syncope in clinical practice at that time.

Therefore, what to do? The solution is the creation of standardized care pathways in which guidelines can be effectively applied. Two recent studies evaluated this new management strategy.

A new management of syncope

The Syncope Evaluation in the Emergency Department Study (SEEDS) evaluated the hypothesis that a designated syncope unit in the emergency department improves diagnostic yield and reduces hospital admission for patients with syncope who are at intermediate risk for an adverse cardiovascular outcome according to the Guidelines on Syncope of the American College of Emergency Physicians. In this prospective, randomized, single-center study, patients were randomly allocated to two treatment arms: syncope unit evaluation and standard care. One hundred and three consecutive patients entered the study. Fifty-one patients were randomized to the syncope unit. For the syncope unit and standard care patients, the presumptive diagnosis was established in 34 (67%) and 5 (10%) patients respectively, hospital admission was required for 22 (43%) and 51 (98%) patients, and total patient-hospital days were reduced from 140 to 64. Thus, the novel syncope unit designed for this study significantly improved diagnostic yield in the emergency department and reduced hospital admission and total length of hospital stay.

Recently the EGSYS-2 validated a new method of management of syncope based on a decision-making approach developed in strict adherence to the recommendations of the updated guidelines of the European Society of Cardiology. In order to maximize its application, a decision making guideline-based software was used and trained core medical personnel were designated – both locally in each hospital and centrally – to verify adherence to the diagnostic pathway and give advice on its correct application. A prospective, controlled, multi-center study was performed in order to verify if this standardized method of care is superior to the usual care. The patients referred from 4 October to 5 November 2004 for emergency to 19 Italian general hospitals were managed according this new standardized care pathway and were compared with those referred from 5 November to 7 December 2001 who were managed according usual practice. There were 929 patients in the usual care and 745 patients in the standardized care group. The baseline characteristics of the two study populations were similar. At the end of the evaluation, the standardized care group had a 17% lower hospitalization rate (39% versus 47%), 11% shorter inhospital stay (7.2 ± 5.7 versus 8.1 ± 5.9 days), and 26% fewer tests performed per patient (median 2.5 versus 3.4). Forty-one percent more of the 'standardized care' patients had a diagnosis of neurally mediated reflex syncope (65% versus 46%), and 66% more of orthostatic syncope (10% versus 6%), while 54% fewer had a diagnosis of pseudo-syncope (6% versus 13%), and 75% fewer remained labeled as unexplained syncope (5% versus 20%). The mean cost per patient was 19% lower (€ 1127 versus 1394) and the mean cost per diagnosis was 29% lower (€ 1240 versus 1753), in the 'standardized care' group. In brief, this study indicated that a standardized care pathway significantly improved diagnostic yield and reduced hospital admissions, resource consumption, and overall costs. Thus, although the results of the EGSYS-2 study are difficult to reproduce in everyday practice, the study shows that ESC guidelines can be implemented in a clinical setting comprising both dedicated trained medical personnel and availability of specifically designed decision making software.

Summary

The publication of guidelines alone does not sufficiently impact clinical care. However, the creation of cohesive, structured syncope facilities incorporating as part of its mandate a well-defined up-to-date set of diagnostic and treatment guidelines, as in the model proposed by the ESC guidelines (see also Chapter 10), may enhance the quality and cost-effectiveness of syncope evaluation and treatment.

Additional reading

Disertori M, Brignole M , Menozzi C *et al*. Management of syncope referred for emergency to general hospitals (EGSYS 1). Europace 2003; **5**: 283–291.

Shen W, Decker W, Smars P *et al*. Syncope evaluation in the emergency department study (SEEDS). A multidisciplinary approach to syncope management. *Circulation* 2004; **110**: 3636–3645.

Brignole M, Menozzi C, Bartoletti A, *et al*. A new management of syncope. Prospective systematic guideline-based evaluation of patients referred urgently to general hospitals (EGSYS 2)(EUR Heart J 2005 (in press)).

Brignole M, Ungar A, Bartoletti A, *et al*. Standardized care pathway versus usual management of syncope referred in emergency to general hospitals (EGSYS 2) (in press)

American College of Emergency Physicians. Clinical policy: critical issues in the evaluation and management of patients presenting with syncope. *Ann Emerg Med.* 2001; **37**: 771–776.

Brignole M, Alboni P, Benditt D, *et al*. Guidelines on management (diagnosis and treatment) of syncope – Update 2004. Europace 2004; **6**: 467–537.

Brignole M, Alboni P, Benditt D, *et al*. Guidelines on management (diagnosis and treatment) of syncope – Update 2004 – Executive summary and recommendations. *Eur Heart J* 2004; **25**: 2054–2072.

Section three:
Specific diagnostic procedures

CHAPTER 12

Ambulatory electrocardiographic monitoring for evaluation of syncope

Adam P. Fitzpatrick and David G. Benditt

Introduction

Syncope is often infrequent and as such it is difficult to document spontaneous symptoms by a diagnostic investigation. Electrocardiographic (ECG) monitoring is one of the most important tools used to establish a basis for syncope by determining a symptom-ECG correlation. However, ECG monitoring is constrained by technologic limitations.

Goals

The goals of this chapter are to:
• review currently available ambulatory ECG (AECG) systems applicable to the evaluation of syncope patients; and
• provide recommendations regarding AECG systems for various circumstances.

AECG monitoring options
Holter monitoring

Monitoring of AECG for evaluation of patients with syncope is most often undertaken using an external 24 or 48 h recorder that uses a cassette magnetic tape or more recently a computer storage media to retain ECG tracings. This device often retains its long-standing name, Holter monitor. The recorder is connected to the patient via external wiring and conventional adhesive ECG patches.

The advantages of this technology are several; it is noninvasive, there is beat-to-beat complete acquisition of the heart rhythm over the period of monitoring (as long as the electrode patches remain secure), the recording device costs are low, and there is relatively high recording fidelity over short time periods.

However, the limitations of this approach include:
• a recurrence of presenting symptoms is unlikely to occur during the relatively limited monitoring period,
• patients may not tolerate adhesive surface electrodes for more than a few days, and
• electrodes may not remain adherent throughout monitoring or during an event.

The vast majority of patients with syncope have a symptom frequency (i.e. interval between events) measured in weeks, months or years, but not days. Consequently, syncope-ECG correlation is rarely achieved with Holter monitoring. The diagnostic yield is variably reported to be between 6 and 20%, but may in fact be much less (see later).

Apart from the limitations noted above, conventional Holter-type AECG monitoring can be additionally problematic in that an asymptomatic arrhythmia detected by Holter is often used to make a diagnosis by inference, but without symptom-ECG correlation. Further, there is potential for symptoms to be inappropriately minimized if monitoring fails to yield any evidence of an arrhythmia. This is particularly likely because many physicians may not understand that given the low likelihood of recording a spontaneous event during the limited Holter recording period (usually 24 or 48 h), such monitoring generally offers a very low diagnostic yield in the syncope evaluation. Our studies and others indicate that the true diagnostic yield of Holter-type AECG monitoring in syncope is about 1%.

Holter monitoring in syncope is inexpensive in terms of set-up cost, but since the diagnostic yield is low, the test is expensive in terms of cost per diagnosis. This is especially the case if a very large number of tapes/storage media must be recorded to yield a symptom-ECG correlation. In this regard, it may be reasonable to avoid unnecessary analysis of 'asymptomatic' tapes, and simply analyze 'symptomatic' tapes. However, while such a strategy may reduce cost in some respects, it nevertheless requires provision of very large numbers of recorders to serve the need, greatly increasing another aspect of cost.

Given the rarity with which an AECG-syncope correlation can be obtained by conventional Holter monitoring, it is highly likely that this monitoring approach will result in frequent false-negative findings. In essence, if syncope does not occur, but certain arrhythmias are detected (e.g. premature ventricular contractions [PVCs] or paroxysmal atrial fibrillation) the physician may be tempted to assume, incorrectly, a diagnostic connection.

Holter monitoring may be of more value in the syncope evaluation if symptoms are very frequent. Single or multiple episodes of loss of consciousness occurring on a daily basis might increase the potential for symptom-ECG correlation. However, experience in these patients (i.e. those with multiple daily events) suggests that it is unlikely that they have true syncope; indeed many of these patients may have psychogenic 'blackouts' (i.e. psychogenic 'pseudosyncope'). On the other hand, in such patients, true negative (i.e. not an arrhythmic origin) findings during Holter monitoring may be useful in ruling out a cardiovascular origin and suggesting a psychogenic underlying cause.

External AECG event monitoring

Most syncope patients experience relatively long asymptomatic periods between events. Consequently, external AECG recorders that are available to the patient over these relatively long time periods would be expected to have a higher diagnostic yield than does a 24- or 48-h recording obtainable with a Holter monitor. These latter AECG recorders are commonly termed 'event recorders' as they are available (in theory) for the patient to use when a symptom 'event' occurs.

Conventional event recorders are external devices equipped with fixed electrodes through which an ECG can be recorded by direct application of the recorder electrodes to the chest wall (or other locations such as the wrist). Provided the patient can comply at the time of symptoms, a high-fidelity recording can be made. Figure 12.1 illustrates a type of widely available event recorder.

Recordings can be prospective (i.e. initiated by triggering the device at onset of symptoms) or retrospective (i.e. a looping memory that retains a period of recording so that it can be triggered after the patient has recovered) or both. Some recorders have long-term cutaneous ECG patch connections facilitating good skin contact for recordings. Newer devices can record every beat over 7 days allowing automatic recording supplemented by patient event

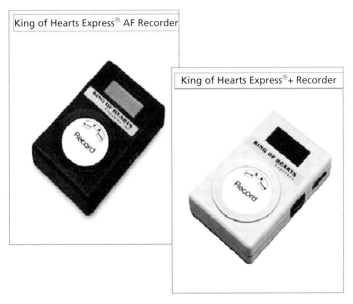

King of Hearts Express® AF Recorder

King of Hearts Express®+ Recorder

Figure 12.1 Figure depicting several typical externally worn AECG event recorders supplied by Instromedix Inc. (San Diego, CA).

notification for longer periods. Often, however, patients consider devices that require long-term cutaneous electrodes to be a substantial inconvenience and they are simply not tolerated. The need for the patient to remove and replace skin electrodes daily (to avoid skin damage) has the potential for considerable adverse impact on patient compliance.

External event recorders often have a limited value in syncope if the patient has to apply the recorder to the chest just prior to or immediately following the period of unconsciousness. In the absence of a very prolonged premonitory warning period or the presence of a very astute bystander, such application is often impossible. Devices that are continuously attached and recording are more useful. Recently, Mobile Cardiac Outpatient Telemetry (MCOT, Cardionet Inc., San Diego, CA) has proven increasingly popular in the United States. This system can be activated by the patient during symptom onset or automatically if a predetermined arrhythmia is detected. Wireless connection via the internet permits the recording to be transmitted almost immediately to a central receiving station and ultimately to the appropriate physician (Figure 15.2)

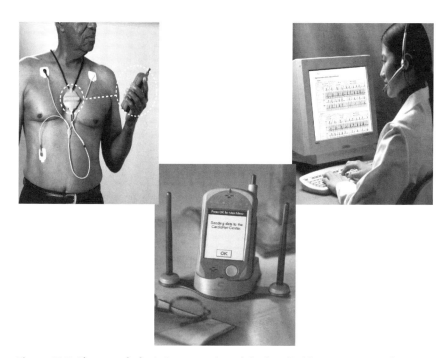

Figure 12.2 Photograph depicting operation of the handheld transmitter used in conjunction with the currently available MCOT system (Cardionet Inc., San Diego, CA). The ambulatory patient's ECG and symptom status are transmitted automatically to the central receiving center (right) either by wireless telephony (left) when away from home or by land line if available (center) when at home.

Inevitably, with long-term external AECG monitoring, if there are no events over quite a long period of time patient compliance drops. In such circumstances, the patient forgets to carry the instrument and the recorder is then not nearby when an event does occur.

Implantable AECG event monitoring

Implantable loop recorders (ILRs) have been available since 1998 (Medtronic Reveal® and RevealPlus® ECG event monitors) (Figure 15.3). These devices are placed in a small subcutaneous pocket analogous to the technique for placement of a conventional pacemaker generator but without the need for vascular access, as there are no leads. The optimal location is usually just to the left of the sternum. However, more discreet locations in the anterior axillary region have also proven effective. The best orientation can be 'mapped' out preoperatively. The procedure is undertaken using local anesthetic and the patient can return home almost immediately thereafter. The battery life is rated at 14 months but the device often operates for 18–20 months.

High-fidelity ILR ECG recordings can be obtained in most patients with relatively little interference from skeletal muscle artifact or extraneous electrical 'noise'. The ILR has a solid state loop memory and the current version can store up to 42 min of continuous ECG. Retrospective ECG allows activation of the device after consciousness has been restored and the RevealPlus® version is capable of both automatic recordings (based on physician-determined recording parameters) and patient-activated recordings. In one series of very symptomatic patients, symptom-ECG correlation was achieved in approximately 90% of patients within 6 months of implantation. Other studies of ILR use in syncope patients have resulted in a diagnostic yield of 25–40% over a 8- to 10-month recording period. Obviously, the more prolonged the monitoring time, the greater the chance of obtaining a useful recording.

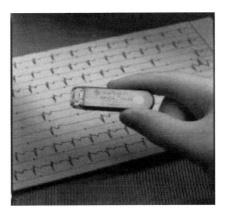

Figure 12.3 Photograph depicting a Reveal® implantable loop recorder (Medtronic Inc., Minneapolis, MN). The small size can be inferred from the fingers holding the device.

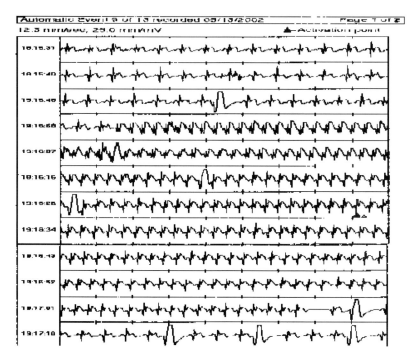

Figure 12.4 ECG recording derived from an ILR in a syncope patient revealing that a supraventricular tachycardia was the cause of symptoms.

The advantages of the ILR include continuous high-fidelity ECG record-ing (Figures 12.4 and 12.5), and a loop memory. The loop memory allows the patient to activate the device after consciousness is restored and thereby retain the critical ECG recording obtained during symptoms. Further, the ILR eliminates certain logistical factors that prevent good ECG recording during symptoms, for example, poor skin contact. The result is a high yield in terms of symptom-ECG correlation. This is because of the very long duration of monitoring, which confers a high likelihood of recording during recurrence of presenting symptoms. Limitations of current ILRs include the need for sur-gical implantation, a lack of recording of any other concurrent physiologic parameter, for example, blood pressure, and the relatively high up-front cost of the device (Table 12.1).

Crude analysis suggests that the ILR carries a high up-front cost. How-ever, if symptom–ECG correlation can be achieved in 90% of patients within 6 months of implantation, then analysis of the cost per symptom-ECG yield would show that the implanted device is far more cost-effective than Holter monitoring. In this regard, we analyzed costs in 200 patients with recurrent syncope. The yield of conventional Holter ECG monitoring was 1%, while a cohort of 186 patients had 90% symptom-ECG correlation at 6 months after ILR implantation. Overall, conventional Holter monitoring costs 3.75 times as

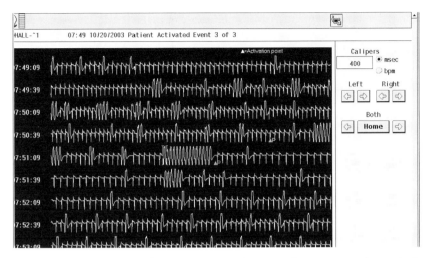

Figure 12.5 ILR ECG tracing from a syncope patient revealing paroxysmal ventricular tachycardia.

Table 12.1 Advantages and limitations of current generation ILRs.

Advantages

Long ECG recording capability (18–20 months)

Loop memory – allows activation after consciousness is restored

Automatic recording – allows automatic acquisition of ECG events, which fall outside
  programmable boundaries

Elimination of technical factors that impair good-quality surface ECG recording during
  symptoms (e.g. poor contact, incapacitated patient)

High symptom-ECG correlation yield (cost-effective) – prolonged recording duration
  increases likelihood of capturing a spontaneous event

Limitations

Need to implant the device surgically

Up-front cost – although proven 'cost-effective' because of improved diagnostic yield

Limited memory storage

Lack of recording of other potentially important physiologic parameters (e.g. blood pressure)

Absence of treatment capability or long-distance communication* should a life-threatening
  rhythm be detected.

---

* Systems are currently in development that will address this limitation.

much per symptom-ECG correlation than did the ILR. Even if the ILR yield proved to be only 30–40%, it would retain a significant cost-effectiveness advantage.

AECG monitoring in syncope – where in the work-up?

The role of AECG monitoring in and the appropriate type of monitor to select for the syncope evaluation cannot be determined in isolation. Physicians should be guided by the clinical history (i.e. frequency and severity of episodes), physical examination, and objective testing. For some situations where evidence is accumulated this way and strongly suggests perhaps a neurally mediated reflex syncope, AECG monitoring may be deemed unnecessary. This might be especially the case if symptoms are infrequent (i.e. Holter monitoring is particularly unlikely to yield a diagnosis) and there is a bias against implantable monitoring (e.g. young patient, patient adverse to procedures, economic issues in the health care system). In other circumstances, where treatment decisions cannot be made without more information, recording a spontaneous event becomes crucial. In the future, as technology allows recording of multiple signals in addition to the ECG (see Chapter 13) greater emphasis will be placed on the features of spontaneous, rather than provoked (i.e. tilt-table or electrophysiologic study [EPS]), syncope.

ILRs will likely become increasingly important in the evaluation of syncope patients. Knowing what transpires during a spontaneous syncopal episode is the gold standard for the syncope evaluation. In some instances, the ILR has taught us definitively the cause of syncope such that any further investigation has become redundant. However, the current ILR represents only a first step. Documentation of blood pressure as well as other physiologic measures (see later) may offer additional insight into syncope mechanisms.

Recommendations

Often the cause(s) of syncope can be identified by application of careful medical history taking and routine low-cost investigations (e.g. resting 12-lead ECG and echocardiography). However, with these tools alone, there remain a high rate of 'unknowns'. AECG monitoring, when used prudently, can be very effective in increasing the diagnostic yield. However, the choice of monitoring strategy requires some thought.

Patients with very infrequent syncope, recurring over months or years, are unlikely to be diagnosed by conventional Holter monitoring or conventional external event recorders, since the likelihood of symptom-ECG correlation during the recording period is very low. Internet-based MCOT systems may provide some advantage in this setting. However, consideration must be given to implanting an AECG loop recorder (ILR). The vast majority of ILR patients provide symptom-ECG correlation within a year of device placement. Consequently, despite the up-front device cost, ILRs have proved to be cost-effective on a diagnostic yield basis when compared to Holter monitoring or even conventional external event monitoring.

Summary

The most powerful investigation in a syncope patient is the one that records a clear abnormality at the time when the presenting symptoms are reproduced. It is important to strive to achieve this with AECG monitoring. Expanded MCOT and ILR use appears to be the most important step forward in this regard. Where symptoms are not reproduced but an ECG abnormality is found, there will always be doubt about the true diagnosis. Nevertheless, sometimes it is necessary to act on the basis of an asymptomatic finding. Future refinements to technology, such as the ability to record systemic pressure and patient posture and activity status, may help remove such doubts.

Additional reading

Crawford MH, Bernstein SJ, Deedwania PC *et al*. ACC/AHA guidelines for ambulatory electrocardiography. *J Am Coll Cardiol* 1999; **34**: 912–948. (Executive summary and recommendations. *Circulation* 1999; **100**: 886–893.)

Ermis C, Zhu AX, Pham S *et al*. Comparison of automatic and patient-activated arrhythmia recordings by implantable loop recorders in the evaluation of syncope. *Am J Cardiol* 2003; **92**: 815–819.

Joshi AK, Kowey PR, Prystowsky EN *et al*. First experience with a mobile cardiac outpatient telemetry (MCOT) system for the diagnosis and management of cardiac arrhythmia. *Am J Cardiol* 2005; **95**: 878–881.

Krahn A, Klein GJ, Yee R, Skanes AC. Randomized assessment of syncope trial. Conventional diagnostic testing versus a prolonged monitoring strategy. *Circulation* 2001; **104**: 46–51.

Krahn AD, Klein GJ, Yee R, Takle-Newhouse T, Norris C. Use of an extended monitoring strategy in patients with problematic syncope. Reveal Investigators. *Circulation* 1999; **99**: 406–410.

Moya A, Brignole M, Menozzi C *et al*. Mechanism of syncope in patients with isolated syncope and in patients with tilt-positive syncope. *Circulation* 2001; **104**: 1261–1267.

Seidl K, Ramekan M, Breuning S *et al*. Diagnostic assessment of recurrent unexplained syncope with a new subcutaneously implantable loop recorder. *Europace* 2000; **2**: 256–262.

CHAPTER 13

Hemodynamic sensors: the future evaluation of syncope

David G. Benditt

Introduction

Outpatient assessment of the cause of syncope has been greatly facilitated by availability of both wearable and insertable (implantable) ambulatory monitoring systems capable of recording and storing clinically relevant ECG data over relatively long periods of time (months to years) (Figure 13.1). In some cases, these devices offer the additional benefit of transmitting critical data immediately via wireless internet connection to a monitor center (Figure 13.2).

However, despite the considerable value of current ambulatory ECG recording systems, some of the most common forms of symptomatic hypotension occur in the absence of clear-cut arrhythmia. Consequently, ECG recordings

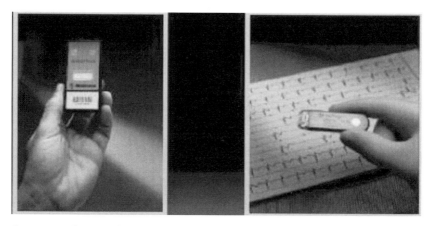

Figure 13.1 Photographs illustrating the insertable loop recorder (ILR) system (Reveal Plus®, Medtronic Inc. Minneapolis, MN). Left hand panel illustrates patient controller used to trigger recording of symptomatic events by the implanted monitor. The device can also be triggered automatically by predesignated abnormal rhythms. Right hand panel depicts the implantable device. The approximate dimensions can be estimated by comparison to the fingers holding the ILR.

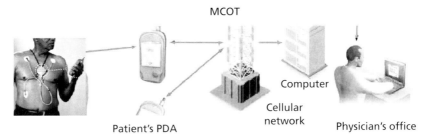

Figure 13.2 ECG electrodes and handheld PDA used in conjunction with an internet-based mobile cardiac outpatient telemetry (MCOT) system (Cardionet Inc., San Diego, CA). The schematic illustrates automatic transmission of ECG and symptom records via the internet to a central receiving station and ultimately to the physician office. (Illustration modified after Ross PE. Managing care through the air. *IEEE Spectrum* 2004; 26–31).

may be unrevealing during symptom events in such patients. Systems capable of detecting changes in blood pressure or blood flow, either directly or by means of some surrogate, may prove desirable in order to fill this important diagnostic gap.

Goals

The goal of this chapter is to examine technologies that may have application for detecting transient periods of diminished systemic blood flow or blood pressure.

Potentially useful markers of an imminent faint

In order to develop wearable or implantable systems for diagnosis and treatment of imminent syncope, diagnostic indicators must be suitable for application in devices that have limited energy supply and are of relatively small size. In the case of neurally mediated reflex faints, the diagnostic targets might include elements of the neural reflex as well as hemodynamic markers suggesting diminished systemic pressure. In the case of other types of syncope (e.g. orthostatic faints, cardiac arrhythmias) hemodynamic markers are the key targets.

Neural targets detecting imminent neurally mediated reflex faints

Direct or surrogate recordings of vagal efferent neural signals
The possibility exists that recognition of altered parasympathetic nervous system activity could be employed as a means of suggesting an imminent faint in susceptible individuals. In theory, direct vagus nerve recording is possible. However, implementation of such a system has yet to be accomplished, and even if it were, there is uncertainty that direct recordings could be effected in

a sufficiently safe and straightforward manner to permit widespread clinical acceptance.

If recognition of changes of vagal nerve traffic have any utility in the identification of imminent neurally mediated reflex events, it is more likely that such changes will be detected through surrogate measures of vagal activity rather than direct recordings. Thus, changes in respiratory pattern or sinus arrhythmia (see heart rate variability later) are candidates. In regard to the former, changes in respiration (rate, tidal volume) may occur either voluntarily or perhaps involuntarily (since respiratory control centers are close to the medullary traffic pattern thought to be relevant in neurally mediated reflex syncope) in an attempt to stabilize the hemodynamic state. Conceivably, respiratory variations may act to improve venous return in tenuous circumstances thereby affecting baroreceptor activity. Alternatively, changes in respiratory pattern may affect processing of baroreceptor afferent signals centrally. In any event, Kurbaan and Sutton have demonstrated the potential for early respiratory changes to be used as a marker for vasovagal syncope. However, apart from the potential respiratory marker, currently there is insufficient information to speculate on the potential utility of any surrogate measures of parasympathetic activity in this setting.

Sympathetic neural efferent activity (vasodepressor response)
Microneurographic recordings from efferent sympathetic nerves have provided important physiological research information. Furthermore, examples exist of such recordings during a spontaneous vasovagal event; however, in the case of the vasovagal faint, sympathetic activity appears to diminish most dramatically only after a considerable preceding period of hypotension. Consequently, despite the intuitive appeal of sympathetic nerve recordings as a potential marker for vasovagal syncope, the clinical utility may be limited due to late changes in nerve activity and the methodology for obtaining these recordings is not yet applicable for use in wearable or implantable systems. For the time being, it seems that a more feasible approach would be to try and obtain surrogate measures of sympathetic nerve activity from nearby skeletal muscle.

Sensors reflecting effects of changes of sympathetic neurohumoral state on the heart
It has long been recognized that increased levels of circulating catecholamine, particularly epinephrine, are characteristic of the presyncope phase in patients with susceptibility to vasovagal faints (Figure 13.3). Therefore, in the absence of practicable techniques for direct *in vivo* measurement of circulating catecholamines, indirect methods suggesting their increase may be useful as part of a diagnostic algorithm. To this end, both changes in myocardial contractile performance as well as catecholamine-induced changes in cardiac conduction intervals may be useful measures.

A vigorous myocardial contraction, presumably resulting from increased circulating catecholamines and diminished central volume (e.g. upright posture,

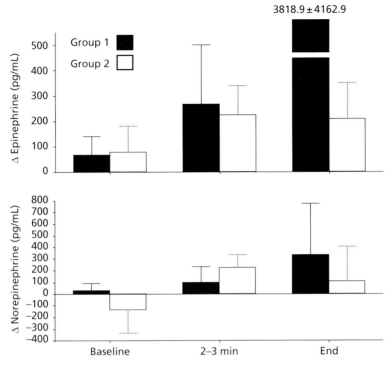

Figure 13.3 Graphs illustrating arterial epinephrine (upper panel) and norepinephrine levels measured during head-up tilt table testing in tilt-positive (Group 1, filled bars) and tilt-negative (Group 2, unfilled bars) subjects. Baseline values (left) were similar in both patient groups. However, by the time of syncope in tilt-positive patients or end-of-study in tilt-negative subjects the epinephrine levels were substantially higher in fainters. (Data from the Cardiac Arrhythmia Center, University of Minnesota Medical School, Minneapolis, MN).

dehydration, fright, etc.), has been closely associated with vasovagal faints. Consequently, recognition of an abrupt increment in contractile activity (especially in the absence of increased physical activity) may be indicative of an imminent faint. To date, changes in right ventricular pressure, preejection index (PEI) and dP/dt, measurements of peak endocardial acceleration (PEA), and related hemodynamic indices have been studied. Of these, the last two appear to offer the most promise currently, but the published experience is limited.

Heart rate
Heart rate variability (HRV) is a recognized accompaniment of evolving vasovagal faints. It is likely that the observed oscillations at least in part reflect attempts by the various vascular baroreceptor systems to fend off the evolving faint. Whether the early recognition of such oscillations can be used to predict

an imminent faint is as yet uncertain. A major limitation is the time it takes to record HRV patterns, undertake the computations and come to a clinical decision.

Hemodynamic sensor targets
The early recognition of diminishing cerebral blood flow could be the most specific indicator of an imminent faint of any origin. Perivascular flow probes, using ultrasonic or perhaps laser Doppler techniques, might be capable of providing such information. However, miniaturizing such systems to both limit power consumption and facilitate implantation seems only a remote possibility.

Blood pressure and blood flow
Technology currently exists to permit noninvasive surrogate assessment of blood flow and by inference systemic blood pressure. As yet, however, these methods have not been miniaturized for use in low-power portable diagnostic devices. Nevertheless, plethysmographic methods may be adaptable for ambulatory use such as in the Portapres system. Similarly, electrical impedance methods may prove applicable if the energy requirement can be minimized.

Oxygen saturation and temperature measurements
Changes in peripheral and central venous oxygen saturation may be feasible for wearable monitors. Similarly, temperature might be used to detect changes in blood flow. However, the energy requirements for long-term measurement of these parameters would need to be substantially reduced and the problem of sensor 'encapsulation' needs to be addressed.

Summary

The evaluation of free-living patients with suspected transient loss of consciousness (TLOC) remains limited by the inability to record both hemodynamic status and ECG findings during symptom events in the outpatient environment. Ultimately, inclusion within wearable or implantable monitors of sensors capable of detecting transient changes in systemic blood pressure or blood flow along with ECG or cardiac electrograms may substantially enhance the ability to document and understand the basis of TLOC in free-living individuals.

Additional reading

Benditt DG, Chen M-Y, Hansen R, Buetikofer J, Lurie KG. Characterization of subcutaneous microvascular blood flow during tilt-table-induced neurally-mediated syncope. *J Am Coll Cardiol* 1995; **25**:70–75.
Kurbaan AS, Erickson M, Petersen ME *et al*. Respiratory changes in vasovagal syncope. *J Cardiovasc Electrophysiol* 2000; **11**:607–611.

Lippman N, Stein KM, Lerman BB. Failure to decrease parasympathetic tone during upright tilt predicts a positive tilt-table test. *Am J Cardiol* 1995; **75**:591–595.

Lurie KG, Benditt DG. Syncope and the autonomic nervous system. *J Cardiovasc Electrophysiol* 1996; **7**:760–776.

Ross PE. Managing care through the air. *IEEE Spectrum* 2004; 26–31.

CHAPTER 14

The basic autonomic assessment

Richard Sutton and David G. Benditt

Introduction

The neurally mediated reflex syncope syndromes (see Chapters 1 and 20 Part 1) are the most frequent of all causes of syncope. Since these conditions reflect a transient functional change in autonomic system function, it is reasonable to utilize tools designed to assess autonomic function as part of the diagnostic assessment in syncope patients.

In regard to identifying susceptibility to the most important of the neurally mediated reflex faints (i.e. vasovagal syncope and carotid sinus syndrome), certain tests are now well established and widely available. The most important of these tests are:

- head-up tilt testing;
- carotid sinus massage.
  Less well delineated in terms of utility are:
- Valsalva maneuver;
- active standing test;
- cold pressor test;
- eyeball compression test;
- response to cough;
- heart rate variability assessment; and
- ATP/adenosine test.

The last two of these tests are discussed in Chapter 16 and will not be considered here.

Goals

The goals of this chapter are to provide a review of the technique, utility, and limitations of:

- head-up tilt-table testing;
- carotid sinus massage;
- Valsalva maneuver;
- active standing test; and
- cough test.

Table 14.1 Recommended tilt test protocols.

Supine pretilt phase of 10 min when no vascular cannulation is performed, and at least
  20 min when cannulation is undertaken
A passive phase of minimum of 20 min and a maximum of 45 min followed by a drug
  challenge phase, if necessary, of 15–20 min
The tilt angle is 60–70°
Either intravenous isoproterenol or sublingual nitroglycerin for drug provocation if needed
The recommended infusion rate for isoproterenol is incremental doses from 1 up to
  3 μg/min in order to increase average heart rate by about 20–25% over baseline,
  administered without returning the patient to a supine position
The dose for nitroglycerin challenge is 400 μg nitroglycerin spray sublingually
A positive endpoint of the test is defined as induction of syncope or reproduction of
  symptoms in association with near-syncope symptoms

Vasovagal syncope and head-up tilt-table testing

Vasovagal syncope may be triggered by any of a variety of factors (see Chapter 20, Part 1). Some of them include unpleasant sights (e.g. sight of blood), pain, extreme emotion, prolonged standing, stuffy rooms, boredom, and recent consumption of alcohol. Typical venues for fainting are churches, hospitals, the sports field (usually in association with injury), parties, standing in queues (i.e. standing in line for prolonged period of time), traveling by air, and restaurants. In general terms, many of these scenarios are characterized by increased susceptibility to dehydration, a feeling of being excessively warm and/or confined, or being in a circumstance that is emotionally upsetting.

Vasovagal syncope is often suspected as a result of the clinical history (see Chapters 6, 7, and 8) ; however, this is not always possible. Consequently, the availability of a test assessing susceptibility to vasovagal syncope, namely the head-up tilt-table test, is of value (Table 14.1).

Detailed discussion of tilt-table testing protocols, test reproducibility, and estimated specificity and sensitivity, are best found in the American College of Cardiology (ACC) Expert Consensus Report and the recent guidelines documents from the European Society of Cardiology (see Additional reading below). As a rule, the first step is 'passive' head-up tilt at 60–70° during which the patient is supported by both a foot-plate and gently applied body straps for a period of not less than 20 min and perhaps as long as 45 min (Figure 14.1). Tilt angles of less than 60 and greater than 80° lead to loss of sensitivity and specificity. Subsequently, if needed, tilt-table testing may be repeated immediately or at a separate time in conjunction with a drug challenge (most often isoproterenol or nitroglycerin).

Drug provocation during head-up tilt-table is particularly important if a short passive phase is used (i.e. 20 to 30 min). Until recently, the most frequently used provocative drug was isoproterenol usually given in escalating

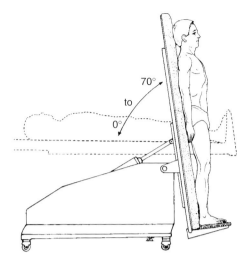

Figure 14.1 Schematic illustrating a typical head-up tilt table test procedure.

doses from 1 to 3 μg/min. However, nitroglycerin intravenously or sublingually has gained favor, in part because it expedites the procedure without adversely affecting diagnostic utility. Additionally, sublingual nitroglycerin can be administered without a parenteral cannula. Other drugs, such as edrophonium or adenosine, have also been reported to be of value in this setting but the reported experience is much smaller.

The head-up tilt-table test is the only readily available test that provides the opportunity to precipitate a typical vasovagal attack under the eyes of the physician (Figure 14.2). As a result, it helps the patient by giving confidence that the physician has witnessed the problem and it also provides the patient with valuable experience that may help in the recognition of impending faints and thereby permit their being able to abort similar events. Nonetheless, tilt-table testing is imperfect. The false-positive rate is approximately 10%. Acute (i.e. same day or within a few days) test reproducibility, in terms of whether syncope is induced or not, is approximately 80–90%. Longer-term reproducibility (i.e. over more than 1 year) is around 60%. Since there is no 'gold standard' for diagnosis of vasovagal syncope, the sensitivity of tilt testing cannot be estimated accurately.

It has been known for some time that head-up tilt testing does not always result in the same hemodynamic picture when repeated in the same patient. Thus, cardioinhibition (i.e. bradycardia) may predominate on one occasion whereas vasodilatation with hypotension may occur at another time. Thus, tilt testing may not be optimal for directing treatment strategy. In this regard, the ISSUE study findings indicate that even when tilt-table testing showed a prominent vasodilatation component to the faint, the subsequent recording of spontaneous faints by means of an implantable loop recorder (ILR) often revealed bradycardic events. Further study of this phenomenon with devices

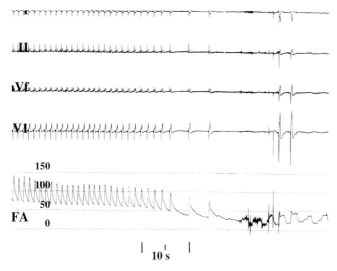

Figure 14.2 ECG and blood pressure recordings during a tilt-table-induced vasovagal faint. Note gradual drop in blood pressure prior to development of a long asystolic pause. Return of the patient to supine posture (not shown) results in prompt termination of the event and restoration of normal hemodynamics.

that can monitor blood pressure (or a surrogate of blood pressure), as well as heart rate is needed (see Chapter 13).

Independent of the protocol employed, certain general measures can be suggested when tilt testing is performed:
• The room where the test is performed should be quiet and with dim lights.
• Patients should fast for at least 2 h before the test.
• Patients should be in a supine position 10 to 45 min before tilting. This longer time interval was proposed to decrease the likelihood of a vasovagal reaction in response to vascular cannulation. The shorter rest periods (e.g. 10 min) are proposed when vascular cannulation is not employed.
• Continuous beat-to-beat finger arterial blood pressure should be monitored noninvasively, if reliable recordings can be obtained. Intermittent measurement of pressure using a sphygmomanometer should be avoided as it is disruptive to the procedure (and autonomic tone), and the frequency of recording is too low. Nevertheless, the latter method continues to be used in clinical practice, especially in children, and when economics dictate.
• The tilt-table should be able to achieve the upright position smoothly and rapidly and to reset to the supine position quickly (<10 s) when the test is completed in order to avoid the consequences of a prolonged loss of consciousness.
• Only a tilt-table of the foot-board support type is appropriate for syncope evaluation. Saddle support should be avoided as it unduly increases the false-positive rate.

• An experienced nurse or medical technician should be in attendance during the entire procedure. A physician should be in proximity and immediately available should a problem arise.
• Resuscitation equipment must be immediately available.

Role of head-up tilt test in treatment selection for vasovagal syncope

In order for any test to be helpful in the evaluation of treatment, it must exhibit a high degree of reproducibility and be predictive of outcomes at follow-up. The overall reproducibility of an initial negative response (85–94%) is higher than the reproducibility of an initial positive response (31 to 92%). In addition, data from controlled trials showed that approximately 50% of patients with a baseline positive tilt-table test became negative when the test was repeated with treatment or with placebo. Moreover, in most cases acute studies were not predictive of the long-term outcome of pacing therapy. Thus, it is generally agreed that head-up tilt-table testing is best reserved for diagnostic testing and is not considered to be of value for assessment of treatment options.

Complications

Head-up tilt test is a safe procedure and the rate of complications is very low. Although asystolic pauses >70 s have been reported, most often the pause is in the range of 8 to 20 s. The presence of a prolonged asystole during a positive response should not be considered a complication, since this is an endpoint of the test.

Rapid return to supine position as soon as syncope occurs is usually all that is needed to prevent or to limit the consequences of prolonged loss of consciousness. Only seldom are brief resuscitation maneuvers required. The mortality rate associated with tilt-table testing is not known. However reports of deaths are exceedingly rare and the mortality rate is likely <1/100 000 tests.

Case reports have documented life-threatening ventricular arrhythmias with isoproterenol in the presence of ischemic heart disease or sick sinus syndrome. No complications have been published with the use of nitroglycerin.

Indications

Head-up tilt-table testing is indicated for diagnostic purposes primarily (Table 14.2). It is not recommended for assessments of treatment efficacy.
Indications for tilt-table testing include:
• unexplained recurrent or single syncope episode in the absence of organic heart disease in high-risk clinical settings;
• unexplained recurrent or single syncope episode in the presence of organic heart disease, after cardiac causes of syncope have been excluded;
• after an etiology of syncope has been established, but where the demonstration of susceptibility to neurally mediated reflex syncope would alter the therapeutic approach.

Table 14.2 Classification of positive responses to tilt testing (based on VASIS group).

Type 1 mixed. Heart rate falls at the time of syncope but the ventricular rate does not fall to less than 40 bpm for less than 10 s with or without asystole of less than 3 s. Blood pressure falls before the heart rate falls

Type 2A cardioinhibition without asystole. Heart rate falls to a ventricular rate less than 40 bpm for more than 10 s but asystole of more than 3 s does not occur. Blood pressure falls before the heart rate falls

Type 2B cardioinhibition with asystole. Asystole occurs for more than 3 s. Blood pressure fall coincides with or occurs before the heart rate fall

Type 3 vasodepressor. Heart rate does not fall more than 10% from its peak at the time of syncope

Exception 1. Chronotropic incompetence. No heart rate rise during the tilt testing (i.e. less than 10% from the pretilt rate)

Exception 2. Excessive heart rate rise. An excessive heart rate rise both at the onset of upright position and throughout its duration before syncope (i.e. greater than 130 bpm)

Tilt testing may also be useful for:

• differentiating syncope with jerking movements from epilepsy;
• evaluating patients with recurrent unexplained falls;
• assessing recurrent presyncope or dizziness;
• evaluating unexplained syncope in the setting of peripheral neuropathies or autonomic failure;
• assessing postexercise-related syncope when an attack cannot be documented by exercise testing;
• educating patients regarding the recognition of premonitory symptoms and strategies for management of incipient events (e.g. leg-crossing, arm pull)

For patients without severe structural heart disease, tilt-table testing can be considered diagnostic and no further tests need to be performed when spontaneous premonitory symptoms and syncope are reproduced as attested to by the patient. For patients with significant structural heart disease, more worrisome arrhythmias should be excluded as a cause of syncope (e.g. by electrophysiological testing, see Chapter 15) prior to considering positive tilt-test results as evidence suggesting neurally mediated syncope. The clinical meaning of abnormal responses other than induction of syncope is unclear.

Carotid sinus syndrome and carotid sinus massage

Carotid sinus syndrome usually presents with syncope without warning. Although rare, a history suggesting that head movements trigger dizziness or syncope supports this diagnosis. As a rule, the condition almost exclusively afflicts older people (>60 years) with substantial male dominance. This is in contrast to vasovagal syncope; the latter tends to affect the sexes equally and occurs at all ages.

It has long been known that pressure at the site where the common carotid artery bifurcates produces a reflex slowing of heart rate and fall of

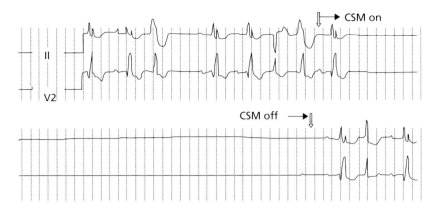

Figure 14.3 ECG recording illustrating a prolonged cardiac asystolic pause induced by carotid sinus massage in an older male patient who presented with several abrupt syncope episodes. A cardiac pacemaker was placed and the patient has been asymptomatic since.

blood pressure. This observation is the basis of the technique of carotid sinus massage (CSM). In some patients with syncope, an exaggerated response to CSM can be observed (Figure 14.3). In the absence of a history of spontaneous syncope attributable to a carotid sinus mechanism (usually based on an appropriate medical history), the exaggerated response is termed 'carotid sinus hypersensitivity'. 'Carotid sinus syndrome' is the term used when the history is compatible with syncope due to carotid sinus hypersensitivity.

Methodology and response to carotid sinus massage

Initially CSM is typically performed with the patient in a supine position. However, it is recommended that CSM be tested with the patient in both supine and upright positions (usually on a tilt-table). Continuous ECG monitoring must be used. Continuous blood pressure monitoring is also desirable as the vasodepressor response is rapid and cannot be adequately detected with devices that do not measure continuous blood pressure. For the latter measurement, a noninvasive device that offers beat-to-beat pressure measurement is often suitable but conventional blood pressure cuff recordings are not.

After baseline measurements, the right carotid artery is firmly massaged for 5 to 10 s at the anterior margin of the sternocleidomastoid muscle at the level of the cricoid cartilage. After 1 or 2 min, a second massage is performed on the opposite side if the first massage failed to yield a diagnostic result. If an asystolic response is evoked, it may be helpful to repeat the massage after intravenous administration of atropine (1 mg or 0.02 mg/kg) in order to assess the contribution of the vasodepressor component (which may otherwise be hidden). Atropine administration is preferred to temporary dual-chamber pacing as it is simple, less invasive, and easily repeatable on other occasions if necessary.

The response to CSM is generally classified as cardioinhibitory (usually an asystolic pause but also severe sinus bradycardia and/or paroxysmal AV block), vasodepressive (fall in systolic blood pressure due to vasodilation), or mixed. This latter response is more difficult to distinguish but is usually diagnosed given the combination of marked bradycardia in conjunction with a decline in systolic blood pressure of 50 mmHg or more from the baseline value. The vasodepressor response can be best appreciated by persistence of hypotension after resumption of a reasonable heart rate (or during cardiac pacing).

Two approaches to the diagnostic use of CSM have been advocated.

Method 1: This is probably the most widely used technique in clinical practice. CSM is performed with the patient supine. Pressure is applied for no more than 5 s. A positive response is defined as a ventricular pause ≥ 3 s and/or a fall of systolic blood pressure ≥ 50 mmHg. Pooled data from four studies performed in elderly patients with syncope show a rate of 35% (235 of 663 patients). Abnormal responses can also be frequently observed in subjects without syncope. The diagnosis may be missed in about one-third of cases if only supine massage is performed.

Method 2: Reproduction of spontaneous symptoms is required during carotid massage. Eliciting symptoms requires a longer period of massage (10 s) performed in both supine and upright positions. In an analysis pooled from three studies, a positive response was observed in 49% of 100 patients with syncope of uncertain origin and in 60% of elderly patients with syncope and sinus bradycardia but only in 4% of 101 control patients without syncope.

Whatever method is chosen, increasing importance is now given to undertaking CSM with the patient in the upright position usually using a tilt-table. Apart from the higher positive diagnosis rate compared to supine massage only, upright CSM better evaluates the magnitude of the vasodepressor component of the reflex; this latter component has been underestimated in the past, and its magnitude may affect the utility of cardiac pacing therapy (i.e. a prominent vasodepressor component may result in persistent symptoms of dizziness even though pacing overcomes bradycardia-related effects).

Complications of CSM

The main complications of CSM are neurologic. In one study, seven neurologic complications were reported among 5000 carotid massages with an incidence of 0.14%. In another study, 16 neurologic complications were reported in 16 000 massages (0.01%). These complication rates apply to 5 s of CSM supine and/or upright.

CSM should be avoided if possible in patients with previous transient ischemic attacks (TIAs) or strokes within the past 3 months (unless carotid Doppler studies convincingly exclude significant carotid artery narrowing), or in patients with carotid bruits. On rare occasion CSM may elicit self-limited atrial fibrillation of little clinical significance.

CSM indications
CSM should be performed as part of the evaluation of syncope in every patient >40 years of age in whom the initial evaluation is negative and in whom there is no evident contraindication.

CSM Summary
CSM is recommended in patients >40 years with syncope of unknown etiology after the initial evaluation if the latter is nondiagnostic.
- In the case of increased risk of stroke due to carotid artery disease (e.g. recent TIA, bruit), the massage should be avoided if possible.
- ECG monitoring and beat-to-beat blood pressure measurement during CSM is mandatory.
- Massage should be of 5–10 s duration and should be performed with the patient both supine and upright.
- A positive outcome to CSM is reported if syncope is reproduced during or immediately after the massage in the presence of asystole longer than 3 s and/or a fall in systolic blood pressure of 50 mmHg or more. Symptom reproduction is rare when the test is done with the patient supine.

Miscellaneous autonomic system tests
A number of additional studies are occasionally used in the laboratory to evaluate autonomic nervous system function in syncope patients, but their clinical value is as yet unclear.

Valsalva maneuver
This test is well known in medicine. Its utility lies in assessment of the integrity of certain vascular reflex responses to induced hemodynamic stress. In this sense it provides an estimate of autonomic nervous system integrity. However, Valsalva maneuver does not directly implicate a mechanism for syncope.

Active standing test
This procedure, as its name implies, has been used in two different ways.
- Assessment of the patient response to active movement from supine to upright posture. This technique may be more useful for evaluating symptoms of orthostatic intolerance than is passive head-up tilt. Normally, active muscle movement is expected to propel more blood toward the central circulation thereby aiding the needed increase in cardiac output. However, active use of lower limb muscles may play a role in aggravating peripheral vascular dilatation and as a result induce greater hypotension. The balance between these physiologic effects of active muscle movement determines the net effect with regard to systemic pressure.

• As a replacement for formal tilt-table testing. In this case (most often reported in children) quiet prolonged standing is used to assess syncope susceptibility.

Cold pressor test

Like the Valsalva maneuver, this test provides insight into autonomic reflex integrity. It has not been used as a means of identifying a specific diagnosis.

Eyeball compression test

This test, previously used to induce a vagal reflex, should be abandoned. Its utility is low and its clinical diagnostic benefit is marginal compared to potential risks.

Cough test

The use of induced cough to assess susceptibility to cough (tussive) syncope has been noted in the literature, but little in the way of supportive data is available. Like carotid massage, it may be most helpful if undertaken with the patient in the upright posture.

Others

Effects of isometric exercise, deep breathing, and heart rate variability (HRV) may be used as part of the overall autonomic assessment, but have as yet no direct diagnostic role in the syncope evaluation.

Summary

Well-established clinical tests are available for evaluation of the status of autonomic function and recognition of transient or more permanent dysautonomias. For the most part, however, only head-up tilt and CSM are of known clinical value in the syncope assessment. These latter two tests are easily performed and have well defined endpoints. They are recommended for diagnosis only and are not recommended for defining treatment options. The remaining tests discussed above may be helpful from time-to-time, but are not adequately substantiated to advocate routine use.

Additional reading

Almquist A, Gornick CC, Benson DW Jr *et al*. Carotid sinus hypersensitivity: evaluation of the vasodepressor component. *Circulation* 1985; **67**: 927–936.

Benditt DG, Ferguson DW, Grubb BP *et al*. Tilt-table testing for assessing syncope. An American College of Cardiology expert consensus document. *J Am Coll Cardiol* 1996; **28**: 263–275.

Benditt DG, Samniah N, Pham S *et al*. Effect of cough on heart rate and blood pressure in patients with 'cough syncope'. *Heart Rhythm* 2005; **2** 807–813.

Brignole M, Alboni P, Benditt DG *et al*. Guidelines on management (diagnosis and treatment) of syncope. *Europace* 2004; **22**: 1256–1306.

Brignole M, Menozzi C, Del Rosso A *et al*. New classification of hemodynamics of vasovagal syncope: beyond the VASIS classification. Analysis of the presyncopal phase of the tilt test without and with nitroglycerin challenge. Vasovagal Syncope International Study. *Europace* 2000; **2**: 66–76.

Moya A, Brignole M, and ISSUE Investigators. Mechanism of syncope in patients with isolated syncope and in patients with tilt-positive syncope. *Circulation* 2001; **104**: 1261–1267.

CHAPTER 15

Electrophysiological testing

Fei Lü and Lennart Bergfeldt

Introduction

The role of invasive electrophysiological study (EPS) in the management of syncope is primarily to determine whether a primary heart rhythm abnormality is the likely cause of the symptoms. This can be accomplished by demonstrating that an arrhythmia or clinically significant conduction disturbance is present, and in the absence of other explanation inferring a relationship between the abnormality and syncope.

Bradycardias or tachycardias may be responsible for syncope and the careful application of EPS techniques by experienced practitioners may be of value in elucidating the most probable cause(s). The most important categories of arrhythmias subject to EPS evaluation include:
- sinus node dysfunction (including bradycardia-tachycardia syndrome),
- atrioventricular (AV) conduction system disease,
- paroxysmal supraventricular tachycardias (including preexcitation), and
- ventricular tachycardias.

In addition, there are a number of other important arrhythmia categories in the evaluation of which EPS practitioners are likely to be of assistance. These include:
- inherited syndromes (e.g. long QT syndrome, Brugada syndrome),
- implanted device (pacemaker, defibrillator) malfunction, and
- drug-induced proarrhythmias.

Goals

The goals of this brief review of EPS techniques and indications in the evaluation of patients presenting with syncope are:
- To summarize the principal indications for EPS in syncope evaluation.
- Review interpretation of common EPS findings and current understanding of the mechanism(s) of specific arrhythmias causing of syncope.
- Examine EPS role in diagnosis and guiding of treatment of specific arrhythmias causing syncope.

Indication

In patients with unexplained syncope, following evaluation of baseline clinical history and noninvasive testing, EPS is commonly used to assess susceptibility

Table 15.1 Indications of electrophysiological testing for syncope.

Class I:

An invasive electrophysiological procedure is indicated when the initial evaluation suggests
  an arrhythmic cause of syncope. Risk factor includes abnormal electrocardiography,
  structural heart disease, syncope associated with palpitations or chest pain, syncope during
  exertion or in the supine position, and family history of sudden death.

Class II:

• To evaluate the exact nature of an arrhythmia which has already been identified as the
cause of the syncope.

• In patients with high-risk occupations, in whom every effort to exclude a cardiac cause of
syncope is warranted.

Class III:

In patients with normal electrocardiograms, no structural heart disease or palpitations, EPS is
  not usually indicated.

---

to a priori suspected sinus node function, AV conduction disturbances, and/or various ventricular and supraventricular tachyarrhythmias (Table 15.1).

As a rule, in patients without evident structural heart disease or abnormal resting electrocardiogram (ECG) undergoing evaluation for syncope associated with palpitations, EPS is best for assessing susceptibility to paroxysmal supraventricular tachycardias as the probable cause. If ventricular arrhythmias are suspected as an etiology of syncope in these patients, ambulatory electrocardiographic monitoring (AECG, see Chapter 12) may be the preferred initial approach since sustained ventricular tachyarrhythmias are rarely inducible in a clinically normal heart. This is also true in the presence of left ventricular hypertrophy and other relatively minor forms of structural heart disease, such as atrial septal defect without significant ventricular dysfunction.

In patients with an abnormal ECG and/or evidence of structural heart disease, particularly in those with coronary artery disease with/without congestive heart failure, ventricular arrhythmias are a greater concern than is the case with individuals who have essentially normal hearts. EPS is often used to confirm the diagnosis of cardiac arrhythmia as an etiology of syncope in these patients.

ECG abnormalities suggesting an arrhythmic syncope are summarized in Table 15.2. In all patients with syncope, however, neurally mediated reflex syncope (in all its forms), and orthostatic syncope need to be carefully considered first as possible causes, regardless of the presence of structural heart diseases. The neurally mediated reflex syncope conditions, along with other possible causes of syncope, are considered in other chapters in this book.

Techniques

For the most part, EPS requires placement of one or more electrode catheters into the heart for recording and stimulation using conventional vascular

Table 15.2 ECG abnormalities suggesting an arrhythmic syncope.

• Bifascicular block (defined as either left bundle branch block, or right bundle branch block combined with left anterior or left posterior fascicular block),
• other intraventricular conduction abnormalities (QRS duration ≥ 0.12 s),
• Mobitz I second degree atrioventricular block,
• asymptomatic sinus bradycardia (<50 bpm), sinoatrial block, or sinus pause ≥3 s in the absence of negatively chronotropic medications,
• preexcited QRS complexes,
• prolonged QT interval,
• right bundle branch block pattern with ST-elevation in leads V_1–V_3 (Brugada syndrome),
• negative T waves in right precordial leads, epsilon waves, and ventricular late potentials suggestive of arrhythmogenic right ventricular dysplasia,
• Q waves suggesting myocardial infarction.

---

access techniques. (Transesophageal EPS is also used from time to time, particularly in children. Since the transesophageal electrode predominantly records and stimulates the atrium, this technique is limited to screening for conditions that primarily involve atrial tissues.) These catheters are usually placed at the high right atrium (HRA) near the sinus node, the tricuspid annulus at the His bundle area (HBE), right ventricle apex (RVA), and occasionally the coronary sinus (CS) vein for left atrial recording and stimulation. Most studies require only venous access (usually the femoral vein). However, arterial access with recording from and stimulation of the left ventricle (LV) is occasionally needed. Further, arterial access allows for the ready monitoring of systemic pressure. The latter can be a distinct advantage when trying to ascertain the hemodynamic importance of an induced arrhythmia (bearing in mind that the study is carried out with the patient supine, whereas most instances of syncope occur in upright individuals). Finally, use of trans-septal puncture in order to access the left atrium directly has become increasingly important for certain procedures (e.g. mapping and ablation of left-sided accessory AV connections, isolation of pulmonary veins for treatment of paroxysmal atrial fibrillation).

Baseline EPS measurements usually include RR interval, AH interval, HV interval, QRS duration, and QT interval (Figure 15.1). The minimum electrophysiological protocol is provided in Table 15.3.

One of the distinct advantages of invasive EPS is the potential to identify and cure certain arrhythmias. In this regard, transcatheter ablation using radiofrequency energy (or other energy delivery systems such as cryothermia) is now an integral part of most EPS laboratory capabilities. Transcatheter ablation can be used to cure several arrhythmias that may cause syncope,

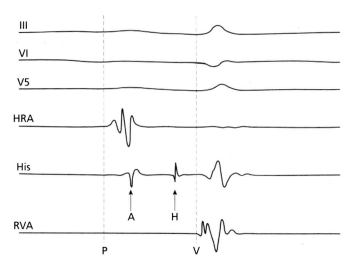

Figure 15.1 Measurements during EPS for evaluation of AV conduction. AH interval, measured from the earliest reproducible rapid deflection of the atrial electrogram in the His recording to the onset of the His deflection, represents conduction time from the low right atrium at the atrial septum through the AV node to the His bundle (AV node function). The HV interval, measured from the beginning of the His deflection to the earliest onset of ventricular activation (either surface leads or intracardiac recordings), represents conduction time from the proximal His bundle to the ventricular myocardium (infra-His conduction function). The tracings here are recorded from a patient with the first degree AV block. The HV interval is relatively long (normal is usually <55 ms, this is >80 ms), indicating the presence of infra-Hisian conduction system disease. III = surface ECG lead III; V1 = surface ECG lead V1; V5 = surface ECG lead V5; HRA = high right atrium; His = His bundle; RVA = right ventricular apex; P = the onset of the P wave; A = the onset of atrial activation; H = the onset of His activation; V = the onset of ventricular activation.

such as:
• preexcitation syndromes such as Wolff–Parkinson–White syndrome (WPW syndrome) and its variants,
• paroxysmal supraventricular tachycardia due to AV nodal reentry,
• ectopic atrial tachycardias,
• atrial flutter and some cases of atrial fibrillation,
• idiopathic ventricular tachycardia arising from the right or left ventricles,
• bundle branch reentry tachycardia, and
• paroxysmal and persistent atrial fibrillation (a developing technique not nearly so advanced as the others).

Diagnostic yield and predictive value of EPS
The gold standard for the diagnosis of arrhythmia-related syncope is the ECG documentation of episodes of spontaneous cardiac arrhythmias causing syncope. Obtaining such documentation is usually attempted by means

Table 15.3 Minimal electrophysiological testing protocol for diagnosis of syncope.

• Measurement of sinus node recovery time and corrected sinus node recovery time by repeated sequences of atrial pacing for 30–60 s with at least one low and two high pacing rates. Suggested low pacing rate is 10–20 beats above sinus rate. Autonomic blockade may be applied if needed.

• Assessment of the His-Purkinje system includes measurement of the HV at baseline and His-Purkinje conduction with stress by incremental atrial pacing. If HV interval is moderately prolonged, pharmacological provocation is recommended unless contraindicated. Suggested drugs include ajmaline 1 mg/kg, procainamide 10 mg/kg, or disopyramide 2 mg/kg.

• Assessment of ventricular arrhythmia inducibility performed by programmed electrical stimulation using up to two extrastimuli (with coupling interval not below 200 ms) from two right ventricular sites (apex and outflow tract) at two drive cycle lengths (100 or 120 bpm and 140 or 150 bpm). A third extrastimuli may be added to enhance sensitivity at the cost of reduced specificity.

• Assessment of supraventricular arrhythmia inducibility by any atrial stimulation protocols.

of various forms of ambulatory ECG recorders (e.g. Holter monitors, event recorders, mobile cardiac outpatient telemetry [MCOT], or insertable loop recorders[ILRs], see also Chapter 12). However, in many patients it is not possible to obtain such documentation due to the infrequency of the rhythm or concerns regarding patient safety should a spontaneous recurrence be associated with a life-threatening circumstance. In such cases, EPS may be warranted in an attempt to obtain at least a plausible cause for the symptoms.

Often, in patients with unexplained syncope, EPS is able to elicit a possible diagnosis of a suspected cardiac arrhythmia. This is particularly the case in those individuals with an abnormal ECG and/or evident underlying structural heart disease in whom the problem is a tachycardia. Nevertheless, when reproduction of symptoms does not occur, the diagnosis remain presumptive. Indications for EPS for evaluation of syncope are summarized in Table 15.2, and the minimum electrophysiological testing protocol for diagnosis of syncope is provided in Table 15.3.

The diagnostic efficiency of EPS is highly dependent on the degree of suspicion of the abnormality (pretest probability), the applied protocols, and the criteria used for diagnosis of clinically significant abnormalities. The diagnostic yield of EPS has not been fully evaluated by assessing concordance with diagnoses determined by AECG monitoring or ILRs. Table 15.4 provides a list of findings during EPS that are highly likely to suggest a correct diagnosis in a syncope patient.

Table 15.4 Diagnostic value of electrophysiological findings.

Class I

• An EPS is diagnostic, and usually no additional tests are required in the following cases:
  • Sinus bradycardia and a very prolonged CSNRT as discussed in the text.
  • Bifascicular block and:
    ○ a baseline HV interval of ≥100 ms, or
    ○ second or third degree His-Purkinje block is demonstrated during incremental atrial pacing, or
    ○ if the baseline EPS is inconclusive, high-degree His-Purkinje block is provoked by intravenous administration of ajmaline, procainamide, or disopyramide.
• Induction of sustained monomorphic ventricular tachycardia.
• Induction of rapid supraventricular arrhythmia, which reproduces hypotensive or spontaneous symptoms.

Class II

• The diagnostic value of an EPS is less well established in case of:
  ○ HV interval of >70 ms but <100 ms,
  ○ induction of polymorphic ventricular tachycardia or ventricular fibrillation in patients with Brugada syndrome, arrhythmogenic right ventricular dysplasia, and patients resuscitated from cardiac arrest.

Class III

• The induction of polymorphic ventricular tachycardia or ventricular fibrillation in patients with ischaemic or dilated cardiomyopathy has a low predictive value.

Note:

• Normal electrophysiological findings cannot completely exclude an arrhythmic cause of syncope; when an arrhythmia is likely, further evaluations (e.g. loop recording) are recommended.

• Depending on the clinical context, abnormal electrophysiological findings may not be diagnostic of the cause of syncope.

EPS Limitations

Although EPS accurately delineates abnormalities in patients with fixed cardiac conduction defects, its sensitivity with conservative criteria for identifying transient rhythm disturbances is low (15%) in syncope patients. Furthermore, false positives are a concern. Thus, abnormal sinus and AV node function unrelated to syncope may be found. Similarly, unrelated supraventricular or ventricular tachyarrhythmias may be induced in many of these patients. These findings may be mistaken as the cause of syncope. However, after neurally mediated reflex syncope and orthostatic syncope have been excluded, evidence of susceptibility to significant bradycardia (i.e. abnormal sinus node or AV node and His-Purkinje conduction function) appears to provide a reasonable

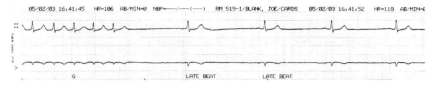

Figure 15.2 ECG recording obtained during elective cardioversion of atrial fibrillation. After atrial fibrillation is terminated by cardioversion shock, there is significant bradycardia. This is commonly seen in patients with bradycardia-tachycardia syndrome. It is also frequent to see prolonged asystole following termination of atrial fibrillation (spontaneously or by cardioversion) before sinus rhythm returns.

diagnosis in a majority of patients (86%) with spontaneous syncope due to sinus arrest or paroxysmal AV block. Recent studies using electrocardiographic monitoring before EPS or monitoring function of a pacemaker after EPS support this observation. Similarly, induction of a sustained supraventricular or monomorphic ventricular tachycardia would be strongly supportive of a basis for syncope.

As noted earlier, EPS tends to be most helpful in patients with known structural heart disease. Thus, ventricular tachycardia was induced in 21% and abnormal indices of bradycardia were found in 34% of patients with organic heart disease or an abnormal ECG. In contrast, abnormal EPS findings are much less frequent (ventricular tachycardia 1% and bradycardia 10%) in patients with an apparently normal heart. Nevertheless, in all cases, the physician must carefully consider whether the EPS findings are consistent with the clinical history or whether they may be a false positive finding. In general, EPS has been less effective in identifying bradycardic causes of syncope than tachycardic causes.

Specific clinical conditions
Suspected sinus node dysfunction
A transient bradycardia due to sinus node dysfunction (SND) (also termed sick sinus syndrome or sinus node disease) should be *suspected* in evaluating a patient with syncope when there is a sinus bradycardia (<50 bpm) or sinus pause >3 s. or a prolonged asystole after spontaneous termination or cardioversion of atrial fibrillation (Figure 15.2). However, although these findings may be very suspicious, they can only be considered as inferential for the cause of syncope in the absence of occurrence of symptoms at the time of the documented arrhythmia.

The EPS assessment of sinus node function should include assessment of sinus node automaticity at baseline (including intrinsic heart rate measured with atropine and beta-blocker pretreatment), and during symptom limited exercise (chronotropic competence), and sinus node recovery time (SNRT).

Other available but clinically less effective measures of sinus node function include sinus node rate variability, sinoatrial conduction time (SACT) and sinus node refractoriness. Of these, only SACT has been well studied, but has proven to be an insensitive indicator of SND (prolonged in 40% of patients with clinical findings of SND) and cannot always be assessed in patients with proven sinus node disease.

All tests designed to search for SND are only indirect and impure measures of sinus node function. Of these, SNRT is the most useful for assessment of sinus node function. SNRT is usually measured after atrial overdrive pacing for 30–60 s or longer at several pacing cycle lengths. SNRT is usually defined as the interval from the last paced beat to the first spontaneous sinus beat. SNRT may be corrected for baseline heart rate (corrected SNRT [CSNRT], equal to SNRT minus baseline sinus cycle length). SNRT >1500–1720 ms or CSNRT >525 is considered abnormal, with sensitivity of 50–80% and specificity of >95%, respectively, for detecting SND.

In general, SNRT is an insensitive measure for SND. This is particularly true in patients with mild or moderate SND. These patients often manifest a transient sinus pause or asystole only when there are certain external factors influencing sinus node function, such as autonomic or electrolyte imbalance or at the termination of paroxysms of atrial fibrillation.

Abnormal SNRT or SACT may be due to either intrinsic sinus node disease or extrinsic autonomic or drug influences. Autonomic blockade by administration of atropine and propranolol is widely accepted for distinguishing between intrinsic and extrinsic SND. When the baseline study is inconclusive, pharmacological interventions may increase sensitivity.

Assessment of sinus node function is more reliable and reproducible after autonomic blockade. *Complete* autonomic blockade can be achieved by administration of intravenous propranolol (0.2 mg/kg) and atropine (0.04 mg/kg). Note, however, that for the elderly the risk for adverse effects of atropine is high. In these patients half of the above doses are advisable. Intrinsic heart rate (i.e. heart rate after complete autonomic blockade) has a linear relationship to age, which is equal to $118.1 - (0.57 \times Age)$. Testing of sinus node function is often positive in patients with abnormal intrinsic heart rate. However, the sensitivity of abnormal intrinsic heart rate is low for diagnosing SND.

SNRT is prolonged in a wide range of patients with suspected SND. The efficacy of pacing on symptoms is associated with a prolonged SNRT. Its predictive value increases with longer SNRT. Patients with a CSNRT of >800 ms have an eight times higher risk of syncope than patients with a CSNRT below this value. It is the opinion of the ESC Syncope Task Force panel that, in the presence of a SNRT >2.0 s or CSNRT >1.0 s, SND may be reasonably surmised to be the cause of syncope if no other diagnostic candidates remain.

Suspected impending high-degree AV block
Transient high-degree AV block should be suspected in patients with syncope in the presence of bundle branch block. Extended ECG monitoring is often needed to document the transient high-degree AV block. The ISSUE study

provides strong evidence of the potential importance of transient AV block as a cause of syncope in patients with bundle branch block on ECG.

The most alarming ECG sign in a patient with syncope is probably alternating complete left and right bundle branch block, or right bundle branch block with alternating left anterior or left posterior fascicular block. This ECG pattern suggests trifascicular conduction system disease and intermittent or impending high-degree AV block. Bifascicular block (right bundle branch block plus left anterior or posterior fascicular block, or left bundle branch block) is also associated with high risk of high-degree AV block in syncope patients.

In these patients, EPS is used mainly to evaluate intra- and infra-His conduction (i.e. the portion of the conduction system below the AV node) (Figure 15.1). A prolonged HV interval is associated with a higher risk of developing AV block. The progression rate to AV block is 2–4% in patients with a normal (<55 ms) or slightly prolonged (55–60 ms) HV interval, and increases to 12% and 24%, when HV interval ≥70 ms and ≥100 ms, respectively. Incremental atrial pacing and pharmacological provocation with sodium channel blocking drugs are often used to increase the diagnostic yield of EPS when HV interval is borderline prolonged.

Development of intra- or infra-His block during incremental atrial pacing (i.e. pacing the atria at progressively more rapid rates to stress the adequacy of the AV conduction system) is rare (<5%) but highly predictive of impending AV block. Progression to complete AV block occurs in ≥30–40% of these patients over 2–4 year follow-up.

In patients with moderate prolongation of HV interval, pharmacological stress testing of the His-Purkinje system may be used to assess His-Purkinje system reserve by acute intravenous administration of class Ia agents (ajmaline 1 mg/kg, procainamide 10 mg/kg, and disopyramide 2 mg/kg). A significant increase of HV interval duration (i.e. a resultant HV >100 ms or the precipitation of second or third degree infra-His block) following pharmacological challenge with or without incremental atrial pacing is highly predictive of subsequent spontaneous AV block during follow-up. Pooled data ($n = 333$) show that pharmacological stress was able to elicit susceptibility to high-degree AV block in 15% of patients studied. Spontaneous AV block developed in approximately 68% of these patients during follow-up for a period of 2–5 years.

In regard to the role of cardiac conduction system disease as a cause of syncope, combining the above mentioned protocols should yield a predictive value of 80% or higher. Pacemaker therapy effectively prevents recurrences of syncope in almost all these patients, indicating the value of EPS in the management of patients with syncope due to conduction system disease. Nevertheless, a small percentage (<20%) of the patients with negative EPS may nonetheless develop AV block during follow-up.

A high incidence of death or sudden cardiac death has been observed in patients with bundle branch block, especially in the presence of structural heart disease. Age, congestive heart failure, and coronary artery disease are associated with higher risk of death. It appears that neither syncope nor a prolonged HV interval is associated with high risk of death. Pacemaker therapy reduces syncope recurrence but does not decrease the mortality risk. The mechanism of sudden cardiac death is believed to be due to ventricular tachyarrhythmia or electromechanical dissociation rather than a bradycardia. A sustained ventricular tachyarrhythmia is frequently induced in patients with bundle branch block (32%).

It is the opinion of the ESC Syncope task force panel that, in patients with syncope and bifascicular block, EPS is highly sensitive in identifying patients with intermittent or impending high-degree AV block. This block is likely the cause of syncope in most cases, but not of the high mortality rate in these patients. The latter seems to be mainly related to underlying structural heart disease and ventricular tachyarrhythmias. Unfortunately, EPS does not seem to be able to correctly identify the high-risk patients and the finding of inducibility of ventricular arrhythmias should be interpreted with caution.

Suspected tachycardias

Paroxysmal supraventricular tachycardia and other supraventricular tachycardias

Paroxysmal supraventricular tachycardia (PSVT) should be suspected in patients with syncope and palpitations in the absence of structural heart disease. PSVT presenting as syncope without accompanying palpitations is relatively rare, but can occur at the onset of an attack or just after its termination when a pause may ensue before normal sinus function is restored. EPS with and without pharmacologic challenge (usually individually titrated doses of intravenous isoproterenol and/or atropine) may be used to both facilitate induction of PSVT and evaluate the hemodynamic effects of tachycardia. In either case, it is important to position the patient in an upright posture (e.g. using a tilt-table) in order to recognize the full hemodynamic impact of the arrhythmia. Recognition of PSVT as a cause of syncope is important, as many cases are curable by radiofrequency ablation as discussed at the beginning of this chapter (Figures 15.3 and 15.4).

In addition to PSVT, other supraventricular tachyarrhythmias can trigger syncope. In the case of atrial fibrillation (Figure 15.5), syncope can be due to insufficient ventricular filling, inadequate reflex vascular compensation at the onset of an episode, or delayed return of normal rhythm at the termination of an episode (Figure 15.2). In certain cases, especially WPW syndrome, syncope may occur due to atrial fibrillation resulting in excessively rapid ventricular rates (Figures 15.6 and 15.7).

In selected atrial fibrillation patients, EPS may be useful to determine whether atrial fibrillation is occurring as a consequence of another treatable rhythm (e.g. PSVT degenerating to atrial fibrillation) or is the primary problem itself. This is particularly the case in younger individuals with so-called lone atrial fibrillation (i.e. without apparent cause for the arrhythmia). Furthermore, atrial fibrillation can be treated by transcatheter ablation in some patients, while in others ablation of the His bundle and placement of a cardiac

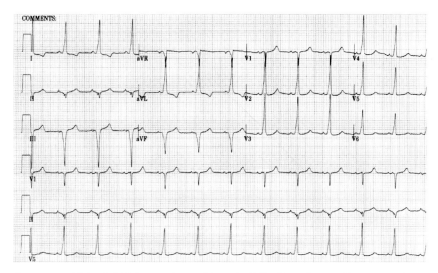

Figure 15.3 12-lead ECG in a patient with typical WPW syndrome. Please note the delta wave (slurred upstroke of the QRS suggesting preexcitation), short PR interval, and wide QRS duration. An experienced ECG reader can often predict the most likely site of the accessory AV connection by careful examination of the delta wave polarity in each lead.

pacemaker can be very effective in preventing excessively rapid heart rates during atrial fibrillation from inducing hypotension and syncope. Finally, EPS may help to identify the infrequent patient in whom an atrial antitachycardia pacemaker can be helpful.

Ventricular tachycardias

Ventricular tachycardia may present as syncope with or without palpitations or other accompanying symptoms such as palpitations, chest pain, and dyspnea. Certain clinical features are useful to the clinician to suspect this arrhythmia as the cause of syncope. The most important risk factors are:
- history of sustained monomorphic ventricular tachycardia,
- history of coronary artery disease, particularly myocardial infarction,
- diminished left ventricular ejection fraction,
- positive signal-averaged electrocardiogram, and
- advanced age.

The major concern with programmed electrical stimulation as part of an EPS for inducing clinically significant ventricular arrhythmia is its uncertain sensitivity and specificity in different clinical settings and stimulation protocols. Generally speaking, programmed electrical stimulation is thought to be a sensitive tool in patients with chronic ischemic heart disease (particularly a prior myocardial infarction) and spontaneous monomorphic ventricular tachycardia. Programmed electrical stimulation has a lower predictive value in patients

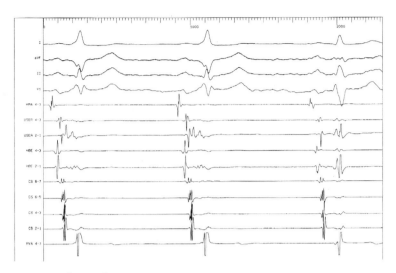

Figure 15.4 Surface and intracardiac electrograms illustrating catheter ablation of a left-sided AV accessory pathway. Please note that the atrial and ventricular signals recorded from distal ablation catheter (USER 1–2) are fused for the first two beats, indicating a rapid conduction from atria to the ventricles over the AV accessory pathway. The atrial and ventricular signals are widely separated from each other in the third beat, indicating that the heart beat only conducts over the AV node after conduction block in the accessory pathway induced by successful transcatheter ablation. I = surface ECG lead I; aVF = surface ECG lead aVF; II = surface ECG lead II; V1 = surface ECG lead V1; HRA = high right atrium; HBE = His bundle; CS = coronary sinus; RVA = right ventricular apex.

with nonischemic dilated cardiomyopathy, but is still useful if monomorphic ventricular tachycardia is triggered.

In ESVEM, a trial composed of ischemic heart disease patients, syncope associated with induced ventricular tachyarrhythmias during EPS indicated a high risk of death similar to that in patients with documented spontaneous ventricular tachyarrhythmias. Polymorphic ventricular tachycardia and ventricular fibrillation, on the other hand, have previously been considered nonspecific findings, a concept that probably needs modification depending on the clinical setting. One example is patients with Brugada syndrome (Figure 15.8), in whom the induction of polymorphic ventricular arrhythmias seems to be the most consistent finding.

Short QT syndrome (QT <280 ms and QTc <300–320 ms) has been recently reported to be an important risk factor for syncope and sudden cardiac death. The short QT syndrome constitutes a new clinical entity that is associated with a high incidence of sudden cardiac death, syncope, and/or atrial fibrillation in young patients and newborns. Patients with this congenital electrical abnormality are characterized by rate-corrected QT intervals of <320 ms. The role of EPS in the evaluation of this condition is uncertain as the worldwide

(a)

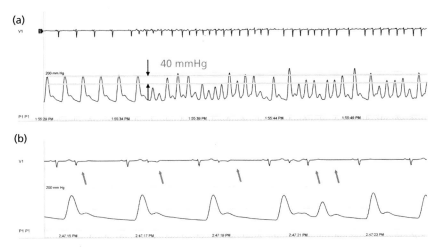

Figure 15.5 ECG tracing and arterial blood pressure recording during a head-up tilt table test in a patient with a clinically normal heart. (a) Atrial fibrillation occurred spontaneously during the tilt test and resulted in an approximately 40 mmHg drop in blood pressure. Under the right circumstances the onset of atrial fibrillation could cause sufficient hypotension to trigger syncope. (b) Futile contraction of ectopic atrial beats is also observed in the same patient. In this circumstance, the patient's 'effective' heart rate has been cut in half, suggesting that even atrial bigeminy could cause cerebral hypoperfusion in some instances. V1 = surface ECG lead V1; P1P1 = arterial blood pressure.

experience is as yet small. The possible substrate for the development of ventricular tachyarrhythmias may be a significant transmural dispersion of repolarization due to a heterogeneous abbreviation of the action potential duration. The implantable cardioverter-defibrillator (ICD) is the therapy of choice in patients with syncope and a positive family history of sudden cardiac death. No antiarrhythmic drug has been shown to be effective for treatment of short QT syndrome. Quinidine may serve as an adjunct to ICD therapy or as a possible alternative treatment, especially for children and newborns.

Advent of ICD with improved documentation of arrhythmic events offers a safe and sensitive tool for the follow-up (and thereby ultimately better understanding) of potentially high-risk populations (Figure 15.9). The ESC syncope task force reviewed seven studies evaluating the utility of ICDs in a small number of highly selected patients with syncope. In 67 patients with unexplained syncope and coronary artery disease (mostly with a prior myocardial infarction and ejection fraction of $37 \pm 13\%$), monomorphic ventricular tachycardia was induced in 43% of these patients. During >1 year follow-up, 41% of the inducible patients received appropriate ICD therapy. ICD therapy was highly effective for preventing recurrence of syncope in these patients. However, the total mortality for patients with inducible monomorphic ventricular tachycardia was significantly higher than for noninducible patients. The respective

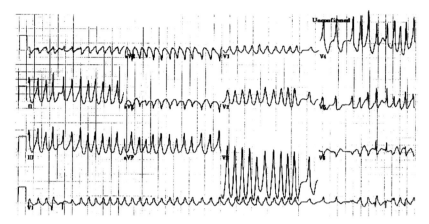

Figure 15.6 Typical 12-lead ECG during preexcited atrial fibrillation in a patient with WPW syndrome. Please note the very rapid and irregular ventricular response with varying QRS morphology depending on the degree to which AV conduction proceeded down the bypass connection versus the AV node. This rapid rate often causes hypotension and syncope, and in some cases may degenerate into ventricular fibrillation leading to death. This ECG was recorded in a 31-year-old pregnant female (11 weeks) with recurrent syncope. The patient had recurrent episodes of rapid conducted atrial fibrillation and resultant syncope requiring emergent electrical cardioversion.

one- and two-year survival rates were 94% and 84% in noninducible patients and 77% and 45% in inducible patients, respectively.

It seems that patients with inducible ventricular tachycardia have similar incidence of ICD discharges (approximately 50%) compared with patients with previously documented spontaneous ventricular tachycardia at 1 year follow-up. A high correlation between recurrence of syncope and ventricular arrhythmias has been observed in patients with inducible ventricular arrhythmias (85%) similar to that in those with spontaneous ventricular arrhythmias (92%). Although ICD has been proven to be effective in primary and secondary prevention of sudden cardiac death, syncope may still recur in some patients due to the time delay in detection of tachycardia and a long battery charge time.

The predictive value of programmed electrical stimulation remains controversial in patients with unexplained syncope and nonischemic dilated cardiomyopathy. In one recent report, preimplant EPS was performed in 41 patients with syncope and/or nonsustained ventricular tachycardia, sustained ventricular tachycardia was induced in 41% of these patients. The sensitivity of EPS for predicting subsequent ICD therapies during a follow-up period of up to 60 months (median 21 months) was 53% with specificity of 88% and positive predictive value of 75% (*p* value <0.01).

In another study in 14 patients with nonischemic dilated cardiomyopathy, unexplained syncope, and negative EPS, the incidence of appropriate ICD

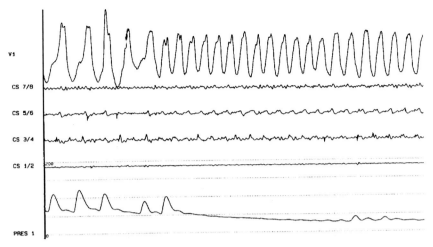

Figure 15.7 Surface and intracardiac electrograms and blood pressure recording in the same patient as in Figure 15.6 with preexcited atrial fibrillation. Her baseline blood pressure was 116/77 mmHg during sinus rhythm at 94 bpm. Radiofrequency ablation was considered after failed drug therapy. Atrial fibrillation was induced prior to ablation in the electrophysiology laboratory. Surface lead V_1, intracardiac recordings from the coronary sinus ($CS_{7/8}$, $CS_{5/6}$, $CS_{3/4}$, and $CS_{1/2}$), and femoral arterial blood pressure (PRES 1) are shown. During atrial fibrillation, blood pressure was dropped from 110/70 mmHg during slow ventricular rates (left) to 35 mmHg during extremely fast ventricular rates (right, shortest RR interval 140 ms) and syncope ensued. A left anteroseptal accessory pathway was successfully ablated using nonfluoroscopic electroanatomic mapping with minimal fluoroscopic guidance in this patient. V1 = surface ECG lead V1; CS = coronary sinus; PRES = arterial blood pressure.

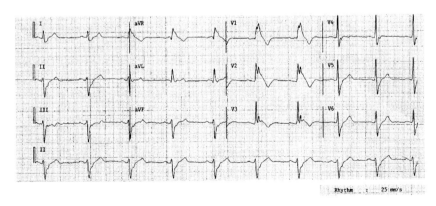

Figure 15.8 ECG tracings of a patient with Brugada syndrome. Tracings show right bundle branch block (RBBB) with coving ST-segment elevation in right precordial leads. There is marked left axis deviation suggesting presence of left anterior fascicular. In presence of RBBB, QTc is prolonged (482 ms).

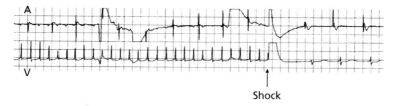

Figure 15.9 Termination of an episode of VT by an ICD shock. The ICD terminates a life-threatening rhythm, but the patient may nonetheless experience syncope or near-syncope during the time it takes the device to detect the arrhythmia and charge the capacitors needed to deliver the shock. A = atrial electrogram; V = ventricular electrogram; Shock = ICD discharge.

therapy was approximately 50% at 2 year follow-up, similar to that in patients with a documented cardiac arrest due to ventricular tachyarrhythmias (42%). The relapse of syncope or presyncope in these patients is primarily due to ventricular fibrillation. Finally, ICD therapy in these patients has been shown to be associated with improved survival.

Summary

EPS with programmed electrical stimulation is generally a helpful diagnostic test for patients with unexplained syncope who have coronary artery disease. Its utility is more questionable for patients with nonischemic dilated cardiomyopathy or valvular heart disease. EPS is of little diagnostic value in patients with normal hearts in the absence of documented (or at least strongly suspected) supraventricular or ventricular tachyarrhythmias.

In selected patients, EPS may be helpful in defining the presence of SND, the nature and severity of an AV conduction disturbance, and the nature of an inducible tachycardia. In these settings, such testing may help to define useful treatment strategies such as the need for cardiac pacemaker or ICD implantation, and the potential for transcatheter ablation to be of value.

Additional reading

Bergfeldt L, Vallin H, Rosenqvist M, Insulander P, Åström H, Nordlander R. Sinus node recovery time assessment revisited: role of pharmacological blockade of the autonomic nervous system. *J Cardiovasc Electrophysiol* 1996; **7**: 95–101.

Bigger JT Jr, Reiffel JA, Livelli FD, Wang PJ. Sensitivity, specificity, and reproducibility of programmed ventricular stimulation. *Circulation* 1986; **73**: 73–78.

Brignole M, Menozzi C, Moya A *et al*. The mechanism of syncope in patients with bundle branch block and negative electrophysiologic test. *Circulation* 2001; **104**: 2045–2050.

Englund A, Bergfeldt L, Rosenqvist M. Pharmacological stress testing of the His-Purkinje system in patients with bifascicular block. *PACE Pacing and Electrophysiology* 1998; **21**: 1979–1987.

Fei L, Trohman RG. Advances in cardiac electrophysiology and pacing. *Crit Care Clin* 2001; **17**: 337–364.

Fonarow GC, Feliciano Z, Boyle NG *et al.* Improved survival in patients with non-ischemic advanced heart failure and syncope with an implantable cardioverter-defibrillator. *Am J Cardiol* 2000; **85**: 981–985.

Gaggioli G, Bottoni N, Brignole M *et al.* Progression to second or third-degree atrio-ventricular block in patients electrostimulated for bundle branch block: a long-term study. *G Ital Cardiol* 1994; **24**: 409–416.

Knight BP, Goyal R, Pelosi F *et al.* Outcome of patients with non-ischemic cardiomyopathy and unexplained syncope treated with an implantable defibrillator. *J Am Coll Cardiol* 1999; **33**: 1964–1970.

Link M, Kim KM, Homoud M, Estes III M, Wang P. Long-term outcome of patients with syncope associated with coronary artery disease and a non-diagnostic electrophysiological evaluation. *Am J Cardiol* 1999; **83**: 1334–1337.

Menozzi C, Brignole M, Garcia-Civera R *et al.* Mechanism of syncope in patients with heart disease and negative electrophysiologic test. *Circulation* 2002; **105**: 2741–2745.

Moya A, Brignole M, and ISSUE Investigators. Mechanism of syncope in patients with isolated syncope and in patients with tilt-positive syncope. *Circulation* 2001; **104**: 1261–1267.

Olshansky B, Hahn EA, Hartz VL, Prater SP, Mason JW. Clinical significance of syncope in the electrophysiologic study vs. electrocardiographic monitoring (ESVEM) trial. *Am Heart J* 1999; **137**: 878–886.

Zipes DP and Jalife J. *Cardiac Electrophysiology. From Cell to Bedside.* 4th edn., W. B. Saunders Company, Philadelphia, 2004.

CHAPTER 16

Miscellaneous diagnostic procedures: when are they indicated

Lennart Bergfeldt and Piotr Kulakowski

Introduction

In a patient with syncope, the presence of structural heart disease with or without other findings indicative of risk for life-threatening ventricular arrhythmias has important prognostic and therapeutic implications. It is against this background that this chapter reviews certain diagnostic tests that have potential value for risk assessment in selected patients.

Echocardiography plays an essential role for assessing the nature and severity of suspected underlying structural heart disease. Other procedures such as exercise testing, coronary angiography, signal-averaged electrocardiography (ECG), and assessment of microvolt T-wave alternans have more limited applications.

Goals

The goals of this chapter are to review the indication for and utility of certain diagnostic procedures applied to assess the nature and severity of underlying structural heart disease in the setting of the syncope evaluation. The following techniques are addressed:

- Echocardiography;
- exercise testing;
- coronary angiography;
- specific ECG analyses;
- pharmacologic tests.

Echocardiography

Echocardiography is frequently used as a screening test to detect and/or quantify the severity of cardiac disease in patients with syncope (Table 16.1). Although numerous case reports have suggested an important role of echocardiography in disclosing the cause and/or mechanism of syncope, larger studies

Table 16.1 Echocardiography – role in syncope patients.

Detection and quantification of cardiac disease
suggesting mechanism of syncope (HCM/HOCM, aortic stenosis, ARVD, atrial myxoma,
  coronary anomaly);
prognostic value (ejection fraction).

Suggesting treatment
surgery: aortic and mitral stenosis, atrial myxoma;
catheter interventions: coronary artery disease, alcohol ablation (HOCM);
implantable devices (ICD and pacemaker): ejection fraction <30% after myocardial
  infarction, HCM and HOCM, ARVD;
specific pharmacologic therapy: primary pulmonary hypertension.

---

have shown that the diagnostic yield is low in the absence of clinical, physical, or ECG findings suggestive of a cardiac abnormality. However, even if echocardiography alone is seldom diagnostic in terms of identifying the basis of syncope, it may provide useful information regarding the type and severity of underlying heart disease. If moderate to severe structural heart disease is found, evaluation is directed toward a cardiac cause of syncope. On the other hand, in the presence of minor structural abnormalities or no structural abnormality, the probability of a cardiac cause of syncope is less and the evaluation may proceed as in patients without structural heart disease (see Chapter 7).

Echocardiography should be part of the initial evaluation when cardiac disease is suspected and/or when syncope is provoked by exercise regardless of the age of the patient. Estimation of left ventricular ejection fraction (LVEF) is essential in the presence of cardiac disease, particularly when the therapeutic strategy includes a decision regarding the use of antiarrhythmic agents or implantation of an ICD. In the former case, proarrhythmic and/or negative inotropic effects of certain drugs might preclude their use in the presence of substantial left ventricular dysfunction. In the case of ICD therapy, LVEF plays a major role in determining which patients are appropriate ICD candidates, even though a low LVEF remains a relatively poor positive predictor of the risk of sudden cardiac death (a normal LVEF, on the other hand, denotes low risk).

Apart from being of value for identifying patients with probable ischemic heart disease (i.e. regional wall motion disturbances) and significant valvular disease, echocardiography may suggest the presence of less common conditions that can be associated with syncope. Important examples include:
• hypertrophic cardiomyopathy (HCM, with or without left ventricular outflow tract obstruction, HOCM), intracardiac tumors,
• dilated cardiomyopathy (whether familial or secondary to identifiable causes such as infections, alcohol, etc.),

Table 16.2 Mechanisms of syncope associated with exercise.

- postexertional form of neurally mediated reflex syncope
- exercise-induced AV block (bradycardia induced syncope)
- exercise-triggered tachycardias (e.g. VT, paroxysmal SVT)
- cardiac ischaemia
  reflex syncope
  arrhythmic syncope
  syncope due to low cardiac output (contractility abnormalities)

- arrhythmogenic right ventricular dysplasia or cardiomyopathy (ARVD), and
- pulmonary hypertension.

Echocardiographic quantification of disease severity is far more precise than can be achieved by physical examination alone. With regard to ischemic heart disease, the echocardiographic diagnostic sensitivity is enhanced by exercise or dobutamine stress ('stress echo'). Valvular heart disease, not identified through the history or by the initial physical examination is probably rare. Nevertheless, certain conditions such as mitral and aortic stenosis may be unappreciated even by skilled examiners, and their relevance to patient symptoms only becomes evident after imaging assessment. MRI is, however, more sensitive (perhaps excessively so) than echocardiography for diagnosing ARVD.

A normal echocardiogram is probably more helpful in the diagnostic evaluation of the middle-aged and older syncope patient, than in the young. In the latter group, neurally mediated reflex faints are the predominant cause of syncope and usually unassociated with structural heart disease.

Exercise testing

Syncope occurring during exercise may be neurally mediated or cardiac in origin (Table 16.2). When it is of cardiac origin, syncope may be associated with significant cardiac disease (e.g. aortic stenosis, HCM, ARVD) or symptomatic arrhythmia (e.g. supraventricular [SVT] or ventricular tachycardia [VT]). Syncope occurring in the immediate recovery phase after exercise (postexertional syncope) is almost invariably due to a neurally mediated mechanism. The diagnostic yield of tilt-testing is equally high in patients with exercise-related and exercise-unrelated neurally mediated reflex syncope.

Exertional syncope in athletes is of particular importance. It has been shown that in the vast majority of such individuals syncope is of neurally mediated origin and the prognosis is very good. However, albeit relatively few cases exhibit cardiac involvement (HOCM, ARVD, congenital coronary artery anomalies), these are crucial to detect as their prognosis may be grave if untreated. Thus, in general, athletes with exercise-associated syncope have a good prognosis but cardiac disease should be excluded before allowing further training. This is particularly important in the presence of a family history of cardiac disease (e.g. HOCM, ARVD, premature coronary artery disease), and/or syncope or sudden cardiac death.

Atrioventricular (AV) block may be provoked as the atrial rate exceeds the ability of the AV conduction system to sustain conduction. This is a rare finding with important prognostic importance. When it occurs, it is usually in a patient with bundle branch block at rest, and it is an ominous sign of transient or impending high degree AV block. Progression to complete AV block is therefore a concern in this setting. Resting ECGs in patients exhibiting exercise-induced AV block usually show an intraventricular conduction abnormality, but not always. Coronary artery disease may be a contributory factor to exercise-induced AV block and warrants further investigation. With the exception of exercise-related syncope, routine exercise testing is not indicated in the evaluation of syncope patients because it is not cost-effective. The exercise test should always be symptom limited, and ECG and blood pressure recordings should be extended throughout the recovery phase.

Apart from identifying ST segment changes suggestive of ischemia or exercise-induced AV block, the heart rate response during exercise provides potentially useful additional information. Chronotropic incompetence observed during exercise may help to explain exertional lightheadedness or syncope. Chronotropic incompetence is part of the spectrum of sinus node disease. Various criteria have been suggested, but as a rough guideline a heart rate >135 bpm should be reached at maximum workload in the absence of treatment with negative chronotropic drugs (e.g. beta-blockers). Further, identification of chronotropic incompetence may signal the presence of other manifestations of sinus node dysfunction (e.g. sinus pauses), although sensitivity of such a test finding is probably low.

Finally, in the presence of heart disease and occasionally even in its absence, maximal or even supra-maximal exercise testing might provoke ventricular arrhythmia, a potentially critical observation of a life-threatening nature.

Coronary angiography

Coronary angiography is seldom necessary in syncope evaluation and is rarely indicated to establish a diagnosis of coronary artery disease (since noninvasive methods are highly effective). Nonetheless, angiography has an obvious place when myocardial ischemia is believed to play a role in the syncopal attack and in decisions related to the need for and feasibility of coronary revascularization. Additionally, in instances when congenital anomalies of the coronary arteries come to mind coronary arteriography is a crucial step in the evaluation process.

Specific ECG analyses

Several methods for ECG analyses in the time and frequency domains exist. They aim at detecting depolarization and/or repolarization abnormalities or altered autonomic tone, and include signal-averaged ECG (SAECG), QT and QT dispersion, T wave alternans, T vector and vector loop analysis, and heart rate variability (HRV), respectively. Currently, these tests have very limited utility in the syncope evaluation. In general, their use is intended to identify those patients with syncope in whom VT may be the underlying mechanism and consequently are at high risk of sudden death. Nevertheless, they are hampered by low positive predictive value (on the other hand a negative test reduces but does not eliminate concern regarding ventricular tachyarrhythmias). Only SAECG has been systematically evaluated in syncope patients. In this regard, the presence of late potentials might suggest inducible VT in ischemic heart disease or support the diagnosis in suspected ARVD.

Pharmacologic tests

Pharmacologic stress testing is applied to enhance the induction of tachycardia, provoke latent cardiac conduction system disease, or facilitate the diagnosis of ischemic heart disease (see echocardiography). Thus, isoprenaline (also termed isoproterenol), and to some extent atropine, are used to facilitate the induction of SVT during invasive or noninvasive electrophysiologic testing. Isoprenaline is sometimes also used to enhance the induction of VT during programmed ventricular stimulation, an invasive procedure.

Pharmacologic inhibition of autonomic tone with atropine and propranolol can be used to evaluate sinus node function, either to increase the sensitivity of sinus node recovery time assessment or to determine the intrinsic heart rate (IHR). While sinus node recovery time (SNRT) requires cardiac pacing (at least on a temporary basis), the assessment of IHR only requires venous cannulation.

Type I antiarrhythmic drugs may be used to stress infra-nodal cardiac conduction system. Sodium channel blockers such as procainamide, ajmaline, and disopyramide have all been applied to detect latent His-Purkinje dysfunction as the mechanism for intermittent AV block, usually in patients with bundle branch block already at baseline. Because prolonged AV block might ensue requiring safe ventricular back-up pacing, such pharmacologic provocation should only be applied in connection with an invasive electrophysiologic procedure including a stable ventricular lead. These agents, as well as flecainide, have also been used to unmask or confirm the Brugada syndrome that may manifest as syncopal episodes due to ventricular tachyarrhythmias.

Bolus injection of ATP (or less desirably adenosine) has been used to unmask propensity to AV block in older individuals with syncope of unknown origin (so-called ATP test). Because the ATP effect is very short-lasting it can be performed without back-up pacing. Initial positive experiences largely reported by Flammang and colleagues have yet, however, to be confirmed in currently ongoing larger studies.

Summary

This chapter has examined the value of certain diagnostic tests that may be useful in the evaluation of selected syncope patients. However, with the exception of echocardiography and possibly exercise testing, most of the tests discussed here have limited utility and are only infrequently indicated.

Additional reading

Ascheim DD, Markowitz SM, Lai H, Engelstein ED, Stein KM, Lerman BB. Vasodepressor syncope due to subclinical myocardial ischemia. *J Cardiovasc Electrophysiol* 1997; **8**: 215–221.

Brignole M, Gaggioli G, Menozzi C *et al.* Adenosine-induced atrioventricular block in patients with unexplained syncope: the diagnostic value of ATP test. *Circulation* 1997; **96**: 3921–3927.

Cheung JW, Stein KM, Markowitz SM *et al.* Significance of adenosine-induced atrioventricular block in patients with unexplained syncope. *Heart Rhythm* 2004; **1**: 664–668.

Colivicchi F, Ammirati F, Santini M. Epidemiology and prognostic implications of syncope in young competing athletes. *Eur Heart J* 2004; **25**: 1749–1753.

Donateo P, Brignole M, Menozzi C *et al.* Mechanism of syncope in patients with positive adenosine tests. *J Am Coll Cardiol* 2003; **41**: 93–98.

Flammang D, Church T, Waynberger M *et al.* Can Adenosine 5'triphosphate be used to select treatment in severe vasovagal syndrome? *Circulation* 1997; **96**: 1201–1208.

Flammang D, Pelleg A, Benditt DG. The adenosine triphospate (ATP) test for evaluation of syncope of unknown origin. *J Cardiovas Electrophys* 2005 (In Press)

Sakaguchi S, Shultz JJ, Remole SC *et al.* Syncope associated with exercise, a manifestation of neurally mediated syncope. *Am J Cardiol* 1995; **75**: 476–481.

Sarasin FP, Junod AF, Carballo D *et al.* Role of echocardiography in the evaluation of syncope: a prospective study. *Heart* 2002; **88**: 363–367.

Steinberg JS, Prystowsky E, Freedman RA *et al.* Use of the signal-averaged electrocardiogram for predicting inducible ventricular tachycardia in patients with unexplained syncope: relation to clinical variables in a multivariate analysis. *J Am Coll Cardiol* 1994; **23**: 99–106.

CHAPTER 17

Neurologic diagnostic procedures in syncope

J. Gert van Dijk

Introduction

In the context of transient loss of consciousness (TLOC), neurologic diagnostic tests may be directed at 4 different fields:

1 cortical function,
2 structural integrity of the brain,
3 the arteries supplying the brain, and
4 the autonomic nervous system.

Corresponding tests for these fields are:

1 the electroencephalogram (EEG) including video-EEG
2 computed tomography (CT) and magnetic resonance imaging (MRI) scanning, and
3 ultrasound investigation of the carotid and vertebral arteries.
4 There is a wide range of tests to investigate the autonomic nervous system, of which the tilt-table test and tests of cardiovascular reflexes are most widely used (see Chapter 14).

Determining which test to order and when, depends on the circumstances of specific attacks. For this reason, a careful history is without doubt the single most important procedure (see Chapters 7 and 8). The testing strategy should be based on the pattern of clinical presentation as discussed below.

Goals

The goals of this chapter are to:

• outline the role of neurologic studies in the diagnostic assessment of syncope; and
• examine appropriate evaluation steps in certain specific neurologic conditions that may cause syncope or syncope-like states.

Laboratory testing in the evaluation of syncope: an overview

In the evaluation of true syncope (defined as in the ESC Syncope Task Force guidelines as a transient, short-lived and self-limited loss of consciousness due to insufficient cerebral blood flow), there is no reason to order an EEG, CT,

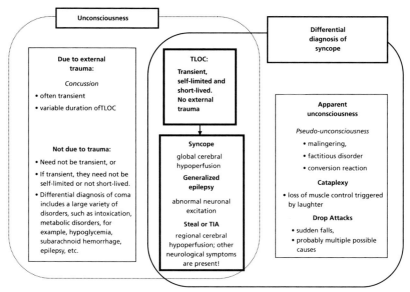

TLOC=transient loss of consciousness (of any etiology)

Figure 17.1 Schematic representation of the relationship of true syncope to other conditions that cause unconsciousness whether of a long-lasting nature or transient (TLOC).

MRI, or ultrasound investigation of the arteries supplying the brain. Unfortunately, numerous and very recent studies on syncope suffer from using a much less strict definition (see discussion in Chapter 2), in which a specific pathophysiologic mechanism leading to loss of consciousness is not stated. The result is that entities such as concussion and seizures may end up (albeit inappropriately) in a syncope group. In such cases, the diagnostic strategy is of necessity different. Most importantly, there becomes a need to encompass within the evaluation of syncope a much broader array of conditions (i.e. apart from just those associated with transiently diminished cerebral perfusion) that may cause loss of consciousness. To prevent confusion, it is best not to use syncope for this broader group, but the phrase 'transient loss of consciousness' (TLOC, see also Chapter 2). This phrase (TLOC) incorporates a range of conditions and can be used until a likely cause has been established, such as syncope, epilepsy, or concussion (Figure 17.1).

Readers may feel that they need a battery of tests simply to make the distinction among various conditions that cause TLOC; however, this is rarely the case. The clinical presentation usually provides enough clues to choose among the main categories. Additional tests should be directed at disorders within the appropriate category. For example, in a patient with exercise-dependent attacks of unconsciousness and antecedent heart disease, syncope is very likely, and the '*a priori*' chances of epilepsy are so low that an EEG is unlikely to change this view.

Testing in specific conditions
Autonomic failure

Syncope in autonomic failure can benefit from ancillary neurologic testing (see Chapters 3, 4, and 20 part 2). In such patients, the faint may occur through an orthostatic hypotension mechanism as well as through postexercise hypotension. In autonomic failure, the neurologic dysfunction is often not restricted to blood pressure regulation, so the history-taking should include sexual function (impotence), sweating (dry skin, sometimes with patches of compensatory hyperhidrosis), bladder function (both incontinence and retention), gastrointestinal function (delayed stomach emptying, constipation, diarrhea), and pupillary function (blurred vision).

History-taking is also important to distinguish between the three main groups of autonomic failure.

• Primary autonomic failure encompasses degenerative diseases such as multiple system atrophy, pure autonomic failure, and autonomic failure, in the context of Parkinson's disease.

• Secondary autonomic failure concerns damage to the autonomic nervous system in the context of other diseases, such as diabetes, kidney and liver failure, and alcoholism.

• In the third group, autonomic failure occurs as a side-effect of medication. Likely culprits are antidepressants, antihypertensives, vasodilators, and beta-adrenergic receptor blocking drugs. In this drug-induced group, autonomic failure may be restricted to orthostatic hypotension.

The differential diagnosis of autonomic failure is complex and establishing the ultimate diagnosis requires considerable expertise. The same holds for the application of cardiovascular or other tests of autonomic function, such as catecholamine studies or isotope studies of the brain and heart. When the more obvious causes, such as diabetes and drug effects have been excluded an expert opinion should be sought.

Syncope mimics

As discussed elsewhere in this book (Chapters 2 and 23), a large number of conditions are often diagnosed as 'syncope', but in reality they do not cause true syncope. Thus we use the term 'syncope mimics'. In this group of conditions, investigations should be chosen based on the *a priori* chance of the disorder in question.

Epilepsy

The EEG has a twofold role in the diagnosis of epilepsy. First, by showing 'epileptiform abnormalities' it may considerably increase the likelihood of epilepsy being present and being the cause of loss of consciousness spells. The detected EEG abnormalities have different weights depending on their nature: some, like 'spike–wave' complexes provide hard evidence, whereas sharp waves and a variety of other waveforms carry considerably less weight. Second, their nature and location help to identify the specific type of epilepsy. For instance, a typical 3 per s run of large spike–wave complexes all over the brain points to 'absence' epilepsy, whereas isolated temporal spike–wave complexes are more often seen in partial complex epilepsy.

In the vast majority of cases, the EEG is recorded interictally (i.e. between seizure events). The chance of detecting abnormalities in epilepsy starts at about 40% for one EEG, and increases to about 60% for three EEGs. Thus, it rarely pays to order another EEG if two or three previous ones did not show epileptiform abnormalities. Photic stimulation (flashing lights), hyperventilation, and sleep deprivation are commonly used procedures that increase the chances of finding epileptiform abnormalities. These abnormalities are highly specific, in that they occur in only about 1% of people without overt epileptic attacks. In some cases it may be necessary to obtain an ictal recording to prove or disprove epilepsy as a cause for attacks. This may be done with ambulatory EEGs on an outpatient basis or by video and EEG observation in a dedicated center.

Brain imaging by CT or MRI is indicated in epilepsy to search for the cause of epilepsy rather than to establish epilepsy itself. Thus, structural abnormalities such as brain tumors may be detected. However, such scans should only be ordered when concrete evidence points to a neurologic disorder, such as probable epilepsy. For probable syncope these scans should be avoided in view of their expense and exceedingly low diagnostic yield. The only exception is syncope due to primary autonomic failure; an MRI can help in the diagnosis of multiple system atrophy. Here too there should be clinical evidence suggestive of the underlying neurologic abnormality other than just the occurrence of syncope.

Subclavian steal syndrome
Syncope-like attacks provoked by physical exercise of the arms point to a steal phenomenon (often termed 'subclavian steal syndrome'). Apart from measuring blood pressure in both arms, ultrasound studies are indicated to search for a steal syndrome. Note that not all steal phenomena result in clinical symptoms, so it is wise to think twice whether or not an observed steal phenomenon is to be blamed for a specific attack.

Strokes and transient ischemic attacks
Transient ischemic attacks (TIAs) obviously need accurate diagnosis and prompt medical attention, but it should be understood that they do not really look like syncope. In carotid TIAs, neurologic deficits such as hemiparesis or aphasia predominate while consciousness is normal. Only TIAs involving a very large proportion of the cortex can impair consciousness. However, even these do not usually go as far as complete loss of consciousness. Further, they last too long to look like syncope and the deficit will be impressive. Vertebrobasilar TIAs are theoretically more likely to mimic syncope, but again loss

of consciousness is not very common and there are a large number of additional signs, such as dysarthria, ataxia, vertigo, and nystagmus to suggest the diagnosis. A vertebrobasilar TIA should be considered most unlikely as the explanation for a loss of consciousness without any such signs.

There is no need to order a CT scan, MRI, or ultrasound studies of the carotid or vertebral arteries for attacks looking like syncope, and in which the history and physical findings clearly point away from a structural neurologic problem, that is, loss of consciousness without neurologic deficit.

To summarize, a TIA represents neurological deficit without loss of consciousness whereas syncope represents loss of consciousness without neurological deficit.

Hyperventilation syndrome
This name was (and sometimes still is) used for attacks of anxiety together with a variety of somatic complaints, such as shortness of breath, a tight sensation in the chest, and tingling fingers. It was built on the theory that hyperventilation induced hypocapnia, which induced cerebral vasoconstriction, leading to cerebral hypoxia and the associated complaints. However, subsequent studies have shown that the attacks also occurred in the absence of hypocapnia, so the presumed pathophysiologic theory was incorrect. This also means that the hyperventilation provocation test aiming for complaint recognition is dubious, as it is not clear what is being tested. Attacks of a similar nature fall under the term 'panic attacks' in the psychiatric nomenclature (see Chapter 18).

Summary

Neurologic disease is rarely the cause of true syncope, although it may cause periods of transient impairment of consciousness (TLOC) or seemingly transient impairment of consciousness that can be mistaken for syncope (e.g. epilepsy). Consequently, ancillary neurologic testing is rarely indicated in the diagnostic evaluation of the cause of syncope and such tests should certainly not be part of the initial assessment of syncope patients. For those patients suspected of autonomic failure, referral to a neurologic specialist is warranted. This also holds when it is not certain that the attack was syncope that is, when dealing with TLOC.

Additional reading

Benbadis SR. The problem of psychogenic symptoms: is the psychiatric community in denial? *Epilepsy Behav* 2005; **6**: 9–14.
Colman N, Nahm K, van Dijk JG, Reitsma JB, Wieling W, Kaufmann H. Diagnostic value of history taking in reflex syncope. *Clin Auton Res* 2004; **14**: 37–44.
Flink R, Pedersen B, Guekht AB *et al*. Guidelines for the use of EEG methodology in the diagnosis of epilepsy. International League Against Epilepsy: commission report.

Commission on European Affairs: Subcommission on European Guidelines. *Acta Neurol Scand* 2002; **106**: 1–7.

Hornsveld HK, Garssen B, Dop MJ, van Spiegel PI, de Haes JC. Double-blind placebo-controlled study of the hyperventilation provocation test and the validity of the hyperventilation syndrome. *Lancet* 1996; **348**: 154–158.

CHAPTER 18

Contribution of psychiatric disorders to apparent syncope

George Theodorakis

Introduction

Psychiatric disorders are known to be associated with and possibly responsible for certain 'apparent' loss of consciousness episodes. However, although psychiatric disturbances may be an important source of syncope mimics (see Chapters 2 and 23), they do not cause true syncope.

Goals

The primary goals of this chapter are;
• to identify the possible roles psychiatric disease may play in patients with apparent syncope; and
• review psychiatric conditions that may result in behavior that mimics syncope (pseudo-syncope).

Do psychiatric conditions cause syncope?

In terms of the relationship between potentially abnormal psychiatric states and apparent loss of consciousness, several clinical scenarios may be relevant. First, syncope of 'unknown etiology' may occur in patients who happen to have a coexisting psychiatric disorder. Most of these cases are probably vasovagal faints. Nevertheless, careful evaluation is needed. Syncope of any etiology may occur in such a patient population as they are not immune to the many causes of syncope discussed elsewhere in this book. Second, syncope-like episodes or syncope mimics are particularly common in association with certain psychiatric conditions (see later). In these latter cases, it is important to keep the definition of syncope in mind; specifically, true syncope is transient loss of consciousness triggered by inadequate cerebral perfusion (see Chapter 2).

In the absence of cerebral hypoperfusion, true syncope is not present, and anything else suggesting transient reversible loss of consciousness is then a syncope mimic (see Chapter 23). Recognition of a mimic is often difficult in these patients, but is based on documenting that blood pressure and heart rate remain stable during the attack. Syncope in association with hyperventilation is a special case in which there are differences of opinion as to whether true syncope can really be induced; some believe that anxiety disorders and other psychiatric states might predispose to hyperventilation and that the consequent hypocapnia and cerebrovascular constriction results in true syncope. However, other evidence refutes this hypothesis; the issue is discussed more extensively in Chapter 17.

Finally, and perhaps most importantly, psychiatric disturbances (particularly anxiety disorders) may develop as a consequence of recurrent syncope episodes. In these cases, the recurring medical problem may be considered to be the source. However, proof of this relationship is difficult and may only be possible after successful control of recurrent syncope ultimately results in resolution of the abnormal psychiatric state.

Association of syncope and psychiatric illness

The most frequent psychiatric disorders that may be associated with or mimic syncope are:
- somatoform disorders,
- mood disorders, and
- anxiety disorders.

Somatoform disorders

Somatoform disorders have been referred to as *hysteria* in the past. They usually present before the age of 30 and extend over a period of several years. Patients who meet the DSM-IV (Diagnostic and Statistical Manual) diagnostic criteria, must have at least four pain, two gastrointestinal, one sexual, and one pseudo-neurologic symptom. Major depressive, panic, and substance-related disorders are frequently associated with this disorder.

Apparent syncope can be one of the manifestations of somatoform disorders. Extreme cases of patients who wander from hospital to hospital feigning serious medical illness with cardiac symptoms and syncope have been characterized as the cardiac Munchausen syndrome. 'Faints' or 'blackouts' in most of these cases are not true syncope and is not associated with changes in blood pressure or heart rate. Further, symptoms are much more frequent (e.g. daily or multiple times daily) than is expected of true faints, even in severely affected 'true' fainters.

Mood disorders

Mood disorders include mania, hypomania, and depression. They are usually easily recognized by loss of interest, weight loss, fatigue, anorexia, sexual dysfunction, and sleep disturbances. Mood disorders and major depression are the most frequent psychiatric conditions diagnosed in patients complaining of syncope. Mood disorders should be differentiated from other medical conditions such as multiple sclerosis, cerebrovascular accidents, and hypothyroidism.

Anxiety disorders

Anxiety disorders are classified as:

- general anxiety disorder,
- panic disorders with or without agoraphobia, and
- epidemic fainting.

General anxiety disorder

This disorder is characterized by the presence of excessive anxiety and worry, associated with three or more symptoms of restlessness, fatigue, difficulty of concentrating, irritability, muscle tension, or sleep disturbance for at least 6 months.

Panic disorders with or without agoraphobia

Panic attacks are characterized by the sense of impending doom and fear. Physical symptoms develop abruptly and frequently and are associated with apparent syncope. These attacks tend to disrupt the patient's life significantly. The mechanism by which anxiety disorders might actually cause syncope is probably hyperventilation, although the vasovagal faint should not be excluded. Accurso *et al.* showed that patients with a phobia for blood or injury often also exhibit a positive tilt test suggesting an autonomic dysregulation similar to vasovagal patients.

Epidemic fainting

This condition is more frequent in females of adolescent age; it usually occurs during periods of uncertainty and social stress. These epidemics have been reported in schools, marching bands, rock concert audiences, and other groups. In some cases, hyperventilation is probably the responsible mechanism for apparent syncope.

In attempting to assess reports of an association between syncope and psychiatric diagnoses it is important to bear in mind that most studies use the term syncope more loosely (see also Chapter 2) than is used in this book or is advised by the ESC Syncope Task Force. Thus, most published reports are difficult to assess as they almost certainly include both true syncope and syncope mimics (Chapter 23). Furthermore, many studies suggesting a frequent relation between psychiatric illness and syncope were published before widespread acceptance of head-up tilt table testing as a diagnostic tool. Consequently, it is likely that many cases of syncope attributed to a psychiatric or psychogenic origin in the early literature, may well have been unrecognized vasovagal faints. Another difficulty in categorizing these patients is that the estimated sensitivity of head-up tilt testing in most laboratories ranges only from 25 to 50%. This means that a number of patients could have been misdiagnosed as having psychiatric disease due to low sensitivity of the tilt test.

Given the important caveats noted above, we can derive only an uncertain sense of the psychiatry-syncope relationship. In this regard, in a study of the association between apparent syncope and psychiatric illness by Kapoor *et al.*, 163 patients suffering from recurrent unexplained syncope episodes were subjected to a diagnostic interview schedule (DIS). The DIS suggested a psychiatric diagnosis in 24.5%, with major depression in 12.3% and somatization, panic, or anxiety disorders in another 14.7%. Compared with syncope patients in whom the cause of the faints were of known etiology, patients with syncope of unknown origin had higher rates of psychiatric disorders, especially panic attacks. Furthermore, patients with any psychiatric disorder had a 35% 1-year recurrence rate for 'syncope' compared to 15% in those without a psychiatric disorder. Similar observations have been reported by Linzer *et al.* They found that psychiatric disorders, in particular panic disorders and major depression, were a common cause of 'syncope' in 24–31% patients with 'unknown etiology' syncope. Most of these patients exhibited positive head-up tilt-testing suggesting that in fact vasovagal syncope may have been the predominant underlying mechanism. However, these findings are subject to the concern that the conditions may be coexisting morbidities (or even laboratory false positives) rather than a causal relationship. It will be necessary to revisit this presumptive diagnosis in the future with more definitive diagnostic tools.

In a study by Kouakam *et al.*, psychiatric disorders were frequent in patients with syncope in a cohort of 40 patients. Twenty-six patients (65%) had at least one psychiatric disorder compared to 14 (35%) control subjects. In the same study, the psychiatric illness did not differ between positive and negative tilt-test patients. Tilt-testing was positive for vasovagal syncope in 63%. It was interesting that the existence of psychiatric disorders was a stronger predictor of syncope recurrence than the tilt-test result. Similar results were found in our laboratory using clomipramine as a challenge drug during head-up tilt-testing. Forty-six percent of patients with positive tilt-tests had abnormal anxiety scores based on DSM IV diagnostic criteria.

A major problem in the evaluation of patients with unexplained syncope is that many of them refuse psychiatric examination. In a report by Ventura *et al.*, psychiatric evaluation was accepted in 26 out of 50 patients with a negative tilt test. In most, (81%) of the patients who accepted, a psychiatric disorder was diagnosed. Specifically, depression was diagnosed in 46%, panic attacks in 15%, and general anxiety and somatization disorder in five patients.

A wide range of disorders from simple emotional stress to psychiatric illnesses can be associated with syncope. However, it is uncertain whether these findings indicate a causal relationship. Central serotoninergic systems have been evaluated with clomipramine and other challenge drugs in patients with psychiatric disorders such as major depression or panic disorders. Most of them have shown a significant increase in prolactin and cortisol in patients with panic disorders compared to normal controls, as a response to drug challenge. The same pattern of response was found in patients with vasovagal syncope implying that an increased response to serotoninergic stimulus exists in these situations and suggesting (but not proving) that there may be a common pathophysiological pathway.

Evaluation of syncope patients with potential psychiatric contribution to symptoms

Medical history

As has been emphasized throughout this book, a detailed medical history and a complete physical examination are essential in order to determine the basis of syncope. This is certainly also the case when it comes to evaluating the possible contribution of psychiatric conditions to apparent syncope. Many times, the history leads to the suggestion that a psychiatric component is present. For example, patients with multiple syncope episodes without injury or those who describe nonspecific symptoms referable to many organ systems, leads one to think of psychogenic pseudosyncope. This latter situation is usually related to psychologic factors causing the patients to manifest unexplained somatic symptoms. Of course, it is essential to evaluate the possibility of a true syncope diagnosis before labeling the disorder as psychogenic. The appropriate evaluation steps are described in other chapters.

Evidence from the patients' relatives is useful. Families with distressed parents exhibit a higher incidence of children's syncope and visits to emergency departments. A preceding episode of anxiety, fear, or various other somatic, stressful, or panic phenomena with apparent hyperventilation suggests a psychogenic cause (i.e. pseudosyncope). In the case of hyperventilation, true syncope may theoretically occur; the basis for this has been thought to be hypocapnia causing constriction of cerebral vessels and thus reduced cerebral blood flow. However, this mechanism is now less certain. In any case, it has not yet been clarified whether hyperventilation is a separate clinical entity or should be incorporated within the group of psychogenic causes of apparent syncope. For example, it was recently reported that syncope masquerading as panic disorder was proven to be a result of prolonged episodes of ventricular asystole detected only after the implantation of a loop recorder (ILR).

Physical examination

The physical examination may be helpful in making the distinction between true syncope and pseudosyncope. First, clinical examination during the syncope attack offers information regarding heart rate or blood pressure fall. In psychogenic pseudosyncope, for example, the heart rate and blood pressure remain relatively stable during the attack. Sinus tachycardia may be expected. Second, in cases of psychogenic pseudo-unconsciousness, patients have a tendency to close their eyes when attempts are made by medical personnel to open them passively. The muscle tone of the patients' limbs is also different than in true syncope. The result is a nonflaccid posture of the limbs in pseudosyncope patients, which is easily recognized by an experienced examiner. Likewise, when the patient's hand is raised above the face and then released it will not drop on the face. Other signs include the observation that the eyes may show stable movements upwards or downwards, or consistently away from the observer.

Certain patients with psychiatric disease may appear to be unconscious for extended periods of time, unlike true fainters in whom the event is usually brief. In patients with prolonged periods of apparent pseudo-unconsciousness on a psychogenic basis, the real diagnosis may be overlooked and confused with syncope by some practitioners. However, the differential diagnosis should more reasonably consider coma rather than syncope.

Additional clinical considerations

Patients with vasovagal syncope frequently have somatization, anxiety, panic disorders, or major depressive disorder. Psychiatrists often rely on the *Diagnostic and Statistical Manual of Mental Disorders* (i.e. *DSM IV*) to evaluate these patients. There are specific criteria that characterize individual psychiatric disorders.

Apart from the psychiatric component contributing to syncope, many patients suffering from psychiatric problems use drugs that may influence vascular tone and blood pressure, or which are potentially proarrhythmic. These should be taken into account as possible triggers of true syncope. Such drugs include phenothiazines, tricyclic antidepressants, and monoamine oxidase inhibitors (Table 18.1). QT interval prolongation, with susceptibility to *torsade de pointes* ventricular tachycardia is a major concern with several of these agents. Overdose is of course another issue of concern in this population.

Table 18.1 Drugs that can cause prolongation of the QT interval and/or *torsade de pointes*.*

Category of the drug	Drugs
Antiarrhythmic	
Class IA	Procainamide quinidine disopyramide
Class III	Amiodarone, sotalol, dofetilide, ibutilide, bretylium
Antimicrobial	Erythromycin, clarithromycin, trimethoprim-sulfamethoxazole
Antifungal	Fluconazole, ketonazole, itraconazole, sparfoxacine
Antimalarial	Chloroquine, halofantrine, qinine mefloquine pentamidine
Psychoactive	Haloperidol, lithium, phenodiazines, tricyclic antidepressants, chloral hydrate.
Gastrointestinal	Cisapride
Antistamine	Diphenhydramine, terfenadine, astemizole
Miscellaneous	Droperidol, vasopressin, tacrolimus, probucol, indapamide, amantadine
Cancer	Arsenic trioxide
Antianginal	Bepridil, ryanodine
Antiemetic	Domperidone
Opiate agonist	Levomethadyl, methadone

*The reader should be aware that this list is incomplete. Several internet websites maintain more comprehensive and up-to-date lists of QT prolonging drugs (e.g. www.longQT.org).

Revision of the patient's medications and/or ease of access to medications may solve the syncope problem.

Tests for psychiatric syncope (psychcogenic pseudosyncope) patients

A number of tests may be useful in an attempt to identify patients with psychogenic pseudosyncope. These include:

1 hyperventilation test;
2 head-up tilt testing;
3 electroencephalogram (EEG) or Doppler cerebral blood flow; and
4 psychiatric diagnostic testing alluded to earlier.

• Hyperventilation test is performed with 3-min open-mouthed forced hyperventilation and (although not without contraversy) is considered useful. It has an estimated, but not well established, positive predictive value of 59% for diagnosing 'psychiatric syncope' in young adults. This test is in need of additional study and is not yet widely accepted. Furthermore, since hyperventilation can rarely provoke angina or heart block, vital signs should be monitored with continuous ECG recording.

• Tilt-table testing is widely used for evaluation of these patients. Most reactions observed are vasovagal (see Chapters 7, 14, and 20, Part 1). However, there is often an overlap between vasovagal syncope and psychiatric illness. The tilt-test can be performed without drug challenge or after provocation with isoproterenol, nitroglycerin, adenosine, or perhaps other agents such as clomipramine.

Patients with psychogenic pseudosyncope during head-up tilt-testing may show an apparent unconsciousness response with intact blood pressure and heart rate. In some cases (not often) such patients warrant a thorough neurologic evaluation to exclude other rare causes of true unconsciousness. However, psychiatric assessment is certainly crucial.

Summary

The term psychogenic or psychiatric syncope is imprecise. This imprecision can be largely attributed to the fact that substantial literature on this topic has usually disregarded the concept that syncope is the result of cerebral hypoperfusion. This same literature has tended to lump anything that appears to be transient loss of consciousness under the term syncope. The result has been unfortunately confusing for practitioners.

A relation between psychiatric illness and apparent syncope-like states (syncope mimics, not true syncope), especially affecting patients mainly with panic attacks, anxiety, or depression may be quite common. Some have suggested that there is a 'vicious circle' where syncope can lead to psychological distress and dysfunction. On the other hand, most psychogenic fainting is neither fainting nor true syncope. In some cases, vasovagal syncope may result from anxiety and depressive disorders and thereby be more common in this population. In any event, the practitioner must carefully exclude causes of true syncope before concluding that the patient has a psychogenic disorder.

Additional reading

Accurso V, Winnicki M, Shamsuzzaman SM, Wenzel A, Jonson AK, Somers V. Predisposition to vasovagal syncope in subjects with blood/injury phobia. *Circulation* 2001; **104**: 903–907.

Kapoor W, Fortunato M, Hanusa B, Schulberg H. Psychiatric illness in patients with syncope. *Am J Med* 1995; **99**: 505–512.

Kouakam C, Lacroix D, Klug D, Baux P, Marquie C, Kacet S. Prevalence and prognostic significance of psychiatric disorders in patients evaluated for recurrent unexplained syncope. *Am J Cardiol* 2002; **89**: 530–535.

Linzer M, Felder A, Hackel A *et al*. Psychiatric syncope: a new look at an old disease. *Psychosomatics* 1990; **31**: 181–188.

Theodorakis GN, Markianos M, Livanis EG, Zarvalis E, Flevari P, Kemastinos DT. Provocation of neurocardiogenic syncope by clomipramine administration during head-up tilt test in vasovagal syndrome. *J Am Coll Cardiol* 2000; **36**: 174–178.

Theodorakis GN, Markianos M, Livanis EG, Zarvalis E, Flevari P, Kremastinos DT. Hormonal responses during head up tilt-table test in neurally mediated syncope. *Am J Cardiol* 1997; **79**: 1692–1695.

Thijs RD, Wieling W, Kaufmann H, van Dijk JG. Defining and classifying syncope. *Clin Auton Res* 2004 Oct; **14**: 4–8.

Ventura R, Maas R, Ruppel R *et al*. Psychiatric conditions in patients with recurrent unexplained syncope. *Europace* 2001; **3**: 311–316.

Section four:
Causes of syncope and syncope mimics, and treatment

CHAPTER 19

Who to treat

Michele Brignole and Rose Anne Kenny

Introduction

Treatment objectives for the 'syncope patient' may be classified into:
• prevention of syncope recurrences, and
• reducing mortality risk.
Multiple factors affect the need for recommending the specific treatment strategy selected for each individual. In this regard, treatment may be broadly viewed as education, nonpharmacologic and pharmacologic treatments directed at syncope susceptibility (including addressing underlying disease state) and lifestyle recommendations.

Goals

The goals of this chapter are to highlight:
• factors determining need for treatment for prevention of syncope recurrences;
• the objective of therapy in various syncope diagnostic categories; and
• issues affecting the 'aggressiveness' of treatment, including the need for addressing underlying diseases.

The need for hospitalization of patients in order to conduct the evaluation and initiate treatment is dealt with in Chapter 9.

Factors affecting decision regarding need for treatment

The need for initiating prophylactic treatment varies depending on specific clinical circumstances. The most important of these are:
• level of certainty that the etiology of the symptoms is known;
• an estimate of the likelihood that syncope will recur;
• the individual's anticipated syncope-associated mortality risk which is, for the most part, determined by the nature and severity of underlying cardiac and cardiovascular disease;
• the occurrence of, or potential risk for, physical or emotional injury associated with recurrent faints;
• the implications of syncope recurrence on occupation and avocation (i.e. individual economic and lifestyle issues);
• the public health risk, such as in the case of motor vehicle operators, pilots, etc.; and

• an assessment of the effectiveness, safety, and potential adverse effects associated with proposed therapies (in particular given comorbidities in the patient being evaluated).

Specific conditions
Neurally mediated reflex syncopal syndromes

Since neurally mediated reflex syncope carries virtually no direct mortality risk, the treatment goals are directed almost exclusively toward primarily prevention of both symptom recurrence and associated injuries and improved quality of life.

Patients who seek medical advice after having experienced a vasovagal faint require reassurance and education regarding the nature of the disease, and ways to minimize exposure to known triggering events. In general, education and reassurance are sufficient for most patients. Modification or discontinuation of hypotensive drug treatment for concomitant conditions is another first line measure for the prevention of syncope recurrences. Treatment is not necessary for patients who have sustained a single syncope and in whom syncope did not occur in a high risk setting (e.g. during driving).

Additional treatment may be necessary when there is a high frequency of episodes that:
• adversely affect the quality of life;
• is recurrent and unpredictable (absence of premonitory symptoms) and exposes patients to 'high risk' of trauma; and
• occurs during the prosecution of a high risk activity (e.g. driving, machine operation, flying, competitive athletics, etc.)

Treatment of vasovagal syncope and related neurally mediated syncope disorders is dealt with in detail in Chapter 20, Part 1. In brief, however, for highly motivated patients with recurrent vasovagal symptoms, the prescription of progressively prolonged periods of enforced upright posture (so-called tilt-training) may reduce syncope recurrence. Isometric counter-pressure maneuvers of the legs (leg crossing) or of the arms (hand grip and arm tensing) are able to induce a significant blood pressure increase during the phase of an impending vasovagal syncope, and thereby allow the patient to avoid or delay losing consciousness in most cases.

Many drugs have been used in the treatment of vasovagal syncope. In general, long-term placebo-controlled prospective trials have failed to show any benefit of most drugs over placebo. To date, with the possible exception of midodrine, there is not sufficient data to support the use of any pharmacological therapy for vasovagal syncope.

Cardiac pacing appears to be beneficial in the carotid sinus syndrome while the role of pacing in vasovagal syncope is less established. It seems that pacing therapy might be effective in some but not in all vasovagal syncope patients. This is not surprising if we consider that pacing is probably efficacious for cardioinhibition (i.e. marked bradycardia) but has no role in combating the hypotension due to vascular dilatation that is frequently a dominant component in vasovagal syncope. Cardiac pacing should be employed as a last resort choice in a very selected small proportion of (usually older) patients affected by severe cardioinhibitory vasovagal syncope. Unfortunately, there are no clear-cut rules on how best to select these patients. Finally, certain forms of presumed neurally mediated syncope (usually in older individuals) are unmasked by adenosine triphosphate (ATP) injection (see Chapter 16). This type of syncope seems to be amenable to pacemaker therapy.

Orthostatic syncope

The treatment goals in individuals with symptomatic orthostatic hypotension are directed to prevention of symptom recurrence and associated injuries and to improve quality of life. Many of these patients are in older age groups and/or are relatively frail due to the presence of multiple concomitant medical conditions (e.g. diabetes, heart and vascular disease, autonomic dysfunction). Iatrogenic factors, as well as poor diet and fluid intake may play a key role in triggering symptoms in such cases.

Syncope due to symptomatic orthostatic hypotension should be treated in all patients. Drug-induced autonomic failure is probably the most frequent cause of orthostatic hypotension. The principal treatment strategy is elimination of the offending agents, mainly diuretics and vasodilators. Alcohol is also commonly associated with orthostatic intolerance Thus, if new-onset orthostatic syncope can be reasonably attributed to a drug being taken by the individual, then its withdrawal should suffice. However, clinical follow-up is still warranted. Additional treatment options, used alone or in combination, are appropriate for consideration on an individual patient basis; these include nonpharmacological and pharmacological methods and are discussed elsewhere in this book.

Cardiac arrhythmias as primary cause

Treatment goals are prevention of symptom recurrence, improved quality of life and reduction of mortality risk.

Treatment for syncope due to cardiac arrhythmias must be appropriate for the specific arrhythmia cause. All patients, even those with single or rare events, warrant careful consideration for treatment. However, absent unusual extenuating circumstances (e.g. poor prognosis due to comorbidity), therapy recommendation should be considered mandatory in all patients in whom the basis for syncope is life threatening and when there is a high risk of injury. The latter is often the case in elderly or frail individuals, those in whom warning is minimal or absent and those whose employment or avocation might result in physical injury to themselves or others.

Antiarrhythmic drugs, cardiac pacing, implantable cardioverter defibrillators (ICDs), and transcatheter ablation are all treatment options to be considered depending on the specific arrhythmia causing syncope. It is important to bear in mind, however, that while pacing or ablation may prevent arrhythmias and thereby eliminate syncope, the ICD-treated patient may remain at risk for fainting. In ICD-treated patients, device intervention is delayed for a period long enough to assure that the rhythm is sustained, that the arrhythmia has been correctly (as best as is possible) diagnosed, and the device's capacitors have had a chance to charge. ICD's only reduce sudden-death risk not syncope risk.

Structural cardiac or cardiopulmonary disease

Treatment goals are prevention of symptom recurrence and reduction of mortality risk. The basis of syncope in these conditions is often multifactorial, including the hemodynamic impact of the specific lesion, as well as that of related arrhythmias and neurally mediated reflex effects. Therefore the decision is not only when to treat but rather to identify the exact mechanism(s) responsible in order to target treatment appropriately.

When the cause of syncope is directly related to a structural lesion(s) that is correctable, the correction is usually indicated (assuming other health factors permit). This is the case for syncope in which there is fixed or dynamic obstruction to left ventricular outflow (e.g. aortic stenosis, hypertrophic obstructive cardiomyopathy [HOCM], atrial myxoma, etc.) where the basis for the faint is at least in part due to inadequate blood flow as a result of the mechanical obstruction. On the other hand, when syncope is caused by certain difficult to treat conditions, such as primary pulmonary hypertension or restrictive cardiomyopathy, it is often impossible to ameliorate the underlying problem adequately.

Coexisting factors may contribute importantly to the development of syncope in the setting of structural cardiovascular disease. Thus, in the case of valvular aortic stenosis, neurally mediated reflex disturbance of vascular control is believed to be an important contributor to hypotension. Similarly, in hypertrophic cardiomyopathy, (with or without left ventricle outflow obstruction) neural reflex mechanisms may also play a role. Furthermore, whenever structural disease is present, the occurrence of cardiac arrhythmias as a contributing cause of syncope must remain a consideration as well. Atrial tachyarrhythmias (particularly atrial fibrillation) or ventricular tachycardia (even at relatively modest rates) are particularly important causes of syncope events in these settings, but bradyarrhythmias (e.g. sinus node dysfunction, transient AV block) should not be overlooked.

Cerebrovascular disease

Cerebrovascular disease is only a very infrequent cause of syncope (see Chapter 20, Part 5). The goals of treatment of syncope associated with cerebrovascular disease are aimed at preventing stroke and improving quality of life.

Subclavian steal is the only commonly recognized condition in this group. There are no well-defined treatment indications, but intervention seems appropriate when the condition is severe enough to cause clinically important symptoms such as syncope or near-syncope.

Carotid vascular disease is almost never a cause of syncope. Recurrent syncope is uncommon in these patients even with bilateral critical carotid artery stenosis or with vertebrobasilar disease. Treatment of these conditions may be indicated to prevent stroke, but a syncope indication would be extremely rare.

Miscellaneous syncope-like conditions (syncope mimics)

Disorders in this category are not true syncope (see Chapter 23), but are part of the differential diagnosis. Treatment goals are primarily aimed at improved quality of life.

Psychiatric disturbances

The importance of psychiatric disturbances as syncope mimics lies in the fact that they are both very common and difficult to diagnose (see Chapter 18). Often, the diagnosis only materializes after considerable time and unproductive laboratory testing. If recurrent 'syncope-like' symptoms are a feature of the patient's presentation then psychiatric referral for treatment is indicated.

Epilepsy

Epilepsy is part of the differential diagnosis of transient loss of consciousness but are rare as causes of syncope (see Chapter 17). Frontal lobe partial complex seizures may be misdiagnosed as true syncope by virtue of their tendency to be abrupt in onset, brief, and often unassociated with postictal confusion. Temporal lobe epilepsy may also mimic (or possibly trigger) vasovagal syncope. Conventional epilepsy therapy under the care of a neurologist is appropriate.

Metabolic disturbances

Apart from the controversial role of hyperventilation as a cause of syncope (see Chapter 17), metabolic disturbances (e.g. hypoglycemic coma, hypoxemia) causing loss of consciousness are best considered as syncope mimics by virtue of the fact that they are not typically self-limited. Treatment is indicated in all cases and may require referral to a specialist in internal medicine.

Intoxication

Various agents, most commonly alcohol but more recently amphetamines and opiods, may induce alterations of consciousness that mimic syncope. As a rule, however, the episode is relatively long lasting and not immediately reversible as is usually expected in true syncope.

Summary

Treatment of syncope patients is critically dependent on establishing the correct diagnosis, and understanding the patient's overall health condition and social circumstances. Apart from the universal requirement that education regarding syncope be provided, various specific issues determine the need for further treatment steps. Certain of these considerations have been summarized in this chapter. More detailed analysis is found in the chapters dealing with individual conditions in detail.

Additional reading

Brignole M, Alboni P, Benditt DG *et al.* Guidelines on management (diagnosis and treatment) of syncope. Update 2004 *Europace* 2004; **6**: 467–537.

Kapoor W. Evaluation and outcome of patients with syncope. *Medicine* 1990; **69**: 160–175.

Sheldon R, Rose S, Ritchie D *et al.* Historical criteria that distinguish syncope from seizures. *J Am Coll Cardiol* 2002; **40**: 142–148.

CHAPTER 20

Specific causes of syncope: their evaluation and treatment strategies

Part 1: Neurally mediated reflex syncope

David G. Benditt and Jean-Jacques Blanc

Introduction

Neurally mediated reflex syncope (see also Chapter 1) encompasses a group of disorders, the best known of which are the vasovagal (or common) faint and carotid sinus syndrome. The former is generally believed to be the most frequent of all causes of syncope in humans. The latter (carotid sinus syndrome) is mainly a problem in older individuals (generally >60 years of age). Postmicturition syncope, defecation syncope, and cough syncope are probably the next most frequently occurring forms of neurally mediated faints. These latter conditions are often also termed situational faints, since they are associated with specific scenarios (e.g. micturition, coughing, straining at stool) (Table 20.1.1).

Goals

The goals of this part of the chapter are to:
• review the most common forms of neurally mediated reflex syncope and their diagnostic features;
• discuss the laboratory studies used to help establish the diagnosis; and
• provide a brief review of treatment options.

Evaluation
Medical history
The strategy for establishing a diagnosis of one of the neurally mediated reflex syncopes relies heavily on obtaining a thorough medical history. Reports of eyewitnesses are particularly important. The reader is referred to Chapters 7, 8, and 9 for specific recommendations regarding the elements of taking and interpreting the medical history. Most important is documentation of the details of

Table 20.1.1 Situational faints.

Postmicturition syncope
Cough, sneeze syncope
'laugh' syncope
Defecation syncope
Postexercise variant of vasovagal syncope
Swallow syncope
Glossopharyngeal neuralgia
Brass or wind instrument playing
Weightlifting

---

patient activity, circumstances of the event, and symptoms immediately prior to the faint and in the period following recovery.

The vasovagal faint may be triggered by any of a variety of factors. In the case of the classic vasovagal faint these include unpleasant sights, pain, extreme emotion, and prolonged standing. Consequently, circumstances surrounding a faint may lead to suspicion of vasovagal syncope as the cause. However, most informed practitioners have come to realize that the so-called classic features of vasovagal syncope are more often than not either absent or not recollected. Therefore, even a detailed medical history undertaken by an experienced individual may not provide a definitive diagnosis. In such cases additional testing is prudent. In this regard, head-up tilt-table testing is the most important readily available supportive test (see later).

Carotid sinus syndrome is considered to be the second most common form of neurally mediated reflex syncope. Spontaneous carotid sinus syndrome may be defined as syncope which:
• by history seems to occur in close relationship with accidental mechanical manipulation of the neck (and presumably the carotid sinuses); and
• can often be reproduced by carotid sinus massage (the role of neck muscle deafferentation as a contributing cause is also of importance, but that discussion lies beyond the scope of this chapter).

Recognition of spontaneous carotid sinus syndrome relies on obtaining a classic history of syncope associated with neck movement or manipulation. Such a correlation, although definitive in terms of diagnosis, is relatively uncommon and thus spontaneous carotid sinus syndrome accounts for only about 1% of all causes of syncope.

Given the rarity of detecting spontaneous carotid sinus syndrome, one can reasonably assume that the importance of the carotid sinus mechanism as a cause of syncope would be substantially underestimated if only the spontaneous form were deemed to be relevant. Thus, in the clinical evaluation of older syncope patients it is often necessary to rely on the so-called induced carotid sinus syndrome (Figure 20.1.1). This latter diagnosis is more broadly defined, and may be accepted to be present even though a close relationship

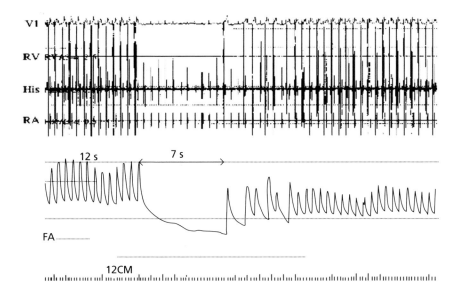

Figure 20.1.1 Prolonged asystolic pause induced by carotid sinus massage in an older patient with multiple abrupt syncope episodes. Note persistence of hyopotension despite resumption of the cardiac rhythm.

between manipulation of the carotid sinus and the occurrence of syncope is not demonstrated. Thus, induced carotid sinus syndrome is diagnosed when patients are found to have an abnormal response to carotid sinus massage (usually an asystolic pause >3–5 s), and an otherwise negative work-up for syncope. Regarded in this way, carotid sinus syndrome is much more frequent being found in 26–60% of patients affected by unexplained syncope. The occurrence of syncope or unexplained 'falls', especially in older persons, should lead to consideration of carotid sinus syndrome.

Situational faints (e.g. postmicturition syncope, cough syncope, etc.) (Figure 20.1.2) are diagnosed primarily by careful history-taking. The 'trigger' events surrounding the faints must be elicited during the patient interview or in discussions with witnesses. Faints during blood drawing, following bladder voiding, inconjunction with a painful experience, or during defecation are among the more common of the situational faints. The clinical overlap of situational and emotion-triggered vasovagal syncope is not surprising and should not cause concern inasmuch as the mechanisms are essentially the same as best we currently understand.

Laboratory studies

To date, the head-up tilt-table test is the only diagnostic tool to have been scrutinized to assess its effectiveness in the diagnosis of vasovagal syncope (see Chapter 14). Such testing, especially when undertaken in the absence of drugs, appears to discriminate well between symptomatic patients and asymptomatic

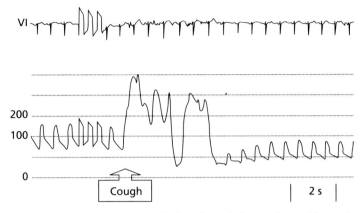

Figure 20.1.2 Hypotensive response to induced cough in a patient with cough syncope.

control subjects. In fact, there is strong evidence to suggest that head-up tilt-table testing at angles of 60–70°, in the absence of pharmacologic provocation, exhibits a specificity of approximately 90%. In the presence of pharmacologic provocation, test specificity may be reduced but nonetheless remains in a range that permits the test to be clinically useful.

Carotid sinus syndrome can also be assessed in the clinical laboratory, although the specificity and sensitivity of the carotid sinus massage procedure has not been rigorously studied. Nevertheless, based on consensus opinion, carotid sinus syndrome may be diagnosed when carotid sinus massage reproduces symptoms in conjunction with a period of asystole (>3–5 s), paroxysmal atrioventricular (AV) block, and/or a marked drop (usually ≥50 mmHg systolic) in systemic arterial pressure (see Chapter 14 for additional methodologic aspects). In many instances, the most convincing results from carotid sinus massage are obtained when massage is undertaken with the patient in the upright position (gently secured to a tilt-table for safety). Continuous arterial pressure and ECG recordings should be obtained throughout. The test is usually contraindicated if a carotid bruit is present or if the patient has symptoms suggestive of transient ischemic attacks.

The situational faints are not readily assessed in the laboratory. Cough syncope may be an exception, but diagnostic criteria for hemodynamic response to induced cough have yet to be determined.

Treatment options

In general, initial 'treatment' of all forms of neurally mediated reflex syncope comprises education regarding avoidance of triggering events (e.g. hot crowded environments, volume depletion, effects of cough, tight collars, etc.), recognition of warning symptoms, and maneuvers to abort the episode (e.g. supine posture, leg crossing, arm-tugging). Additionally, if possible, strategies should address trigger factors directly (e.g. suppressing the cause of cough in cough syncope). Specific thoughts regarding younger patients are found in Chapter 21.

Vasovagal syncope and situational faints

In the vast majority of cases, patients who seek medical advice after having experienced a vasovagal faint require principally reassurance and education regarding the nature of the condition. Patients should be informed that vasovagal syncope is common in humans, and that in most people its occurrence is infrequent with only one or two events in a lifetime. However, certain individuals have greater susceptibility and multiple random recurrences are not uncommon in such cases. In regard to treatment options, most have not been subjected to rigorous study and recommendations are largely based on 'expert consensus' at this time.

Initial advice should include review of the types of environments in which faints are more common (e.g. hot, crowded, emotionally upsetting, etc.), and provide insight into the typical warning symptoms (e.g. hot/cold feeling, sweaty, clammy, nauseated, etc.) that may permit many individuals to recognize an impending episode and avert the faint. Thus, avoiding venipunture may be desirable when possible (e.g. not volunteering for blood donation), but psychologic conditioning may be necessary. Additional common sense measures such as keeping well hydrated and avoiding prolonged exposure to upright posture and/or hot confining environments should also be discussed. With regard to these latter treatment concepts, formal randomized studies are not available.

Patients should be taught that certain physical maneuvers may help abort imminent faints and thereby give them an opportunity to seek a safe posture (i.e. seated or supine) until the risk has passed. In this regard, based on the fact that muscular contractions induce an increase in blood pressure, it has been observed that voluntary contractions of muscles of the legs (such as with 'leg crossing') or arms (i.e. arm-tensing) may be helpful. Of course, the effective application of such counter-maneuvers depends on the presence and recognition of premonitory symptoms. Nevertheless, it has been demonstrated that blood pressure could increase by a value of 30 to 40 mmHg and thus avoid or delay the syncope.

These counter maneuvers could be considered as an adjunct to other treatment strategies.

In recent short-term trials in patients with syncope induced by tilt test, drinking water was shown to prevent a positive outcome on a subsequent tilt test. This observation suggests that it is reasonable to recommend drinking before exercising. Whether conventional tap-water or bottled water are as effective as beverages containing electrolytes (e.g. sport drinks) is currently unknown, but likely the latter would be preferable.

When a more aggressive treatment strategy is needed, 'volume expanders' (e.g. increased dietary salt and electrolyte intake with fluids such as 'sport'

Tilt-training methodology

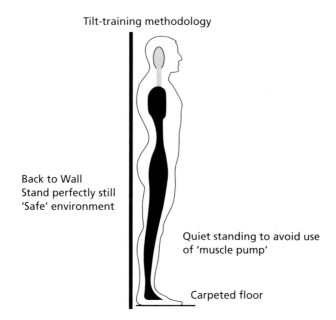

Back to Wall
Stand perfectly still
'Safe' environment

Quiet standing to avoid use
of 'muscle pump'

Carpeted floor

Figure 20.1.3 Schematic illustrating methodology of tilt-training.

drinks or salt tablets) or moderate exercise training appears to be safe and reasonable recommendations. Additionally, in highly motivated patients with recurrent vasovagal symptoms, the prescription of progressively prolonged periods of enforced upright posture (so-called tilt training) may reduce susceptibility to syncope recurrence. Tilt-training has anecdotally proven highly effective if undertaken twice daily for periods of 8–12 weeks, with subsequent maintenance 3–4 times weekly thereafter, However, patient compliance is a clearcut limitation. This technique, devised by Ector and colleagues in Belgium, consists of performing progressively longer periods of stationary upright posture. The patient stands with upper back positioned lightly against a wall or a corner (Figure 20.1.3) without moving their arms or legs. Initially starting at 5 min twice daily, over a period of 6 to 8 weeks the tilt training period is gradually increased to as much as 30 to 40 min twice daily. The physiological objective is to 'train' the nervous system to better tolerate supporting gravitational stress by more efficient vasoconstriction.

Clinical investigations from Kitakyushu in Japan, examined the efficacy of orthostatic tilt training in a group of patients with recurrent syncope and a positive tilt table evaluation. Patients were randomized to treatment with propranolol, the vagolytic antiarrhythmic agent disopyramide or tilt training. On repeat tilt table test, pharmacologic therapy was poor at preventing syncope (only 32% with propranolol and 26% with disopyramide). In contrast, orthostatic tilt-training was highly efficacious and prevented syncope in 92% of patients. Others have also observed excellent results with tilt-training for

30 min once a day, with one report indicating that follow-up tilt table tests were rendered negative in almost 90% of patients.

Some concern has been raised about the long-term efficacy of tilt-training, as patients who become asymptomatic may not remain compliant with the protocol. The longest term follow-up reported for a series of patients assigned to a tilt-training program is 43 months. In that study, 76.3% of the patients had abandoned tilt-training by the time of reevaluation. Despite this, 82% remained free of recurrent syncope.

Many drugs have been used in the treatment of vasovagal syncope (beta-blockers, disopyramide, scopolamine, clonidine, theophilline, fludro-cortisone, ephedrine, etilephrine, midodrine, clonidine, serotonin inhibitors, etc.). While the results have often been satisfactory in uncontrolled trials, placebo-controlled prospective trials have been unable to show a benefit of most of these drugs. For example, the recently reported POST trial showed no benefit of metoprolol over placebo, with the possible exception of some benefit in older subjects. The principal exception is midodrine, a prodrug that is metabolized into a predominantly veno-constrictor agent.

Since failure of appropriate vasoconstriction of peripheral blood vessels is common to all of the neurally mediated reflex faints, vasoconstrictors may be employed. The alpha adrenergic-stimulating agents etilephrine and midodrine have both been studied in a placebo-controlled fashion. Etilephrine was studied as a segment of the randomized placebo-controlled VASIS trial, and proved to be ineffective. On the other hand, studies from Newcastle (United Kingdom) and Cleveland (United States) on short-term outcomes with midodrine in vasovagal syncope have shown a beneficial effect. This drug is generally well tolerated in doses of 2.5 to 10 mg three times daily. The principal adverse effect is scalp tingling and/or 'goose bumps' due to the drug's action on pilo-erector muscles.

Head-up tilt laboratory findings have generally reported that pacing fails to prevent vasovagal syncope, although it may prolong the premonitory warning phase. Nevertheless, unlike most other treatment avenues in this condition, pacing has been the subject of a number of both small single/multiple-center studies and major multicenter randomized controlled trials demonstrating effectiveness in select highly symptomatic patient populations. In this regard, the strongest supportive evidence comes from three randomized controlled trials: the North American vasovagal pacemaker study (VPS1), the European VASIS trial, and the SYDIT report. For example, in the case of the North American trial, the actuarial 1-year rate of recurrent syncope was 18% for pacemaker patients and 60% for controls. The results of the pacing arm of the VASIS trial were similar; 5% of patients in the pacemaker arm experienced recurrence of syncope compared with 61% in the no-pacemaker arm during a mean follow-up of 3.7 years. However, these studies failed to account for the potential 'placebo' effect of pace-maker implantation since unpaced patients did not have a device implanted. In this regard, the VPS2 trial indicated that when both groups (paced and not paced) undergo pacemaker implantation, the pacing benefit appears to be less impressive than had been anticipated, at least during in the first 6 months of follow-up. Whether the latter observation will change with longer follow-up remains to be seen. In any case, the VPS2 observations tend to be supported by findings from the SYNPACE study, in which all patients received pacemakers. Consequently, current opinion tends to down-play the value of implantable pacemakers in vasovagal syncope.

Carotid sinus syndrome

Cardiac pacing appears to be beneficial in carotid sinus syndrome except in the relatively rare exclusively vasodepressor form and is acknowledged to be the treatment of choice when bradycardia has been documented. For the most part, dual-chamber cardiac pacing is preferred. Medical therapy for carotid sinus syndrome has largely been abandoned.

The relationship between carotid sinus syndrome and spontaneous, otherwise unexplained, syncope has been demonstrated by pre/post comparative studies, two controlled trials, and a prospective observational study. Pre/post comparisons were done by analyzing the recurrence rates of syncope in patients treated by pacing in several nonrandomized studies. These studies show fewer recurrences at follow-up. Nonrandomized comparative studies of patients receiving a pacemaker and untreated patients showed syncope recurrence rates to be lower in paced than nonpaced patients. Brignole *et al.* undertook a randomized study in 60 patients; 32 patients were assigned to the pacemaker arm and 28 to the 'no treatment' group. After a mean follow-up of 36 ± 10 months, syncope recurred in 9% of the pacemaker group versus 57% in the untreated patients ($p < 0.0002$). Finally, patients implanted with a pacemaker especially designed to monitor cardiac rhythm to detect asystolic episodes, showed long pauses (>6 s) in 53% after a 2-year follow-up, suggesting that a positive response to carotid massage predicts the occurrence of spontaneous asystolic episodes during follow-up.

As yet, there are no randomized studies examining treatment of carotid sinus syncope in which hypotension is predominantly of vasodepressor origin. Certain therapies used for vasovagal syncope may be expected to be of some benefit; vasoconstrictors and salt are the most likely in this regard, but the development of supine hypertension as a consequence of long-term treatment is a concern.

Situational faints

Treatment of most forms of neurally mediated situational syncope relies heavily on avoiding or ameliorating the trigger event. However, this may be difficult. For example, the 'cough' trigger in cough syncope (for instance due to chronic obstructive pulmonary disease or asthma) is readily recognized, but suppressing it (the ideal treatment) is not easily accomplished. In other cases, avoidance of the 'trigger' may have economic or avocation implications (e.g. syncope associated with blowing a wind instrument). In yet other cases, it is impossible to avoid exposure to the trigger situation (e.g. unpredictable emotional upset or painful stimuli, bowel movement in defecation syncope, bladder emptying in postmicturition syncope).

In conditions where trigger avoidance is not entirely feasible, certain general treatment strategies may be advocated. These include: maintenance of central volume; protected posture (e.g. sitting during micturition rather than standing); slower changes of posture (e.g. waiting after a bowel movement before arising); and recognition of increased risk when getting out of a warm bed (a common predisposing factor in patients with postmicturition and defecation syncope). In specific conditions, certain additional advice may be helpful. Thus, use of stool softeners may help in patients with defecation syncope. Avoidance of excessive fluid intake (especially alcohol) just prior to bed-time may reduce risk in postmicturition syncope. Elimination of excessively cold drinks or large boluses of food may help in 'swallow' syncope patients.

The role of cardiac pacing in situational faints must be considered on a case-by-case basis. As a rule, the value of pacing will likely depend on the relative importance of the cardioinhibitory component of the faint. Anecdotal reports of pacing utility have been published but randomized studies are not available.

Guideline recommendations for treatment

Treatment is usually indicated when syncope or near-syncope:
• is accompanied by severe physical injury or motor vehicle or other accident;
• occurs in a 'high-risk' setting (e.g. commercial vehicle driving, machine operation, flying, window washing, competitive athletics), or may result in substantial economic hardship, such as due to loss of employment or employment opportunity, or restricted lifestyle; or
• is sufficiently severe or frequent as to impair the patient's quality of life to a point, which is unacceptable to the patient.
Treatment may sometimes be justified in patients with recurrent falls, or falls associated with physical injury when clinical aspects suggest the possibility of neurally mediated hypotension bradycardia (especially carotid sinus hypersensitivity) as a cause.

Treatment is not necessary for patients with single (or infrequent) syncopal episode(s) without injury and not in a high-risk setting and/or in which there are no over-riding economic or lifestyle concerns. When pharmacologic or pacemaker treatment is considered, a general prerequisite is to attempt to understand the relative importance of the cardioinhibitory and vasodepressor components of the reflex in causing syncope. To do this, the documentation of a spontaneous episode by means of ECG monitoring (including implantable loop recorder, ILR) or its provocation by means of carotid sinus massage or tilt testing is recommended. The tilt-table may also be used to assess the vasodepressor component, that may not respond to pacing.

Summary

Neurally mediated reflex syncope encompasses a wide variety of clinical scenarios. The vasovagal faint and carotid sinus syndrome are the most commonly encountered of these conditions but the various forms of situational faints are not rare. A detailed medical history is usually sufficient to obtain a diagnosis. Treatment may vary from education and reassurance, to physical maneuvers (e.g. leg crossing, tilt training), and finally drugs. As noted above, pacemaker therapy is of considerable value in most forms of carotid sinus syndrome. However, this does not seem to be the case as a general rule in other types of neurally mediated reflex syncope. If in these latter conditions, pacing intervention appears to be necessary, careful assessment by a consultant experienced in the evaluation of such patients is warranted.

The general physician, if confident of the diagnosis, should feel comfortable initiating the treatment program for most forms of neurally mediated syncope. Speciality referral is needed when the diagnosis is uncertain, or more aggressive therapy (e.g. drugs, devices) is thought to be necessary, or economic issues (e.g. occupation eligibility) become relevant.

Additional reading

Abe H, Kohsi K, Nakashima Y. Home orthostatic self-training in neurocardiogenic syncope. *PACE* 2005; **28**: S246–248.

Almquist A, Goldenberg IF, Milstein S *et al*. Provocation of bradycardia and hypotension by isoproterenol and upright posture in patients with unexplained syncope *N Engl J Med* 1989; **320**: 346–351.

Brignole M, Menozzi C, Gianfranchi L *et al*. A controlled trial of acute and long-term medical therapy in tilt-induced neurally mediated syncope. *Am J Cardiol* 1992; **70**: 339–342.

Connolly SJ, Sheldon R, Roberts RS, Gent M, Vasovagal pacemaker study investigators. The North American vasovagal pacemaker study (VPS): A randomized trial of permanent cardiac pacing for the prevention of vasovagal syncope. *J Am Coll Cardiol* 1999; **33**: 16–20.

Ector H, Reybrouck T, Heidbuchel H, Gewillig M, Van de Werf F. Tilt training: a new treatment for recurrent neurocardiogenic syncope or severe orthostatic intolerance. *PACE* 1998; **21**: 193–196.

Healey J. Connolly SJ. Morillo CA. The management of patients with carotid sinus syndrome: is pacing the answer? *Clin. Autonomic Research.* 2004; **14**: 80–86.

Kenny RA, Ingram A, Bayliss J, Sutton R. Head-up tilt: a useful test for investigating unexplained syncope. *Lancet* 1986; **1**: 1352–1355.

Kerdiet CTP, van Dijk N, Linzer M, van Lieshout JJ, Wieling W. Management of vasovagal syncope: controlling or aborting faints by leg crossing and muscle tensing. *Circulation* 2002; **106**: 1684–1689.

Melby DP. Cytron JA. Benditt DG. New approaches to the treatment and prevention of neurally mediated reflex (neurocardiogenic) syncope. *Current Cardiology Reports.* 2004; **6**: 385–390.

Moore A. Watts M. Sheehy T. Hartnett A. Clinch D. Lyons D. Treatment of vasodepressor carotid sinus syndrome with midodrine: a randomized, controlled pilot study. *J. Am. Geriatrics Society.* 2005; **53**: 114–118.

Numata T, Abe H, Nagatomo T, Sonoda S, Kohshik, Nakashima Y. Successful treatment of malignant neurocardiogenic syncope with repeated tilt training program. *Japanese Circulation J* 2000; **64**: 406–409.

Reybrouck T, Heidbuchel H, Van De Werf F, Ector H. Long-term follow-up results of tilt training therapy in patients with recurrent neurocardiogenic syncope. *PACE* 2002; **25**: 1441–1446.

Sutton R, Brignole M, Menozzi C *et al.* Dual-chamber pacing is efficacious in treatment of neurally mediated tilt-positive cardioinhibitory syncope. Pacemaker versus no therapy: a multicentre randomized study. *Circulation* 2000; **102**: 294–299.

Wieling W. Colman N. Krediet CT. Freeman R. Nonpharmacological treatment of reflex syncope. *Clin. Autonomic Research.* 2004; **14**: 62–70.

Wieling W, Van Lieshout JJ, Van Leeuwen AM. Physical maneuvers that reduce postural hypotension in autonomic failure. *Clin Autonom Res* 1993; **3**: 57–65.

CHAPTER 20

Specific causes of syncope: their evaluation and treatment strategies

Part 2: Orthostatic syncope

Angel Moya and Wouter Wieling

Introduction

Orthostatic faints are those associated with movement from a more gravitationally neutral position (e.g. supine position) to one in which gravitation tends to further diminish cerebral blood flow (e.g. upright posture). Thus, the orthostatic faint is most readily identified by a careful medical history in which the association with postural change is documented (i.e. syncope occurring shortly after moving from a lying or sitting to a standing position).

Although even healthy individuals may experience a tendency to orthostatic hypotensive symptoms when they stand up (e.g. transient 'gray' out or 'blackout'), the groups most susceptible to orthostatic syncope are:
• older frail individuals,
• patients with other underlying medical problems (e.g. diabetes, alcoholic neuropathy),
• persons who are dehydrated from hot environments, diuretics, or inadequate fluid intake,
• individuals taking certain commonly prescribed medications such as diuretics, antidepressants, and antipsychotics, vasodilators like nitroglycerin and alpha-adrenergic blockers, and beta-adrenergic blockers.

Goals

The goals of this chapter are to review:
• pathophysiology of orthostatic syncope;
• clinical features;
• approach to diagnosis;
• treatment options for orthostatic hypotension and syncope.

Pathophysiology of orthostatic hypotension
Patients with orthostatic hypotension have an inability to maintain arterial blood pressure when standing up (Figure 20.2.1). As a result, a significant and

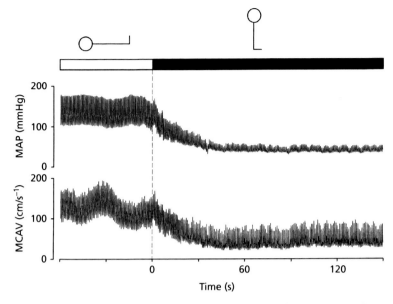

Figure 20.2.1 Changes in blood pressure and cerebral blood flow in the middle cerebral artery in a 54 year old patient with pure autonomic failure (Reproduced after Harms MP, Colier WN, Wieling W, *Stroke* 2000; **31**: 1608–1614 with permission of the editor).

persistent decrease in systemic pressure may occur leading to characteristic features as a result of retinal and/or cerebral ischemia, including:

• visual disturbances ('gray out' or 'blackout'),
• lightheadedness, or 'dizziness',
• loss of consciousness (i.e. orthostatic syncope).

Symptoms resulting from impaired perfusion of muscle tissue causing symptoms such as pain in the neck region ('coat-hanger' distribution), lumbar pain, and angina pectoris may also occur. Typically symptoms develop on standing and resolve on lying down.

A mismatch between intravascular volume and required cardiac output upon standing is a common cause of orthostatic hypotension (Table 20.2.1). In a minority of cases, however, orthostatic hypotension results not from volume depletion but from impairment of autonomic reflex responses required for maintaining blood pressure in the upright position. In essence, orthostatic hypotension, especially early after movement to the upright posture, may be caused by one or more of the following:

• impaired capacity of sympathetic nerves to increase vascular resistance due to primary nervous system disease, or secondary to other diseases that can affect autonomic nervous system or the effect of certain drugs or toxins (Table 20.2.1),
• relative volume depletion,

Table 20.2.1 Classification of orthostatic hypotension.

Volume depletion
hemorrhage
diarrhea
salt-losing nephropathy
Addison's disease
diuretics
Autonomic failure
primary autonomic failure syndromes (e.g. pure autonomic failure, multiple system atrophy, Parkinson's disease with autonomic failure, acute pandysautonomia)
Secondary autonomic failure syndromes (diabetic neuropathy, amyloid neuropathy, chronic renal failure, alcohol, spinal cord transection, brain tumors)
Drugs (other than diuretics)
sympatholytic medications (alpha-blockers, antidepressants)
beta-adrenergic blockers

• downward pooling of venous blood and a consequent reduction in stroke volume and cardiac output,
• conditions that affect arterial baroreflex control of sympathetic activation of resistance vessels; for example, in patients with deafferentation of carotid sinus baroreceptors after neck surgery (impairment of afferent pathways) and in subjects receiving clonidine (blockade of central pathways),
• impaired diastolic relaxation, especially of the aged or hypertrophied heart, causing failure to generate an adequate stroke volume when preload is reduced during movement to upright posture.

Diagnosis

In elderly nonvolume depleted patients, in whom central or peripheral autonomic nervous system diseases have been excluded, the prevalence of orthostatic hypotension is about 9% over the age of 80 and about 12% over the age of 85. It is a significant independent predictor of all-cause mortality.

Orthostatic syncope can be diagnosed when there is documentation of orthostatic hypotension associated with syncope or presyncope. Carefully measuring blood pressure with a sphygmomanometer with the patient supine and again after standing suffices for the routine assessment of orthostatic blood pressure control in the office or at the bedside. However, for purposes of establishing the diagnosis of 'orthostatic hypotension', arterial blood pressure must be measured when the patient adopts the standing position after 5 min of lying supine. Orthostatic hypotension is defined as a decline in systolic blood pressure of at least 20 mmHg, and/or a diastolic fall of 10 mmHg within 3 min standing, regardless of whether or not symptoms occur. If the patient does not tolerate standing for this period, the lowest systolic blood pressure during the upright position should be recorded. Measurements should be continued after 3 min of standing if blood pressure is still falling at 3 min.

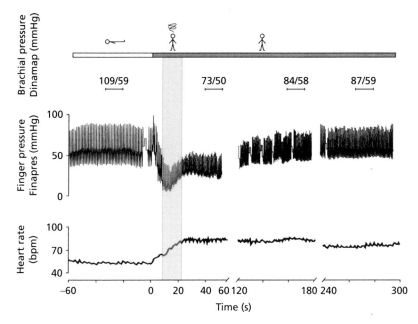

Figure 20.2.2 Tracing obtained in a patient with recurrent unexplained syncope upon standing. Continuous monitoring of finger blood pressure documented an abnormally large transient initial fall in pressure. A combination of medications known to impair orthostatic blood pressure control was responsible for the abnormality (Revised after Wieling W, Harms MPM, Kortz RAM, Linzer M. *Clin Autonom Res* 2001; **11**: 269–270 with permission of the editor).

Initial (i.e. immediately after postural change) orthostatic hypotension is difficult to assess with conventional measurement of blood pressure using a cuff and stethoscope as the blood pressure changes occur very rapidly at this time (Figure 20.2.2). Continuous noninvasive blood pressure measurement (e.g. by Portapres) upon standing is needed to document this abnormality. Of course, in most cases a carefully documented medical history will strongly suggest that this condition is likely to be present.

There are some patients with syncope in whom there is a history suggestive of impaired orthostatic blood pressure control, but in whom measurements in upright position may be normal. In these patients additional tests after major provocative stimuli (e.g. food ingestion, exercise) may be needed to unmask the abnormality. An alternative approach is use of a 24-h or longer ambulatory blood pressure recording during daily living circumstances. These devices offer the potential to capture spontaneous events but are often ineffective unless beat-to-beat blood pressure is obtained.

Establishing the specific underlying 'causative' diagnosis is of particular importance for patients with orthostatic hypotension. First, it is important to identify nonneurogenic potentially reversible causes of orthostatic hypotension such as volume depletion, adrenal insufficiency (not common), and the effect of medications (very common). Second, if there is evidence for a neurological cause, it is important that the patient be appropriately informed of its nature and prognosis.

The most frequent drugs associated with orthostatic syncope are vasodilators and diuretics. Alcohol can also be associated with orthostatic syncope, not only causing orthostatic intolerance but also because it can induce autonomic and somatic neuropathy (see Chapter 17). Elimination of the responsible drug or offending agent usually is enough to improve symptoms. However, reversible causes often coexist with neurogenic mechanisms and this complexity must be appreciated for optimal treatment.

Treatment
The most substantial experience with treatment of orthostatic hypotension has been obtained in patients with chronic primary autonomic failure. These individuals have a relatively consistent failure of circulatory control and consequently experience severe symptomatic orthostatic hypotension. As a result, it has been possible to obtain valuable information about the pathophysiology of abnormalities of orthostatic blood pressure regulation and its treatment.

General measures
The initial treatment (Table 20.2.2) in patients with orthostatic syncope includes advice and education about factors that can aggravate or provoke hypotension upon assuming the upright posture. These factors include avoiding sudden head-up postural change (especially on waking in the morning), standing still for a prolonged period of time, and straining during micturition and defecation. Other less common yet important considerations are high environmental temperature (including hot baths, showers, and saunas) that might lead to dehydration, large meals (especially with refined carbohydrates), and severe exertion. In addition, male patients with symptomatic orthostatic hypotension should also be advised to empty their bladders in a sitting position.

Iatrogenic factors are critically important in many orthostatic syncope patients. The patients are often older individuals who are being treated for a number of commonly occurring comorbidities such as hypertension, coronary artery disease, and benign prostatic hyperplasia. As a result, they may be prescribed drugs such as diuretics, vasodilators, and beta-adrenergic and alpha-adrenergic blockers. Each of these can aggravate any predisposition to hypotension upon standing and in some instances (e.g. excessive diuresis) may induce orthostatic symptoms.

Some patients with autonomic failure exhibit postprandial hypotension. In these patients, symptoms typically begin about 30 min after food ingestion and can last, even while supine, for several hours. Carbohydrate load appears to be a particular problem. Alcohol can exert an additional effect by causing splanchnic vasodilatation. Consequently, advice should include the recommendation that affected patients eat frequent smaller meals with reduced carbohydrate content and avoid alcohol.

Table 20.2.2 General treatment principles and recommendations.

To be avoided
• Sudden head-up postural change (especially on waking)
• Standing still
• Prolonged recumbence during daytime
• Straining during micturition and defecation, hyperventilation
• High environmental temperature (including hot baths and showers)
• Severe exertion
• Large meals (especially with refined carbohydrate)
• Alcohol
• Drugs with vasodepressor properties
• Diet and cold preparations containing sympathomimetic amines

To be introduced
• Salt intake of at least 8 g (150 mmol) a day
• 2–2.5 L fluid/day
• Small frequent meals with a reduced carbohydrate content
• Head-up sleeping ($\geq$ 25 cm head-up elevation)
• Judicious exercise (including swimming)
• Physical counter-maneuvers
• Air-conditioning or fan in summer

To be considered
• Abdominal binders
• Elastic stockings
• Support garment
• Portable chairs
• Impedance threshold device (ITD)

Pharmacological treatment
• Fludrocortisone
• Sympathomimetics: midodrine
• Specific targeting: desmopressin, erythropoietin, octreotide

---

Patients with orthostatic hypotension should be encouraged to have a high dietary salt intake if there are no contraindications (e.g. concomitant hypertension, or heart failure). At least 8 g of salt a day is advised, with liberal use of salt at mealtimes, by eating foods with a high salt content, or even with the use of salt tablets. Additionally, patients should drink 2 to 2.5 L of fluids every day, focusing when possible on electrolyte containing beverages. Elderly patients may have a decreased sense of thirst and may need to be encouraged to increase fluid intake. This latter point is particularly important as many older individuals tend to avoid fluids to prevent urinary frequency or incontinence.

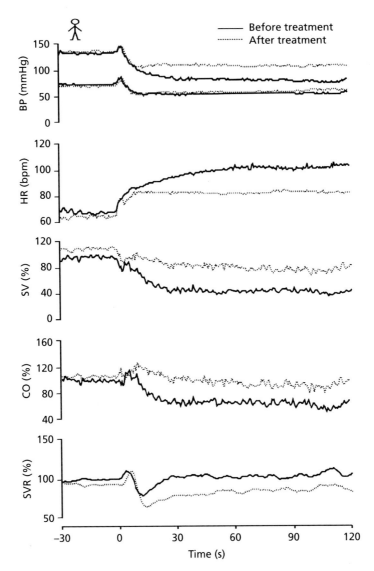

Figure 20.2.3 Average heart rate, systolic and diastolic pressure, stroke volume, cardiac output and systemic vascular resistance responses to standing in 6 patients with autonomic failure before (continuous line) and after (dotted line) treatment with head-up sleeping, high salt diet and fludrocortisone medication. Blood pressure was measured with a Finapres device. Relative changes in stroke volume were computed by arterial pulse wave analysis (From Ten Harkel AD, Van Lieshout JJ, Wieling W. *J Int Med* 1992; **232**: 139–145 with permission of the editor).

Volume expansion can improve orthostatic tolerance markedly, with relatively small increases in arterial pressure (Figure 20. 2. 3). This discrepancy between symptoms and the level of blood pressure can be explained by the fact that treatment shifts mean arterial pressure from just below to just above the critical level of perfusion of the brain.

Nonpharmacological treatment strategies

In patients with orthostatic hypotension in whom, despite the general measures discussed above, orthostatic symptoms persist, several nonpharmacological strategies can be applied.

Head-up sleeping at night

There is evidence that in patients with autonomic failure, sleeping with the head somewhat elevated increases the extracellular fluid volume and improves orthostatic tolerance. Two possible mechanisms accounting for the effectiveness of this intervention have been suggested:

• Head-up tilt reduces renal arterial pressures and promotes renin release with consequent angiotensin II formation and aldosterone release. The result is increased extracellular fluid and circulating blood volume.

• sleeping with the upper part of the body and head tilted upward ('head-up sleeping') increases extracellular fluid volume in the lower extremities. This may result in an increased tissue pressure that prevents venous pooling. The fact that head-up sleeping became effective coincidentally with the appearance of slight edema in lower limbs supports this hypothesis.

Effective head-up tilt sleeping can be achieved by elevating the head of the bed about 20–25 cm. To avoid sliding down while sleeping, a hard pillow under the mattress at the level of the buttocks can be used.

Physical counter-maneuvers

In most patients with orthostatic intolerance, immobility can worsen symptoms whereas bending forward, sitting, or moving around can improve them. Based on these observations, several physical maneuvers that reduce venous pooling have been described (Figure 20.2.4). The changes in blood pressure induced by these maneuvers can immediately be demonstrated to a patient by showing the finger blood pressure tracing from a Finapres or similar device on a video monitor screen. Patients can thereby be trained to apply the maneuvers effectively.

Patients are advised to apply the physical maneuvers described below as soon as symptoms begin. Unfortunately, however, for patients with severe motor disabilities, balance problems, or excessive frailty, it may prove impossible to use counter-maneuvers effectively.

Leg crossing. Crossing one leg over the other at thigh level while standing or sitting is an effective and easy maneuver that increases blood pressure. The beneficial effects of leg crossing have been attributed to mechanical compression of the venous vascular beds in the legs, buttocks and abdomen.

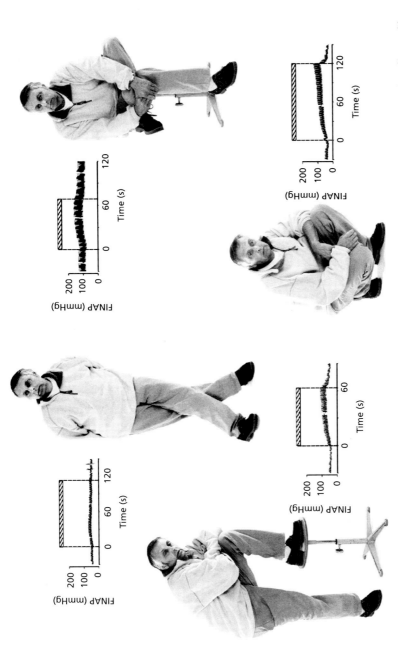

Figure 20.2.4 Physical counter-maneuvers using isometric contractions of the lower limbs and abdominal compression. The effects of leg crossing in standing and sitting position, placing a foot on a chair and squatting on finger arterial blood pressure (FINAP) in a 54 year old male patient with pure autonomic failure and invalidating orthostatic hypotension (same patient as Figure 20.2.1). The patient was standing (sitting) quietly prior to the maneuvers. Bars indicate the duration of the maneuvers. Note the increase in blood pressure and pulse pressure during the maneuvers. (Unpublished from Harms MPM and Wieling W with permission of the patient).

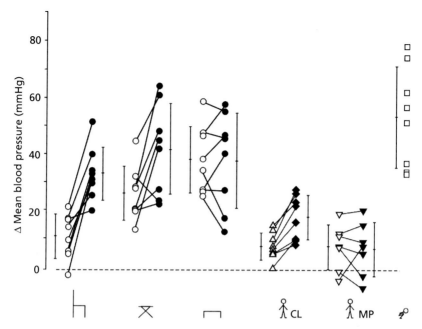

Figure 20.2.5 Effect of sitting, crossing legs, muscle pumping, and squatting to improve orthostatic hypotension in autonomic failure. Mean finger arterial blood pressures are expressed as the blood pressure change during the intervention from the premaneuvre standing blood pressure. From left to right; sitting on a derby chair (height 48 cm), a fishing stool (height 38 cm), and a foot stool (height 20 cm), without (○) and with crossed legs (●); standing in crossed-legs position (CL) without (△) and with (◆) contraction of lower extremity musculature; standing while muscle pumping (MP), marching on the spot (△) and toe-raising (▲); and squatting (□). The vertical line represents mean and standard deviation. (Revised after Smit AAJ, Halliwill JR, Low PA, Wieling W. *J Physiol* 1999; **519**: 1–10 with permission of the editor.)

Leg-crossing has the advantage that it can be performed casually without much effort and without drawing attention to the patient's problem. Muscle tensing during leg-crossing increases the beneficial effect of this counter-maneuver on blood pressure considerably (Figure 20.2.5). Patients may need to 'casually' support themselves by leaning on a wall or piece of furniture in order to accomplish this maneuver safely.

Squatting. This is a highly effective maneuver that increases venous return rapidly and produces an important increase in systolic and diastolic arterial blood pressure (Figure 20.2.5). It can be used as an emergency maneuver to prevent loss of consciousness when presyncopal symptoms develop rapidly. Bending over, as to tie one's shoes, has similar effects and may be simpler to perform by elderly patients. In addition, sitting in the knee-chest position and placing one foot on a chair while standing are comparable with squatting.

When arising from the squatting position muscle tensing should be advised in order to prevent reoccurrence of hypotension.

Bending forward. Lowering the head between the knees is a useful maneuver in fainting patients with autonomic failure. Lowering the head to the heart level is also a rapid way to enhance cerebral perfusion by decreasing the hydrostatic column between the heart and brain.

Skeletal muscle pumping. Maneuvers that use skeletal muscle pumping, such as toe-raising or repeated knee flexion, have less reproducible effects in patients with autonomic failure, and as a consequence are clinically less effective (Figure 20.2.5 far right).

Additional measures. Other measures that decrease dependent pooling that can be used in patients with orthostatic hypotension includes the use of portable folding chairs (Figure 20.2.5) and various types of antigravity pressure garments. Unfortunately, the latter tend to be uncomfortable, hot, and difficult to put on (especially for frail patients).

Pressor response to water drinking
Ingestion of a substantial amount of water is an intervention that is reported to be effective in combating orthostatic intolerance in patients with autonomic failure. After rapid drinking of about half a liter of water an increase in blood pressure is apparent within several minutes. The maximum effect (20–30 mmHg increase of seated and standing systolic blood pressure) is reached after approximately 30 min and the effects are sustained for about 1 h (Figure 20.2.6).

For patients with autonomic failure, water ingestion is also effective to combat postprandial hypotension. Drinking of water also increases blood pressure substantially in healthy elderly but not in healthy young subjects or patients with Parkinson's disease. The mechanisms underlying the rapid pressor response elicited by water drinking is debated. Sympathetic activation resulting in increased vasoconstrictor tone has been reported. Others have emphasized that the time course of the blood pressure response is unusually slow for sympathetic activation. These authors have suggested that minor elevations of intra- and extravascular fluid volume might be involved in patients with autonomic failure, who are extremely sensitive to changes in fluid balance. The afferent signal that activates the sympathetic system through water drinking remains to be fully elucidated.

Impedance threshold device
Improvement in cardiac output and blood pressure can be achieved by enhancing venous return by use of an impedance threshold device (ITD). This device, which the patient breaths through for 30–40 s before standing, provides some resistance to inspiratory effort but not to expiration. Thus, the patient is forced to develop greater negative intrathoracic pressure during

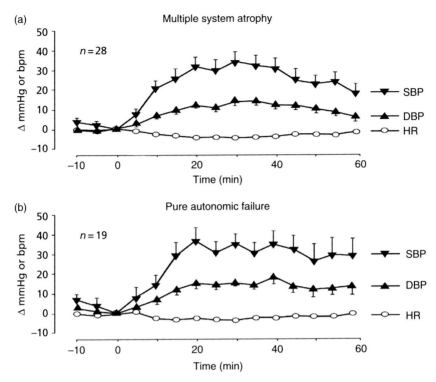

Figure 20.2.6 Changes in systolic blood pressure (SBP), diastolic blood pressure (DBP), and heart rate (HR) induced by drinking of 480 mL of tap water in patients with multiple system atrophy [(a) upper panel] and pure autonomic failure [(b) lower panel]. Patients started drinking at 0 min. The blood pressure increase was evident within 5 min of drinking water, reached a maximum after approximately 20–30 min, and was sustained for more than 60 min (From Jordan J, Shannon JR, Black BK, *et al. Circulation* 2000; **101**: 504–509).

inspiration than is usually the case. The greater negative pressure 'sucks' more venous blood from the periphery to the central circulation and increases cardiac output (Figure 20.2.7). The ITD is available in Europe and North America (Advanced Circulatory Systems Inc., Eden Prairie, MN), and has been mainly used for improving circulatory support during cardiopulmonary resuscitation (CPR). Its value in orthostatic hypotension has only very recently been the subject of clinical study but appears to be promising.

Pharmacological treatment
When nonpharmacological treatments are not effective and symptoms persist, drugs are indicated. The most important of these drugs are:

Fludrocortisone. Fludrocortisone for some time has been the drug of first choice in treatment of patients with orthostatic symptoms due to autonomic failure. It is a potent synthetic mineralocorticoid with minimal glucocorticoid effect.

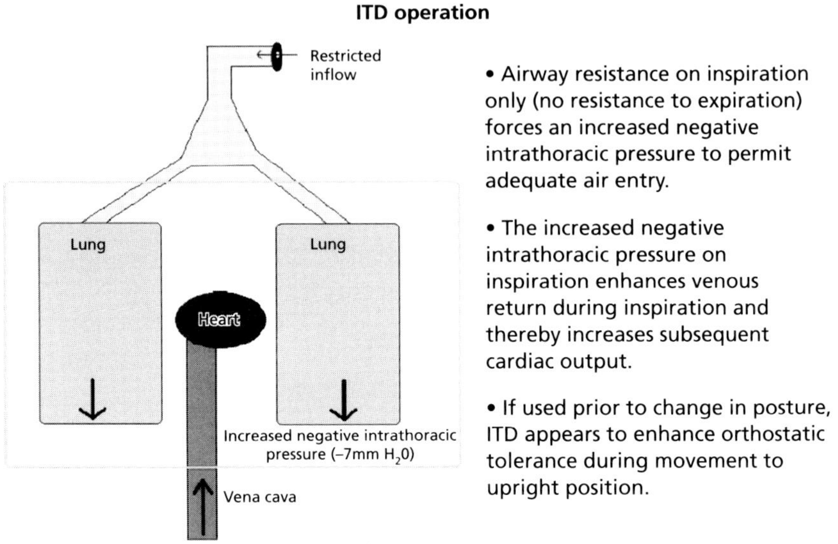
ITD operation
Restricted inflow
Lung
Lung
Heart
Increased negative intrathoracic pressure (–7mm H_2O)
Vena cava
• Airway resistance on inspiration only (no resistance to expiration) forces an increased negative intrathoracic pressure to permit adequate air entry.
• The increased negative intrathoracic pressure on inspiration enhances venous return during inspiration and thereby increases subsequent cardiac output.
• If used prior to change in posture, ITD appears to enhance orthostatic tolerance during movement to upright position.

Figure 20.2.7 Schematic illustrating the mechanism of action of the ITD.

It has several potentially beneficial pharmacological effects for patients with autonomic failure like:
- expansion of intravascular and extravascular body fluid,
- sensitization of vascular receptors to pressor amines, and
- an increase in fluid content of vessel walls that makes them more resistant to stretching.

Usually fludrocortisone treatment is begun with a dose of 0.1 mg once a day. It can be increased by 0.1 mg at 1–2 weeks intervals up to 0.3 mg daily, if needed. The pressor action is not immediate and takes some days to be manifest. The full benefit requires a high dietary salt intake. A weight gain of 2–3 kg is reasonably good clue for adequate volume expansion.

Side-effects of fludrocortisone are primarily accounted for by its expected pharmacological action. Mild dependent edema can be expected. Patients on fludrocortisone may develop hypokalemia within 2 weeks, and foods high in potassium such as fruits, vegetables, poultry, fish, and meat should be advised. Occasionally potassium supplements may be needed. Headaches are other possible side effect of fludrocortisone. Cataracts have also been reported.

Midodrine. Midodrine is a prodrug that is converted to its active metabolite desglymidodrine after absorption. It acts on α-adrenoreceptors to cause constriction of both arterial resistance and venous capacitance vessels, with the predominant effect being on the venous side. It does not cross the blood-brain barrier and consequently it has little in the way of undesirable central stimulant effects.

Midodrine is administered in doses of 2.5–10 mg, three times daily. Supine hypertension is a common but not often serious side-effect. Scalp tingling is a very frequent effect. Midodrine may be of particular value in patients with severe postural hypotension and in those with peripheral neurological lesions, as in pure autonomic failure. For unclear reasons, some patients on midodrine get worse. In such patients, there may be a reduction in intra- and extravascular fluid volume as manifested by weight loss. Midodrine may also aggravate urinary retention.

Others. If the combination of fludrocortisone and sympathetic vasoconstrictor drugs does not produce the desired effect, selective targeting is then needed depending on the pathophysiological abnormalities These patient needs to be referred to a specialized unit with experience in interventions such as:
• desmopressin may be of value in patients with nocturnal polyuria,
• octeoride may benefit patients with postprandial hypotension, and
• erythropoietin.

Summary

Orthostatic hypotension is a common phenomenon as individuals move from a gravitationally neutral position to one in which they become more dependent upon vascular compensatory mechanisms to prevent hypotension and cerebral hypoperfusion. If a significant fall of systemic of pressure occurs, orthostatic hypotension can lead to orthostatic syncope. The key factors affecting susceptibility to these types of faint include prescribed drugs, older age, dehydration, and inadequate nervous system responsiveness (e.g. peripheral neuropathy). Treatment may be difficult, and relies on education, salt/volume replacement, physical maneuvers, and drugs.

Additional reading

Claydon VE, Hainsworth R. Salt supplementation improves orthostatic cerebral and peripheral vascular control in patients with syncope. *Hypertension.* 2004; **43**: 809–813.

Melby DP, Cytron JA, Benditt DG. New approaches to the treatment and prevention of neurally mediated reflex (neurocardiogenic) syncope. *Current Cardiol Rep* 2004; **6**: 385–390.

Omboni S, Smit AA, van Lieshout JJ, Settels JJ, Langewouters GJ, Wieling W. Mechanisms underlying the impairment in orthostatic intolerance after nocturnal recumbency in patients with autonomic failure. *Clin Sci* 2001; **101**: 609–618.

Schatz IJ. Orthostatic hypotension predicts mortality. Lessons from the Honolulu heart program. *Clin Auton Res* 2002; **12**: 223–224.

Smit AAJ, Halliwill JR, Low PA, Wieling W. Topical Review. Pathophysiological basis of orthostatic hypotension in autonomic failure. *J Physiol* 1999; **519**: 1–10.

van Dijk N, de Bruin IG, Gisolf J *et al.* Hemodynamic effects of leg crossing and skeletal muscle tensing during free standing in patients with vasovagal syncope. *J Applied Physiol* 2005; **98**: 584–590.

Wieling W, Harms MPM, Kortz RAM, Linzer M. Initial orthostatic hypotension as a cause of recurrent syncope: a case report. *Clin Auton Res* 2001; **11**: 269–270.

Wieling W, van Lieshout JJ, Hainsworth R. Extracellular fluid volume expansion in patients with posturally related syncope. *Clin Auton Res* 2002; **12**: 243–249.

Wieling W, van Lieshout JJ, van Leeuwen AM. Physical manoeuvres that reduce postural hypotension in autonomic failure. *Clin Auton Res* 1993; **3**: 57–65.

CHAPTER 20

Specific causes of syncope: their evaluation and treatment strategies

Part 3: Cardiac arrhythmias and conduction system disease as a primary cause of syncope

Angel Moya

Introduction

Cardiac arrhythmias are an important cause of syncope. In some cases, the arrhythmia may be secondary to other conditions, such as in the case of brady-arrhythmias associated with the various forms of neurally mediated reflex syncope (e.g. vasovagal syncope, see Chapter 20, Part 1). These secondary circumstances are dealt with elsewhere in this volume. This section is devoted to those circumstances in which cardiac arrhythmias are thought to be the primary cause of symptoms. It details the most common rhythm disturbances to keep in mind when considering arrhythmia as the potential cause of syncope in an individual patient. The role of electrophysiologic study (EPS) is alluded to as part of this discussion (Table 20.3.1), but the reader is also referred to Chapter 15 for a more a detailed analysis of the value and limitations of EPS in syncope evaluation.

Goals

The goals of this part of the chapter are to:
• review the most common forms of syncope in which cardiac arrhythmias are the primary cause;
• provide an approach to establishing the specific diagnosis; and
• summarize clinical features of certain important but less frequent 'arrhythmogenic' syndromes that are known to be associated with syncope.

Bradyarrhythmias

Bradyarrhythmias causing syncope encompass both sustained slow heart rates that may diminish both cardiac output and cerebral blood flow sufficiently to

Table 20.3.1 Minimal recommended EPS protocol for assessment of syncope.

- Measurement of sinus node recovery time (SNRT) and calculation of corrected SNRT by repeated sequences of atrial pacing for 30–60 s each.
- Assessment of AV node and His-Purkinje conduction (including HV interval measurement) at baseline sinus cycle length and during atrial pacing at progressively faster rates until AV Wenkebach conduction is achieved. If these studies are inconclusive, and AV conduction disease remains suspected, the study should be repeated after infusion of antiarrhythmic drug unless contraindicated (ajmaline 1 mg/kg iv. or procainamide 10 mg/kg iv).
- Assessment of susceptibility to inducible supraventricular tachycardias by atrial extrastimulus testing (adding atropine and/or isoproterenol if necessary).
- Assessment of susceptibility to ventricular tachyarrhythmias by ventricular extrastimulus testing at two RV sites, with two basic pacing frequencies, and employing up to two extrastimuli with progressively decreasing coupling intervals until ventricular refractoriness is achieved or the shortest coupling interval is 200 ms.*

---

* A third extrastimulus may be added to increase sensitivity and occasionally infusion of isoproterenol is warranted. The latter is particularly warranted when attempting to reproduce a tachycardia previously documented to have occurred spontaneously.

cause syncope, as well as pauses in the cardiac rhythm during which cardiac output transiently stops and the brain is without nutrient flow for that period of time. Bradycardias may occur secondarily to autonomic or drug-induced effects, or primarily due to underlying disturbances of cardiac pacemaker or cardiac conduction system function. Neurally mediated reflex bradycardias are discussed in Chapter 20, Part 1. The primary bradyarrhythmic causes of syncope discussed in this chapter are principally those due to sinus node disease and/or AV conduction disease.

Sinus node dysfunction

Sinus node dysfunction (SND) is characterized by any of several types of rhythm disturbances, including sinus or junctional bradycardia, sinus pauses, and episodes of supraventricular tachyarrhythmia (most commonly paroxysmal atrial fibrillation but also other primary atrial tachycardias). Syncope can be caused by severe bradycardia (e.g. sinus pauses or sinus arrest) or may be associated with tachycardia. In the latter case, the faint may occur at the beginning of the paroxysm of atrial fibrillation (before blood vessels have had a chance to constrict adequately). Alternatively, it is not uncommon for syncope to be due to a long asystolic pause occurring at the end of an episode of atrial fibrillation (before the sinus pacemaker has an opportunity to resume at a relatively normal rate) (Figure 20.3.1).

In patients with syncope of unknown origin, SND can be suspected in the presence of severe sinus bradycardia (heart rates persistently <40–50 bpm), long asystolic pauses due to sinus arrest, or episodes of sinoatrial block

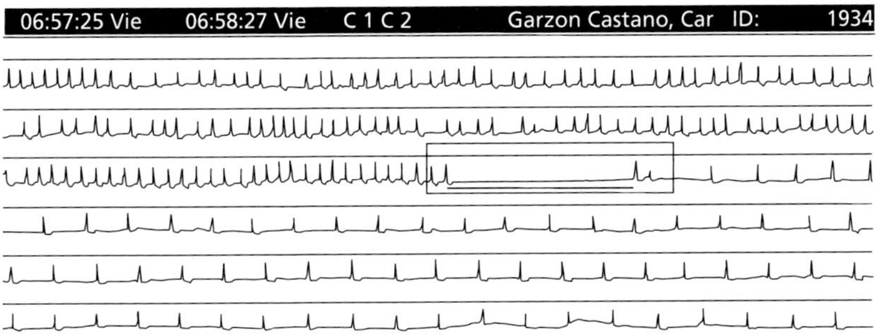

| 06:57:25 Vie | 06:58:27 Vie | C 1 C 2 | Garzon Castano, Car ID: | 1934 |

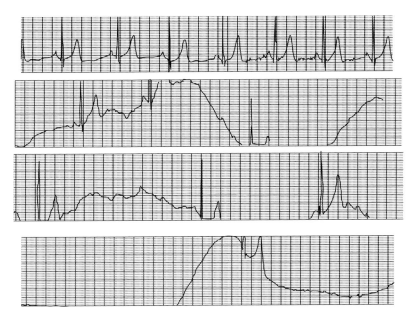

Figure 20.3.1 Holter recording from a patient with syncopal episodes and sinus node dysfunction. Recording shows a period of atrial fibrillation with a rapid ventricular response that terminates abruptly. A 6-s asystolic pause was recorded before a regular rhythm resumes at approximately 50 bpm.

Figure 20.3.2 ECG monitor recording illustrating evolution of sinus bradycardia into sinus pause in a patient with syncope and suspected SND.

(Figure 20.3.2). The role of electrophysiologic testing for the diagnosis of SND as a cause of syncope is limited. The tests used to evaluate the function of sinus node (sinus node recovery time [SNRT] and sinoatrial conduction time [SACT]) exhibit good specificity, but they are relatively insensitive and may miss many affected individuals. Furthermore, with the possible exception of a very prolonged corrected sinus node recovery time (CSNRT), they do not provide direction regarding the appropriate treatment strategy for the patient.

The diagnosis of SND as the cause of syncope is best established when a clear correlation of symptoms with arrhythmia (usually bradycardia) is documented. In the absence of such correlation, severe sinus bradycardia <40 bpm, repetitive sinoatrial block, or sinus pauses >3 s in duration are highly suggestive of symptomatic SND. Ambulatory ECG 'event' recorders or implanted loop recorders (ILRs) have the best chance of making the diagnosis by virtue of their long recording periods. In particular, newer generation 'event' recorders and mobile cardiac outpatient telemetry (MCOT) (see Chapter 12), have the capability of automatic activation in the presence of a serious rhythm disturbance.

In patients with SND and syncope due to bradyarrhythmia, pacemaker implantation improves symptoms. In these patients, physiologic pacing (atrial or dual chamber) is generally considered to be superior to single chamber ventricular (VVI or VVIR) pacing especially if the patient is likely to be pacing frequently. Further, since many of these patients also exhibit inappropriate chronotropic response (i.e. so-called chronotropic incompetence), the use of rate-adaptive pacing is recommended.

In patients with paroxysmal atrial tachycardias associated with SND, anti-arrhythmic drug therapy or even mapping and transcatheter ablation may be needed. In such cases, however, if drugs are chosen, unsuspected susceptibility to bradycardia may be provoked by drug administration. Once again, assuming alternative drugs or ablation are not available, pacing may be a necessary element of therapy.

Atrioventricular conduction disorders

Chronic or paroxysmal atrioventricular (AV) block can be the cause of syncopal episodes. AV block may be a congenital or an acquired disease. As suggested by the ISSUE study results, paroxysmal AV block is not infrequently the cause of 'syncope of unknown origin' in older patients. Establishing the diagnosis may be difficult and use of implantable (insertable) loop recorder, ILR recorders, may be essential to confirm clinical suspicions.

Patients with congenital AV block can be symptomatic early in life or may remain asymptomatic for a long period of time. Previously, congenital AV block was considered a relatively benign condition. This is no longer the case. Follow-up studies have demonstrated that such patients, especially if they have suffered syncope, have an increased mortality (particularly if unpaced). Consequently, it is now believed that these individuals are best advised to undergo pacemaker implantation at an earlier age than was previously thought appropriate. In most cases this would be early adulthood.

Bradycardia due to intermittent AV block is among the more important causes of syncope. The presence of Mobitz II type second degree AV block, third degree AV block, or alternating left and right bundle branch block can be considered as diagnostic findings. In absence of these, there are other findings that can suggest that syncope may be due to AV block, but these

other findings are inferential only, and are not considered definitively diagnostic. Nonetheless, although further investigation should be performed to confirm a relationship to syncope, the suspicion of AV block as the cause is important in directing the subsequent diagnostic strategy. Such observations include:
• presence of bifascicular block (left bundle branch block or right bundle branch block associated with left anterior or left posterior fascicular block);
• other intraventricular conduction abnormalities with a QRS duration longer than 120 ms; or
• documented Mobitz I second degree AV block in older individuals.
In the evaluation of patients suspected of having paroxysmal AV block, conventional 24-h ambulatory ECG (AECG) monitoring has limited diagnostic yield since the chance of recording an event is low. An 'event' recorder, and especially an ILR, markedly extends the ECG monitoring time and thereby improves the chance of detecting an abnormality (see Chapter 12). AECG findings can be considered diagnostic when a correlation between syncope and AV block is obtained. In the absence of such correlation, the presence of ventricular pauses >3 s when the patient is awake or periods of Mobitz II or third degree AV block can be considered diagnostic even in the absence of symptoms.

For patients with syncope of unknown origin and bifascicular block, or intraventricular conduction defects, an electrophysiologic study (EPS) is usually indicated (Table 20.3.1). EPS in these patients should analyze not only the properties of conduction system but also the inducibility of ventricular arrhythmias. The latter is particularly important in patients with structural heart disease. The assessment of the His-Purkinje system during EPS should include the measurement of baseline HV interval, effects of incremental atrial pacing and, if baseline study is inconclusive, pharmacologic provocation with ajmaline, procainamide, or disopyramide to stress further the integrity of the intracardiac conduction system.

Findings that are considered sufficiently diagnostic in terms of suggesting a basis for syncope include:
• HV interval >100 ms,
• presence of second or third degree infra-His AV block with progressively rapid atrial pacing, or
• high-degree AV block after intravenous administration of ajmaline, disopyramide, or procainamide.
There is a difference of opinion regarding the significance of HV intervals of between 70 and 100 ms duration. In such cases, there may be suspicion that AV conduction disease is the source of the problem but it would be prudent to seek additional supportive information (e.g. drug provocation study, AECG monitoring).

The absence of abnormal EPS findings in patients with syncopal episodes and bundle branch block does not exclude an arrhythmia as a possible etiology of syncope. In these patients, implantation of an ILR may be justified.

Recent findings from the ISSUE trial strongly suggest that with prolonged recording periods (often 5 to 10 months is needed) it is ultimately possible to detect correlation between arrhythmia (often paroxysmal AV block) and syncope.

Tachyarrhythmias
Supraventricular tachyarrhythmias

Although syncope is seldom due to supraventricular tachycardias, the recognition of these arrhythmias, and especially the paroxysmal supraventricular tachycardias (PSVTs), as a potential cause of fainting has importance as most of them can be successfully treated (including cure by transcatheter ablation techniques). More often, patients with supraventricular tachycardias experience palpitations and perhaps lightheadedness, but not frank syncope.

In those patients who develop syncope associated with supraventricular tachycardia, transient loss of consciousness usually appears at the beginning of the episodes before adequate vascular compensation is achieved. Some faints occur at the end of episodes, when an asystolic pause may occur before sinus rhythm resumes. In any case, the cause of syncope for patients with supraventricular tachycardias is usually multifactorial. Syncope is related not only to the increased heart rate, but also to an abnormal vasomotor response (i.e. delayed vasoconstriction) at the onset of an arrhythmia episode that leads to more severe transient hypotension than would otherwise be expected. Susceptibility to syncope may also be increased in the presence of underlying SND. The latter predisposes to long posttachycardia pauses and consequent transient hypotension at termination of the tachycardia episode.

PSVT due to AV nodal or accessory pathway reentry (AVNRT, AVRT)
Except in those cases in which PSVT is documented in relation to syncopal episode, the recognition of an arrhythmic origin of syncope in these patients can be difficult. Most of these patients have no structural heart disease and, except in those patients with preexcitation syndrome (e.g. Wolff–Parkinson–White syndrome), the baseline ECG is usually normal. Patients may recall palpitations, usually immediately before loss of consciousness; however, in many instances there is no recollection of unusual heart action. In those patients in whom PSVT is suspected, EPS is indicated. The induction of PSVT, especially if it provokes hypotension or reproduces clinical symptoms (this may not happen with the patient lying supine in the laboratory), can be considered diagnostic. More often than not, hypotension and symptom reproduction is only achieved if tachycardia is induced with the patient in an upright posture such as on a tilt-table. In any case, if tachycardia with a rapid rate consistent with the potential for hypotension is observed, transcatheter ablation (typically using radiofrequency or cryoablation methodology) is the treatment of choice.

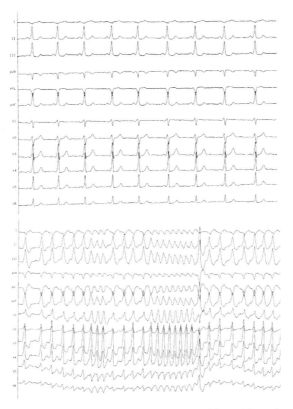

Figure 20.3.3 ECG recording obtained from a patient with WPW syndrome. The top panel trace is sinus rhythm with preexcitation pattern suggesting a left lateral accessory connection. The bottom panel shows a period of atrial fibrillation with a very fast ventricular response and varying degrees of preexcitation. The rapid rate was associated with hemodynamic compromise sufficient to cause syncope.

Patients with evidence of preexcitation on baseline ECG (e.g. WPW syndrome) have additional clinical risks that may contribute to syncope (or even sudden death on rare occasion). In these patients, apart from paroxysmal AV reentrant tachycardias (i.e. paroxysmal tachycardias using an accessory AV connection as part of their reentrant circuit), episodes of atrial fibrillation with very fast ventricular response (due to conduction over the accessory connection) can not only cause hypotension and syncope, but may also induce ventricular fibrillation leading to sudden death (Figure 20.3.3, a similar example is also shown in Chapter 15). In these patients, transcatheter ablation of the accessory connection is clearly the treatment of choice.

Atrial fibrillation and atrial flutter
Patients susceptible to paroxysmal atrial fibrillation may also develop syncopal episodes. As noted earlier, syncope most often occurs at the beginning of the

tachycardia episode (before the vascular system has had a chance to compensate by constricting). However, it may also occur at the end of the episode (especially in patients with concomitant SND) when there may be a long asystolic pause before a regular heart rhythm resumes (Figure 20.3.1).

It has also been shown that patients susceptible to syncope due to paroxysmal atrial fibrillation often have an abnormal vasomotor response at the beginning of the arrhythmia. As discussed earlier, delayed vasoconstrictor compensation may play an important role in the development of symptomatic hypotension. Finally, it is important to keep in mind certain special situations in which paroxysmal atrial fibrillation can cause acute hemodynamic deterioration leading to syncope. These high-risk situations include patients with advanced age, patients who are dehydrated or exposed to hot environments, individuals with left ventricular outflow obstruction (e.g. hypertrophic cardiomyopathy, severe aortic stenosis), and patients with accessory AV connections (see earlier discussion).

Patients with atrial flutter have many of the same risks for syncope as do those with atrial fibrillation. However, two important additional considerations are important to consider. First, exertion in patients with atrial flutter can lead to very rapid ventricular rates (e.g. 1 : 1 AV conduction). At such rapid rates, hypotension may ensue. Second, it has been reported that the use of class IC antiarrhythmic drugs in patients with atrial flutter, and even with atrial fibrillation, can slow the cycle length of the atrial tachyarrhythmia. Paradoxically, this slowing may reduce the degree of physiologic block offered by the AV node. The result is even greater propensity to 1 : 1 AV conduction. Although the atrial rate may be somewhat 'slower' than before the drug, the net ventricular rate is much faster due to 1 : 1 transmission. The result may be a sufficiently fast ventricular rate to cause severe hemodynamic compromise and syncope.

When contemplating the use of antiarrhythmic drugs for treatment of atrial flutter (or similar atrial ectopic tachycardias) it is essential to try and avoid the risk of setting the stage for 1 : 1 AV conduction. Protection can usually be achieved by concomitant administration of drugs that slow AV conduction, such as beta-blockers or calcium channel blockers. Alternatively, in the case of many forms of atrial flutter, atrial ectopic and reentrant tachycardias, and some cases of paroxysmal atrial fibrillation, transcatheter ablation can eliminate susceptibility to the underlying arrhythmia thereby avoiding the treatment problem entirely.

Ventricular tachycardias

Ventricular tachycardias (VTs) most often occur in patients with structural heart disease, especially those with either ischemic heart disease or dilated cardiomyopathy. However, approximately 10 to 15% of patients who are diagnosed with VT have no structural heart disease. Ventricular tachycardias in patients without structural heart disease are often classified as idiopathic ventricular tachycardias (see later).

Ventricular tachycardias associated with structural heart disease

Ischemic heart disease

Ventricular tachyarrhythmias have been reported to be responsible for syncope in up to 20% of patients referred for electrophysiologic assessment. Tachycardia rate, status of left ventricular function, and the efficiency of peripheral vascular constriction determine whether the arrhythmia will induce syncopal symptoms.

Nonsustained ventricular tachycardia (NSVT) is a common finding during AECG monitoring, especially in patients with ischemic heart disease and dilated cardiomyopathies. Consequently, such a finding during the assessment of a syncope patient has not in the past been considered very helpful in the absence of documented concomitant symptoms. However, this view is changing especially in patients with ischemic heart disease and severely diminished left ventricular function (i.e. ejection fractions <35%), given the MUSTT and MADIT2 results. These studies suggest that such patients have a high mortality rate and that implantable cardioverter defibrillator (ICD) therapy can be effective in diminishing mortality risk. Therefore, in the absence of other causes of syncope, the potential role of nonsustained ventricular tachycardia raises concern. In fact, based on the combined findings of MUSTT and MADIT2, it can be argued that ICD therapy may be warranted without undertaking an EPS in ischemic heart disease patients with poor ejection fractions. However, although ICD therapy may prevent premature death, syncope may remain a problem (since hypotension may develop before the ICD 'fires'). Prevention of the latter scenario often requires concomitant use of antiarrhythmic drugs (especially sotalol or amiodarone). Furthermore, the role of NSVT in causing the syncope was at most presumptive (not certain).

Dilated cardiomyopathy

Until very recently, there was uncertainty regarding the appropriate approach to be taken when syncope occurs in patients with severe underlying left ventricular dysfunction due to dilated cardiomyopathy. The SCD-HEFT results suggest that prophylactic placement of an ICD can also be indicated in patients with heart failure and severe underlying left ventricular dysfunction due to dilated cardiomyopathy. According to these data, ICD can be considered to be indicated in patients with syncope and dilated cardiomyopathy. However, even if the faint were due to VT, once again the ICD protects against sudden death but often may not prevent syncope. The latter is particularly the case when a 'shock' is needed. In such instances, a period of time is required to detect the tachyarrhythmia, charge capacitors, reconfirm the arrhythmia, and discharge the shock. Loss of consciousness may have already developed by that time. As discussed in the previous paragraph, concomitant antiarrhythmic drug therapy is often needed in such cases.

Left ventricular outflow obstruction including hypertrophic (obstructive) cardiomyopathy

Syncope may be a presenting feature in conditions in which there is fixed or dynamic obstruction to left ventricular outflow such as valvular aortic stenosis or hypertrophic obstructive cardiomyopathy (HOCM). The basis for the faint is in part inadequate blood flow due to the mechanical obstruction. However, especially in the case of valvular aortic stenosis, ventricular mechanoreceptor-mediated bradycardia and vasodilatation is thought to be an important contributor to the degree of hypotension. In HOCM, neural reflex mechanisms may also play a role. However, symptoms may also be provoked by physical exertion and may even develop in the setting of an otherwise relatively benign arrhythmia (e.g. atrial fibrillation). Even a slow ventricular tachycardia may cause syncope in such cases.

Recurrent unexplained syncope episodes are of considerable prognostic concern when they occur in a young population in association with exercise. In such patients, valve replacement is indicated if valvular aortic stenosis is present. In HOCM patients the implantation of an ICD is indicated. Once again, it should be kept in mind that ICDs act to prevent sudden arrhythmic death but other measures (e.g. beta-blockers, antiarrhythmic medications) may be needed to reduce syncope risk.

Arrhythmogenic right ventricular dysplasia (cardiomyopathy)

Arrhythmogenic right ventricular dysplasia/cardiomyopathy (ARVD) is a hereditary disease in which conventional teaching has been that right ventricular myocardium is replaced to varying degrees by fatty infiltration. The extent of infiltration can range from minimal ventricular wall involvement to a massive right ventricular replacement in the more severe forms of the disease. In some cases, the left ventricle is affected as well but rarely as a solitary finding. Recent thought suggests that ARVD may better be considered a problem of intercellular communication. Future studies will undoubtedly further clarify the pathophysiology.

The clinical picture ranges from asymptomatic patients to symptoms secondary to ventricular tachyarrhythmias or right ventricular failure. In ARVD patients, ventricular arrhythmias are usually triggered by adrenergic stimulation and can range from isolated premature ventricular beats to nonsustained or sustained life-threatening VT. The outcome may vary from palpitations, to syncopal episodes, or even sudden death. Syncope related to exercise should bring this diagnosis to mind, especially in individuals without evident underlying structural heart disease.

ARVD should be suspected in those patients with syncope of unknown origin with family history of premature sudden death or unexplained syncope, or when baseline ECG shows certain suggestive abnormalities such as:
• epsilon waves (a finding of a small late signal analogous to 'late' potentials in ischemic heart disease, found in the ST segment, most often in V1 lead),

- low amplitude and localized prolongation of the QRS complex in leads V1 to V3,
- inverted T waves in right precordial leads in the absence of right bundle branch block.

In addition, some of these patients have frequent ventricular premature beats with a pattern of left bundle branch block suggesting a right ventricular site of origin.

Once suspected, confirmation of the diagnosis of ARVD remains somewhat controversial. Until recently the diagnosis was thought to be best confirmed by imaging techniques, such as echocardiography, right ventricular angiography, or magnetic resonance, imaging (MRI). These images can show dyskinetic areas, dilatation, or depressed right ventricular function and on occasion (in the case of the MRI) fatty replacement in the right ventricular wall. Moving image MRI (cine-MRI) is probably the most sensitive diagnostic tool currently available, but suffers from being expensive, not universally available, and perhaps from being overly sensitive. Myocardial biopsy may be the most specific test, but is difficult to justify in many cases and may 'miss' the affected regions. EPS may be helpful in inducing the ventricular arrhythmia and confirming the site(s) of origin.

An optimum treatment strategy for patients with ARVD and syncope has not been fully established. In some instances it has been suggested that antiarrhythmic drugs, specifically sotalol, and even radiofrequency catheter ablation can be effective. However, drug therapy is not well proven, and ablation success may be hard to predict by virtue of the potential for many regions of the heart to be affected and thereby become arrhythmogenic sites. Consequently, in those patients with syncope in whom the presence of malignant ventricular arrhythmias can be demonstrated (either during a spontaneous recording or induced at EPS) an ICD is the safest treatment approach currently from a mortality perspective (see the earlier discussed caveat regarding the role of ICDs for syncope prevention).

Idiopathic ventricular tachycardias and syncope
Right ventricular outflow tract tachycardia

Idiopathic right ventricular outflow tract (RVOFT) tachycardia is the most frequent type of idiopathic VT (Figure 20.3.4). It represents approximately 80% of all idiopathic VT and about 10% of all patients that are evaluated for VT. RVOFT tachycardia can be present at any age, but it is most frequently seen between the second and fourth decade of life. It originates in the RVOFT and appears to be due to cyclic AMP-mediated 'triggered activity'. Typically RVOFT tachycardia can be terminated by adenosine administration but this is of course only a temporizing step. The arrhythmia will recur if a more permanent solution is not provided (e.g. transcatheter ablation).

RVOFT ventricular tachycardia is usually provoked by physical exercise. Patients with RVOFT tachycardia may be totally asymptomatic or they can experience palpitations, dizziness, or on occasion syncope. Furthermore,

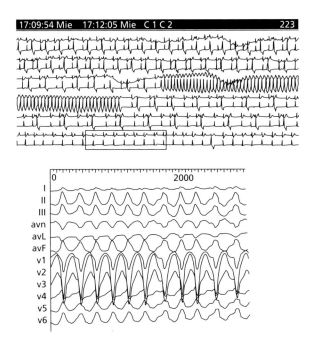

Figure 20.3.4 Recordings obtained from a patient with sudden syncope, no apparent heart disease, and a normal ECG and echocardiogram. The top panel was obtained from a Holter recording showing sinus rhythm and frequent premature ventricular beats, followed by a rapid nonsustained ventricular tachycardia at 200 bpm. The bottom panel is a 12-lead ECG during isoproterenol infusion. The ventricular tachycardia has a left bundle branch block morphology suggestive of a RVOFT origin. Radiofrequency ablation eliminated susceptibility to recurrent tachycardia.

although some sporadic cases of sudden death have been described, most often this tachycardia has a benign course from a mortality perspective. On the other hand, its associated symptoms may have a very negative impact on patient lifestyle.

The baseline ECG in RVOFT patients usually has a normal QRS. Some patients have frequent premature ventricular beats with the same morphology of tachycardia (i.e. a QRS that appears to have a left bundle branch block appearance but relatively narrow with a vertical or rightward frontal axis) (Figure 20.3.5). Tachycardia in these patients can manifest as episodes of nonsustained VT, repetitive monomorphic VT interrupted by short periods of sinus rhythm, or episodes of paroxysmal sustained VT.

By definition, RVOFT tachycardia patients have no evident structural heart disease, but some minor abnormalities in the RV outflow tract have been described based on MRI techniques. As the morphology of this tachycardia can be similar to tachycardia observed in patients with the more worrisome ARVD/cardiomyopathy, it is important that the second of these two conditions be excluded in each case.

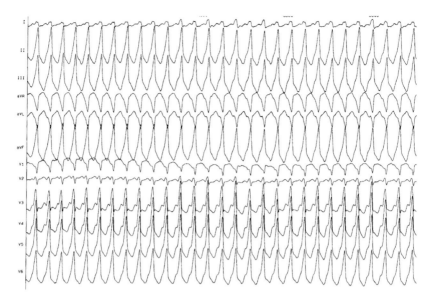

Figure 20.3.5 Ventricular tachycardia in a patient without structural heart disease. The QRS has an inferior axis (i.e. positive QRS in inferior leads II, III, and aVF), and a left bundle branch block morphology, but with 'r' waves from V2 suggesting an origin from the left ventricular outflow tract. Endocavitary mapping confirmed the activation site and radiofrequency ablation was successful.

In patients with syncope of unknown origin and no structural heart disease, ROVFT tachycardia should be suspected when syncope episodes are associated with palpitations or when frequent premature beats or runs of nonsustained VT with left bundle branch block and inferior (i.e. vertical or rightward) axis are recorded. Further diagnostic tests, such as repeated 24 to 48-h ambulatory monitoring, longer-term MCOT or EPS may be helpful in confirming the suspected diagnosis. During EPS, the arrhythmia is typically induced during isoproterenol infusion with rapid atrial or ventricular pacing. Induction by programmed electrical stimulation alone is less reproducible.

Treatment is indicated in symptomatic patients with palpitations or syncope. Beta-blockers have been considered as the first-choice drug for the treatment of these patients. Other drugs that have been used effectively include calcium channel blockers, and class I and class III antiarrhythmic drugs. However, drug therapy has limited efficacy and is often associated with troublesome side-effects. Furthermore, most of these patients are diagnosed at a relatively young age and are not optimal candidates for decades of drug treatment. Fortunately, transcatheter ablation of the arrhythmia site of origin has been used with a success rate of approximately 85%. Complications are uncommon but include perforation of the RV wall leading to tamponade.

Idiopathic left ventricular outflow tract tachycardia

Idiopathic left ventricular outflow tract (LVOFT) tachycardia is less common than but analogous to RVOFT tachycardia. It exhibits subtle variations in QRS morphology during tachycardia consisting mainly of the presence of an R wave in V1 and V2 leads. It has been shown, by intracavitary mapping techniques, that the QRS morphology of the VT may not only suggest LVOFT but may assist in defining the site of origin even more precisely (Figure 20.3.5).

In these patients, as in those with RVOFT tachycardia, syncope can be a clinical manifestation of the arrhythmia. In those cases, treatment with drugs may be considered but radiofrequency catheter ablation is preferred.

Idiopathic left posterior fascicular tachycardia

This is the most frequent form of idiopathic left ventricular (LV) tachycardia. Although it can be present at any age, idiopathic LV fascicular tachycardia is most frequently seen in patients between the second and fourth decade of life and it predominates in males. The mechanism of tachycardia seems to be a reentry in the left posterior fascicle. During EPS, the arrhythmia can usually be induced and stopped by programmed ventricular stimulation. Isoproterenol infusion does not typically facilitate induction and the tachycardia is not affected by adenosine. Usually it can be easily terminated by verapamil infusion (although long-term oral verapamil is not generally effective for prevention of recurrences).

The most frequent form of presentation is as paroxysmal VT, with a QRS pattern of right bundle branch block and left axis deviation. Occasionally, similar right bundle branch block but with right axis deviation can be seen suggesting that reentry arises from the left anterior fascicle. Clinically, these patients may be asymptomatic but when they have symptoms they usually experience palpitations, dizziness, or syncope. Baseline ECG does not show specific abnormalities.

As in RVOFT tachycardia, the prognosis in left fascicular tachycardia is generally benign but some cases of sudden death have been reported. Consequently, symptomatic patients should be treated. Although this tachycardia responds to intravenous verapamil administration, chronic oral treatment is less effective, and in most of these patients transcatheter ablation can be performed safely and effectively.

Long QT syndromes (primary, secondary)

The long QT syndromes may be a primary disorder or secondary to other factors (most commonly various drugs, Table 20.3.2). Recently there has been considerable interest in the molecular biology of primary long QT syndromes and related conditions (e.g. Brugada syndrome, see later). The interested reader is referred to the growing comprehensive literature on this subject. It is only possible to provide a brief overview here.

Table 20.3.2 Drugs implicated in QT prolongation and
*torsades de pointes.**

Antiarrhythmic agents
Class IA
  Quinidine
  Procainamide
  Disopyramide

Class III
  Sotalol
  Ibutilide
  N-acetylprocainamide (NAPA)
  Dofetilide
  Amiodarone (relatively low risk)

Antianginal agents
Bepridil (removed from market in the United States)

Psychoactive/antidepression agents
Phenothiazines
Thioridazine
Amitriptyline
Imipramine

Antibiotics
Erythromycin
Pentamidine
Fluconazole

Nonsedating antihistamines
Terfenadine (removed from market in the United States)
Astemizole

Miscellaneous
Cisapride (removed from market in the United States)
Arsenic
Droperidol

---

* Only the more commonly used agents are listed here.
A complete list is obtainable from the World Wide Web
(see text).

Primary long QT syndromes The primary long QT syndromes comprise a group of disorders, generally familial in nature, and characterized by a prolongation of ventricular repolarization (i.e. long QT interval). Although, the most characteristic alteration at baseline ECG is an abnormal prolongation of QT interval it has been recognized that there are some patients who have normal baseline QT interval duration. However, in many of these cases other abnormalities can be observed, such as T wave alternans or abnormalities in T wave morphology. These conditions predispose to *torsade de pointes* (Figure 20.3.6).

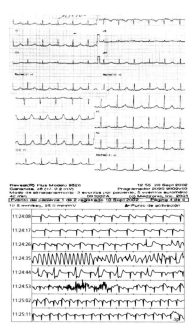

Figure 20.3.6 The top panel is the baseline ECG from a patient with long QT syndrome and recurrent syncope. The faints were associated with triggers suggestive of a vasovagal etiology. The lower panel, obtained from an ILR placed subcutaneously in this patient, revealed a polymorphous ventricular tachycardia (*torsade de pointes*) to be the cause of a near-syncope event.

Syncope is one of the most common clinical presentations but sudden death is also a substantial risk.

Two main forms of 'clinical' (phenotypic) presentation have been described for primary long QT syndrome. The most common is the so called Romano–Ward syndrome, which has an autosomal dominant pattern of transmission, and the second one is the so-called Jervell and Lange–Neilsen syndrome, which is inherited in an autosomal recessive pattern. Up to five different gene mutations have been identified for the Romano–Ward syndrome. These mutations appear to correlate with different patterns of clinical presentation.

Clinical manifestations may consist of syncopal episodes or sudden death. Syncope tends to begin at an early age, usually between 5 and 15 years. In the most common form of long QT syndrome, syncopal episodes are usually triggered by an adrenergic stimulus such as exercise or stressful situations. However, other forms of long QT syndrome may result in *torsades* being triggered by bradycardia.

In patients with syncope of unknown origin, the presence of long QT syndrome must be suspected when there are abnormalities of repolarization, or family history of long QT syndrome, syncope or sudden death. There are several findings that when present seem to enhance further the risk of sudden death. These are:

- the presence of previous cardiac arrest;
- syncope at young age;
- family history of sudden death;
- a very prolonged corrected QT interval (QTc) (>600 ms); and
- the presence of the recessive form of so-called Jervell and Lange–Neilsen syndrome (i.e. long QT with hearing impairment).

As a rule, patients was described with long QT syndrome should be advised to avoid vigorous exercise. They should also not be exposed to drugs that can further prolong QT interval (Table 20.3.2). For patients with a first syncopal episode and no other risk factors, treatment with beta-blockers is considered as a first-line treatment. When bradycardia-triggered syncope is implicated, the use of implanted cardiac pacemakers is justified. In patients that have other risk factors in addition to syncope (see earlier discussion), or those who have syncope recurrences in spite of beta-blockers, implantation of an ICD is indicated. A strong family history of sudden death is probably a strong indicator for an ICD.

Secondary long QT syndrome Secondary forms of long QT syndrome may be the result of drug effects, electrolyte disturbances, bradycardic states or a combination of these. Drug-induced long QT syndrome is by far the most frequently encountered of these conditions, and is far more common than is primary long QT syndrome. New drugs capable of inducing the problem are being identified each year. The result is increased risk of iatrogenic syncope or even sudden death secondary to polymorphous ventricular tachycardia (*torsade de pointes*). Given the substantial public health hazard associated with drug-induced long QT, physicians must be very attentive to the risk. Internet sites such as www.torsades.org are helpful in terms of maintaining relatively up-to-date lists of drugs associated with triggering *torsades*.

Eliminating the offending agent is the key to treatment of drug-induced *torsades*. In an emergent situation (i.e. recurrent *torsades*) infusion of magnesium sulfate, restoration of normal electrolyte status, and prevention of bradycardia are important therapeutic steps.

Brugada syndrome

In 1992, a group of eight patients was described who had experienced recurrent episodes of aborted sudden death without any apparent structural heart disease and who had a distinct pattern at ECG. Further observations have resulted in this entity being recognized as a hereditary disease, characterized by an ECG pattern of right bundle branch block and ST elevation in V1 to V3 (Figure 20.3.7). These individuals are at risk of developing episodes of polymorphous ventricular tachycardia that can present as syncope.

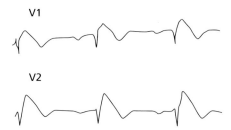

Figure 20.3.7 'Classic' coved ST-T segments in leads V1 and V2 associated with Brugada syndrome.

It has been observed that the ECG of Brugada syndrome can change over time in the same patient from a strictly normal ECG to the full characteristic pattern. In those patients with suspected Brugada syndrome who have an apparently normal ECG, intravenous administration of a Class I antiarrhythmic drug (e.g. ajmaline, procainamide) can provoke the typical QRS-ST segment changes, thereby confirming the diagnosis.

In patients with syncope of unknown origin the diagnosis of Brugada syndrome must be suspected when:
• there is a family history of established Brugada syndrome,
• there is a family history of sudden death or unexplained syncope, or
• when baseline ECG shows the typical pattern.
Although the risk of sudden death in asymptomatic patients with Brugada syndrome is not well known, it is now agreed that those patients who have had syncope or an aborted sudden death are at increased risk of sudden death. Currently available antiarrhythmic drugs are not useful in preventing arrhythmia recurrences in Brugada syndrome. Consequently, symptomatic patients or those with a strong family history of premature sudden death should be treated with an ICD.

Short QT syndrome
Recently, a new hereditary syndrome characterized by a short QT interval on baseline ECG has been described in few families. Clinical manifestations include syncope, palpitations, paroxysmal atrial fibrillation, and sudden death. Characteristically, the corrected QT interval is shorter than 320 ms. In these patients, programmed ventricular stimulation from RVOFT is usually able to induce ventricular fibrillation. However, given the limited experience with this syndrome to date, it would be prudent to track closely the future literature.

At the present time it appears that short QT syndrome is accompanied by high risk of sudden death. Consequently, implantation of an ICD has been suggested as treatment of choice in these patients. Additionally, it has been suggested that the administration of quinidine prolongs the QT interval and decreases the risk of recurrent ventricular arrhythmias. Its administration can be useful in very young patients at high risk of sudden death and in whom an ICD is not feasible or in those patients with frequent appropriate ICD discharges due to recurrent ventricular arrhythmias. It may also be helpful to diminish syncope risk, since as has been emphasized earlier, ICD therapy alone may not be as effective for syncope prevention as it is for reducing sudden death risk.

Summary

Cardiac arrhythmias are important causes of syncope particularly in patients with structural heart disease. Documentation of an arrhythmia in conjunction with syncope is the diagnostic gold standard for establishing the basis of symptoms. However, where this is not possible or clinically prudent EPS may be warranted. However, EPS results may be misleading and findings must be interpreted with care.

In many subgroups of patients in whom ventricular arrhythmias are the apparent cause of syncope, ICD therapy is indicated. However, while sudden death risk is diminished ICDs alone may not prevent syncope in such cases. Concomitant treatment strategies must be carefully considered in such cases.

Additional reading

Brignole M, Menozzi C, Moya A *et al*. Mechanism of syncope in patients with bundle branch block and negative electrophysiological test. *Circulation* 2001; **104**: 2045–2050.

Brignole M, Gianfranchi L, Menozzi C *et al*. Role of autonomic reflexes in syncope associated with paroxysmal atrial fibrillation. *J Am Coll Cardiol* 1993; **22**: 1123–1129.

Brugada J, Brugada P. Further characterization of the syndrome of right bundle branch block, ST segment elevation and sudden cardiac death. *J Cardiovasc Electrophysiol* 1997; **8**: 325–331.

Ermis C, Zhu AX, Pham S *et al*. Comparison of automatic and patient-activated arrhythmia recordings by implantable loop recorders in the evaluation of syncope. *Amer J Cardiol* 2003; **92**: 815–9.

Fox WC, Lockette W. Unexpected syncope and death during intense physical training: evolving role of molecular genetics. *Aviation Space & Environ Med* 2003; **74**: 1223–30.

Gaita F, Giustetto C, Bianchi F *et al*. Short QT syndrome: pharmacological treatment. *J Am Coll Cardiol* 2004; **43**: 1494–9.

Gaita F, Giustetto C, Bianchi F *et al*. Short QT Síndrome. A Familial Cause of Sudden Death. *Circulation* 2003; **108**: 965.

Gann D, Tolentino A, Samet P. Electrophysiologic evaluation of elderly patients with sinus bradycardia: a long-term follow-up study. *Ann Intern Med* 1979; **90**: 24–29.

Gregoratos G, Abrams J, Epstein AE *et al*. ACC/AHA/NASPE 2002 guideline update for implantation of cardiac pacemakers and antiarrhythmia devices: summary article. *Circulation* 2002; **106**: 2145–2161.

Knight BP, Goyal R, Pelosi F *et al*. Outcome of patients with non-ischemic dilated cardiomyopathy and unexplained syncope treated with an implantable defibrillator. *J Am Coll Cardiol* 1999; **33**: 1964–1970.

Krahn AD, Klein GJ, Yee R, Skanes AC. Detection of asymptomatic arrhythmias in unexplained syncope. *Am Heart J* 2004; **148**: 326–32.

Leitch JW, Klein GJ, Yee R, Leather RA, Kim YH. Syncope associated with supraventricular tachycardia. An expression of tachycardia rate or vasomotor response? *Circulation* 1992; **85**: 1064–1067.

Link MS. Hellkamp AS. Estes NA 3rd *et al.* MOST Study Investigators. High incidence of pacemaker syndrome in patients with sinus node dysfunction treated with ventricular-based pacing in the Mode Selection Trial (MOST). *J Amer Coll Cardiol* 2004; **43**: 2066–71.

Moss AJ, Schwartz PJ, Crampton RS *et al.* The long QT syndrome: prospective longitudinal study of 328 families. *Circulation* 1991; **84**: 1136–1144.

Scheinman MM, Peters RW, Morady F, Sauve MJ, Malone P, Modin G. Electrophysiologic studies in patients with bundle branch block. *PACE* 1983; **6**: 1157–1165.

Schwartz PJ, Zaza A, Locati EH, Moss AJ. Stress and sudden death: the case of the long QT syndrome. *Circulation* 1991; **83**(Supp II): 71–80.

Seidl K, Drogemuller A, Rameken M, Schneider S, Zahn R, Senges J. Two year follow-up in 643 patients with non-invasively unexplained syncope and therapy guided by electrophysiologic study. *Zeit Kardiol* 2003; **92**: 852–61.

Silvetti MS, Grutter G, Di Ciommo V, Drago F. Paroxysmal atrioventricular block in young patients. *Ped Cardiol* 2004; **25**: 506–12.

Weerasooriya R, Jaïs P, Hocini M, *et al.* Effect of catheter ablation on quality of life of patients with paroxysmal atrial fibrillation. *Heart Rhythm* 2005; **2**: 619–23.

CHAPTER 20

Specific causes of syncope: their evaluation and treatment strategies

Part 4: Structural cardiac and pulmonary causes of syncope

Jean-Jacques Blanc and Jan Janousek

Introduction

Structural cardiac, vascular, or pulmonary diseases are not often the direct cause of syncope. More often, the relationship of structural cardiopulmonary abnormalities to syncope is indirect operating through increased susceptibility to tachy- or bradyarrhythmias or hypotension of other cause (e.g. low cardiac output, acute myocardial infarction, acute aortic dissection etc.). Additionally, in many of these cases a neural reflex mechanism contributes to the faint (e.g. syncope associated with acute myocardial ischemia, severe aortic stenosis, or pulmonary hypertension). On the other hand, whether structural disease is a 'direct' or 'indirect' participant, syncope associated with severe structural heart disease is a serious matter with a substantial mortality risk, and warrants immediate and thorough evaluation. Careful consideration needs to be given to hospitalizing these patients (see Chapter 9) on an ECG-monitored cardiac station for the diagnostic evaluation and often for initiation of therapy (especially if it entails use of antiarrhythmic medications).

Goals

The goals of this part of the chapter are to summarize:
• a scheme for risk stratification of syncope patients with structural cardiopulmonary disease; and
• the manner in which the diagnostic evaluation strategy differs from patients without underlying structural disease.

Risk stratification

Many different forms of structural cardiac and pulmonary disease may be associated with syncope. The most common are listed in Table 20.4.1.

Table 20.4.1 Common structural cardiac and pulmonary disease conditions associated with syncope.

Condition	Most common mechanism(s) excluding arrhythmias
Acute myocardial infarction or ischemia	Reflex, reduced CO, VT
Chronic ischemic heart disease	VT, AV block
Aortic stenosis	Reflex
Atrial myxoma	Transient blood flow obstruction
Acute aortic dissection	Reflex
Pulmonary embolism	Reflex
Primary pulmonary hypertension	Reflex
Pericardial disease	Inflow obstruction, reduced CO
Dilated cardiomyopathy	VT
ARVD	VT
HOCM	Outflow obstruction, VT

Note: AV = atrioventricular; ARVD = arrhythmogenic RV dysplasia/cardiomyopathy; CO = cardiac output; HOCM = hypertrophic obstructive cardiomyopathy; Reflex = neural reflex vasodepressor/bradycardia; VT = ventricular tachycardia

One study has developed and validated a clinical prediction rule for risk stratification of patients with syncope. This study used a composite outcome of having cardiac arrhythmias as a cause of syncope or death (or cardiac death) within 1 year of follow-up. Four variables were identified and included:

1 age > 45 years,
2 history of congestive heart failure,
3 history of ventricular arrhythmias, and
4 abnormal ECG (other than nonspecific ST changes).

Arrhythmias or death within 1 year occurred in 4 to 7% of patients without any of the risk factors and progressively increased to 58 to 80% in patients with three or more risk factors. The critical importance of identifying cardiac causes of syncope is that many of the arrhythmias and other cardiac diseases are now treatable with drugs and/or devices.

Most frequent causes

Structural cardiac or cardiopulmonary disease is often present in older syncope patients. However, in these cases it is more often the arrhythmias associated with structural disease that are the cause of syncope rather than the structural disease itself (see Chapter 20, Part 3).

In terms of syncope directly attributable to structural disease, probably the most common is that which occurs in conjunction with acute myocardial ischemia or infarction. Other relatively common acute medical conditions associated with syncope include pulmonary embolism and pericardial tamponade. The basis of syncope in these conditions is multifactorial, including both the hemodynamic impact of the specific lesion as well as neurally mediated reflex effects leading to inappropriate bradycardia and peripheral vascular dilatation. The latter is especially important in the setting of acute ischemic events. One of the most commonly observed examples is the atropine-responsive bradycardia and hypotension often associated with inferior wall myocardial infarction.

Syncope is of considerable concern when it is associated with conditions in which there is fixed or dynamic obstruction to left ventricular outflow (e.g. aortic stenosis, hypertrophic obstructive cardiomyopathy [HOCM], prosthetic valve malfunction). In such cases, symptoms are often provoked by physical exertion, but may also develop if an otherwise benign arrhythmia should occur (e.g. atrial fibrillation). The basis for the faint is in part inadequate blood flow due to the mechanical obstruction. However, especially in the case of valvular aortic stenosis, neurally mediated reflex disturbance of vascular control is an important contributor to hypotension.

In hypertrophic cardiomyopathy, with or without left ventricle outflow obstruction, neural reflex mechanisms may also play a role. However, in HOCM, the occurrence of atrial tachyarrhythmias (particularly atrial fibrillation) or ventricular tachycardia (even at relatively modest rates) may be important causes of syncopal events.

Other important but less common causes of syncope associated with clinically important cardiopulmonary disease include:
• acute aortic dissection,
• left ventricular inflow obstruction in patients with mitral stenosis or atrial myxoma,
• right ventricular outflow obstruction, and
• right-to-left shunting secondary to pulmonic stenosis or pulmonary hypertension.
The mechanism of the faint may once again be multifactorial, with hemodynamic, arrhythmic, and neurally mediated origins in need of evaluation.

Vascular steal syndromes are rare causes syncope. Subclavian steal syndrome, albeit very uncommon, is perhaps the most important of these conditions and can reasonably be incorporated in the context of either cardiopulmonary disease or cerebrovascular disease (see Chapter 20, Part 5). Subclavian steal may occur on a congenital or acquired basis. Low pressure within the subclavian artery due to a stenosis in its most proximal portion near the aorta causes retrograde flow to occur in the ipsilateral vetebral artery (especially during upper arm exercise). The result is a diminution of cerebral blood flow due to 'steal' from the Circle of Willis. Syncope is typically associated with upper extremity exercise. Direct corrective angioplasty or surgery is usually feasible and effective. Other forms of vascular steal, particularly within the cranium, are recognized as potential causes of syncope but are virtually impossible to diagnose.

A final consideration, although not precisely a conventional form of structural heart disease, is failure of implanted pacemaker or defibrillator systems.

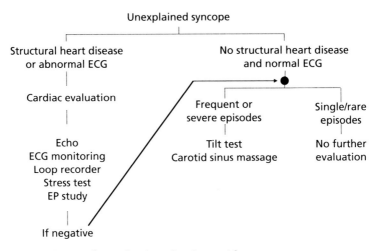

Figure 20.4.1 Strategy for evaluation of patients with syncope.

Thus, intermittent failure to pace due to lead fracture, device failure or battery depletion, or a loose set screw in the connector block may cause syncope in a pacemaker-dependent individual. Similarly, an ICD may trigger syncope by failing to pace appropriately or by inappropriately introducing burst pacing.

Evaluation

Apart from identifying the nature and severity of any underlying cardiopulmonary disease in a patient with syncope, the cause of the faint needs special consideration (Figure 20.4.1). The same disease may induce syncope by different mechanisms. For example, acute myocardial infarction may result in cerebral hypoperfusion by initiating ventricular tachycardia or AV block or even a neurally mediated reflex ventricular asystole (particularly in the case of inferior wall infarction). Similarly, faints during exertion in patients with severe valvular aortic stenosis can be due to inadequate cardiac output or an inappropriate vascular response resulting in transient systemic hypotension. The latter is thought to be the more important in most cases. Syncope in patients with HOCM can also be the consequence of several mechanisms. Hypotension may again be due to direct obstruction to left ventricular ejection, but transient ventricular and atrial tachyarrhythmias as well as neural reflex causes are probably more common.

As has been emphasized throughout this book, it is of major importance to consider whether structural cardiopulmonary disease is present in every patient with syncope. Usually the medical history and a few readily available tests (e.g. ECG, echocardiogram) are sufficient in this regard. Two possibilities can be defined: cardiopulmonary disease is known to be present; or cardiopulmonary disease is not known to be present.

Cardiopulmonary disease is known to be present

In those patients in whom cardiopulmonary disease is known to be present and its severity is not thought to be critical, then only the mechanism of the syncope has to be determined. This aspect is readily solved if an arrhythmia has been registered during or immediately after the syncope episode. Conversely, and much more commonly, it is more difficult when there is no prior arrhythmia documentation. In such cases, a complete hemodynamic assessment of the structural disturbance becomes essential along with selection of appropriate tests to assess potential rhythm disturbances (see Chapters 12,15, and 20 Part3).

In cases where the presence of cardiopulmonary disease is known, but its severity has not previously been characterized, referral for selected noninvasive (e.g. echocardiogram, exercise testing, radionuclide imaging) and possibly invasive (e.g. angiography, hemodynamic measurements) evaluation is recommended. An arrhythmia or neural reflex event may have been the cause of the faint but prognosis depends on the severity of the underlying disease.

Cardiopulmonary disease is not known to be present

When the structural cardiopulmonary disease is previously unknown two different circumstances need to be considered:

1 In an emergency setting (e.g. cardiogenic shock, acute severe prosthetic valve occlusion or regurgitation, acute chest pain) syncope is only one component of a complex clinical presentation. The presence of structural cardiopulmonary disease may now be obvious but its nature may be uncertain. Highest priority must be given to establishing the basis for the acute decompensation and initiating appropriate treatment (e.g. acute pulmonary embolism, aortic dissection, myocardial infarction, papillary muscle, or chordal rupture).

2 In the second scenario, syncope is the only symptom, but ancillary factors such as patient age, medical history, family history, and physical examination suggest the possibility of underlying structural cardiopulmonary disease. In such cases, it is reasonable to undertake straightforward low-risk noninvasive assessment to confirm (or set aside) the clinical suspicion. An ECG (probably already obtained as part of the 'initial evaluation', see Chapter 7) and echocardiogram are appropriate starting points. Depending on these findings and the physician's comfort in assessing cardiovascular risk, referral for additional selected noninvasive (e.g. exercise testing, radionuclide imaging) and invasive (e.g. angiography, hemodynamic measurements) evaluation may be prudent.

Treatment
Addressing underlying structural disease as the treatment of syncope

The treatment of syncope in the setting of structural cardiopulmonary disease is dependent on the nature and severity of the underlying structural

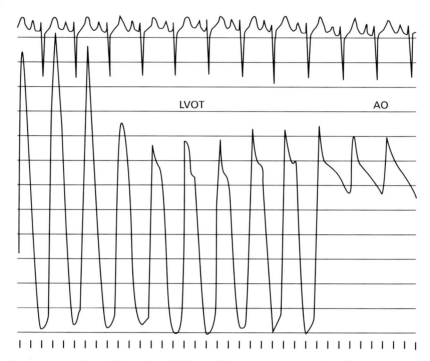

Figure 20.4.2 Figure illustrating fall in systolic pressure associated with dynamic subaortic obstruction in a HOCM patient. The lower pressure could cause syncope, especially during exertion or in the presence of vasodilator drugs. However, various cardiac arrhythmias as well as neurally mediated reflex vasodilation and bradycardia are perhaps even more important contributors to syncope in such patients.

abnormalities and the apparent mechanism (i.e. arrhythmia, hemodynamic abnormality) leading to syncope. In an emergency situation, the underlying structural disturbance must be treated first (e.g. acute myocardial infarction, severe aortic stenosis). Referral to a facility experienced in and capable of dealing with the problem is recommended. In nonemergency circumstances, treatment of the structural disease should be considered if feasible (e.g. aortic valve replacement in the case of severe aortic stenosis).

In syncope associated with acute myocardial ischemia, pharmacologic therapy, and/or revascularization is clearly the appropriate strategy in most cases. Similarly, when syncope is closely associated with surgically addressable lesions (e.g. valvular aortic stenosis, atrial myxoma, congenital cardiac anomaly, implanted device malfunction), a direct corrective approach is often feasible. There are no convincing data on the effect of reducing outflow gradient on relief of syncope relapses in HOCM (Figure 20.4.2). Nevertheless, it would seem reasonable to consider such a step using medications and/or pacing, and on occasion surgical intervention.

Addressing underlying structural disease is not feasible or adequate
When syncope is caused by certain difficult-to-treat conditions such as in many instances of severe left ventricular dysfunction, primary pulmonary hypertension, or restrictive cardiomyopathy, it is often impossible to ameliorate the underlying problem adequately. In such cases it is reasonable to turn attention to determining the cause of syncope (e.g. ventricular tachycardia in dilated cardiomyopathy) and focusing on its treatment (e.g. antiarrhythmic drugs, ICD, etc.). In addition, it should be emphasized that for patients with structural cardiopulmonary disease, additional factors could participate in the triggering of a syncope event. For instance, electrolyte disturbances, increasing heart failure, or worsening oxygenation may all aggravate susceptibility to arrhythmia initiation leading to syncope. Hypokalemia occurring as a side-effect of diuretic therapy is one of the most common scenarios to keep in mind. It is of course of crucial importance to recognize these triggering factors as their reversal can eliminate the symptoms.

Summary

Structural cardiac, vascular, or pulmonary diseases are relatively uncommon direct causes of true syncope, but contribute to increasing susceptibility to faints by virtue of the increased risk of tachy- or bradyarrhythmias, or systemic hypotension of other causes. In any event, syncope associated with severe structural heart disease has a worrisome prognosis, and warrants immediate and thorough evaluation of the underlying problem. Consideration needs to be given to hospitalizing these patients on an ECG-monitored cardiac station for their diagnostic evaluation and often for initiation of therapy. As a rule, treatment is best directed at amelioration of the specific structural lesion or its consequences.

Additional reading

Colivicchi F, Ammirati F, Santini M. Epidemiology and prognostic implications of syncope in young competing athletes. *Eur Heart J* 2004; **25**:1749–1753.
Dixon MS, Thomas P, Sheridon DJ. Syncope as the presentation of unstable angina. *Int J Cardiol* 1988; **19**: 125–129.
Fox WC, Lockette W. Unexpected syncope and death during intense physical training: evolving role of molecular genetics. *Aviation Space & Environmental Medicine* 2003; **74**:1223–1230.
Gosselin C, Walker PM. Subclavian steal syndrome. Existence, clinical features, diagnosis, management. *Semin Vasc Surg* 1996; **9**: 93–97.
Gregoratos G. Abrams J. Epstein AE *et al.* American College of Cardiology/American Heart Association Task Force on Practice Guidelines/North American Society for Pacing and Electrophysiology Committee to Update the 1998 Pacemaker Guidelines. ACC/AHA/NASPE 2002 guideline update for implantation of cardiac pacemakers and antiarrhythmia devices: summary article: a report of the

American College of Cardiology/American Heart Association Task Force on Practice Guidelines (ACC/AHA/NASPE Committee to Update the 1998 Pacemaker Guidelines). *Circulation* 2002; **106**:2145-2161.

Johnson AM. Aortic stenosis, sudden death, and the left ventricular baroreceptors. *Br Heart J* 1971; **33**: 1–5.

Manganelli F, Betocchi S, Ciampi Q *et al.* Comparison of hemodynamic adaptation to orthostatic stress in patients with hypertrophic cardiomyopathy with or without syncope and in vasovagal syncope. *Amer J Cardiol* 2002; **89**:1405–1410.

Maron BJ. Hypertrophic cardiomyopathy. *Circulation* 2002; **106**: 2419–2421.

Nienaber CA, Hiller S, Spielmann RP, Geiger M, Kuck KH. Syncope in hypertrophic cardiomyopathy: multivariate analysis of prognostic determinants. *J Am Coll Cardiol* 1990; **15**: 948–955.

Shen WK, Decker WW, Smars PA. Syncope Evaluation in the Emergency Department Study (SEEDS): a multidisciplinary approach to syncope management. *Circulation* 2004; **110**: 3636–3645.

CHAPTER 20

Specific causes of syncope: their evaluation and treatment strategies

Part 5: Cerebrovascular disorders as the primary cause of syncope

J. Gert van Dijk

Introduction

As has been emphasized throughout this volume, neurological disease is rarely the cause of true syncope. Neurologic disturbances may cause other forms of loss of consciousness, such as in the case of epilepsy, or in the setting of head trauma causing loss of consciousness by way of concussion. However, syncope (i.e. transient loss of consciousness due to inadequate cerebral perfusion) should not typically lead to a search for a neurological etiology.

Goals

The goals of this part of the chapter are to:
• review the few important cerebrovascular conditions potentially associated with syncope; and
• emphasize the diagnostic differences between transient ischemic attacks (TIAs) and true syncope.

Transient ischemic attacks

Transient ischemic attacks (TIAs) may resemble syncope in terms of being transient and self-limited. The similarity ends there, however. TIAs commonly last longer, and are associated with transient localizing neurological signs and symptoms. However, an even more important difference lies in the symptomatology (Table 20.5.1). Syncope basically entails loss of consciousness without focal neurological deficit; TIAs are the exact opposite: focal neurological deficits without loss of consciousness. This holds without restrictions for carotid TIAs. Consequently, these two types of presentation do not cause any diagnostic confusion in neurology.

Vertebrobasilar TIAs are more likely to cause unconsciousness than are TIAs arising from the carotid circulation. However, once again, the symptomatology provides evidence for distinguishing this condition from true syncope.

Table 20.5.1 Clinical findings: syncope versus carotid or vertebrobasilar ischemia.

	Consciousness	Vision	Focal deficits
Syncope	Lost	May be impaired just before unconsciousness	None
Carotid TIA	Normal	Hemianopia or amaurosis fugax	Hemiparesis, hemianesthesia, aphasia, dysarthria, other higher cortical functions
Vertebrobasilar TIA	Rarely lost (not as isolated symptom)	Hemianopia	Hemiataxia, diplopia, hemiparesis, dysarthria, vertigo, cranial nerve symptoms

Vertebrobasilar TIAs are accompanied by focal neurologic deficits such as hemianopsia or ataxia, symptoms and signs that prove their nature as TIAs. The presence of such symptoms would be highly unlikely in the case of true syncope.

Subclavian steal

The subclavian steal syndrome may cause loss of consciousness. This relatively rare condition refers to the circumstance in which a luminal stenosis occurs at or near the origin of the subclavian artery (usually on the left), proximal to the origin of the vertebral artery. If the stenosis is sufficiently severe, exercise of the affected limb (a process that reduces vascular resistance in the muscle bed to enhance nutrient flow), may cause reversal of flow in the vertebral vessel. Reversal of flow pulls (steals) blood from the Circle of Willis in order to provide sufficient arm muscle blood flow. The net effect is diminution of blood flow to the brain, the prerequisite for true syncope. Subclavian steal syndrome can be detected by asking about the circumstances provoking the attack. Physical exercise involving an arm suggests this entity, and should be followed by measuring blood pressure in both arms and ultrasound studies if necessary. Relief of the stenosis by angioplasty or surgery eliminates the problem and susceptibility to syncope.

Migraine

In individuals who suffer from migraine, syncope of an orthostatic nature occurs statistically more often than in nonmigraineurs. These attacks do not occur at the same time as the migraine attacks, however, and so they can usually be distinguished without additional diagnostic confusion.

A rather rare type of vertebrobasilar migraine does involve impaired consciousness, but this lasts too long to cause confusion with true syncope. Nevertheless, making the diagnosis can be a challenge for most practitioners.

Consequently, when migraine-related syncope is being considered, referral to a specialist experienced in these conditions is prudent.

Summary

Cerebrovascular disorders are only rarely the cause of syncope. Consequently, in the absence of focal neurologic signs or symptoms suggesting such a possibility, their evaluation should be considered a low priority. In essence, any testing directed toward cerebrovascular disease should be reserved for those instances in which the contribution of more likely potential causes of syncope have been excluded.

Additional reading

Devuyst G, Bogousslavsky J, Meuli R, Moncayo J, de Freitas G, van Melle G. Stroke or transient ischemic attacks with basilar artery stenosis or occlusion: clinical patterns and outcome. *Arch Neurol* 2002; **59**: 567–573.

Savitz SI, Caplan LR. Vertebrobasilar disease. *N Engl J Med* 2005; **352**: 2618–2626.

Shechter A, Stewart WF, Silberstein SD, Lipton RB. Migraine and autonomic nervous system function. A population-based, case-control study. *Neurology* 2002; **58**: 422–427.

Wasson S, Bedi A, Singh A. Determining functional significance of subclavian artery stenosis using exercise thallium-201 stress imaging. *Southern Med J* 2005; **98**: 559–560.

CHAPTER 21

Syncope and other causes of transient loss of consciousness in children, teenagers, and adolescents

Wouter Wieling, Karin S. Ganzeboom, and Jan Janousek

Introduction

Transient loss of consciousness (TLOC) is common in young subjects. It is a dramatic event not only for the patients involved but also for other children, parents, and teachers. The main causes of TLOC in the young are:
• syncope, a sudden transient fall in systemic blood pressure resulting in a decrease in cerebral perfusion below a critical level necessary for maintenance of consciousness. Vasovagal syncope also called the common faint is by far the most common cause of TLOC in young subjects;
• neurological disorders, in particular epilepsy;
• psychiatric disorders mimicking true loss of consciousness, in particular conversion reactions (rare); and
• metabolic disorders (very rare).

Goals

The goals of this chapter are to review:
• epidemiology of TLOC, and syncope in particular, in children, teenagers, and adolescents;
• initial approach to diagnosis;
• subsequent work-up; and
• therapy of syncope and certain other important causes of TLOC.

Epidemiology

In children <6 years of age, TLOC is unusual; breath-holding spells, cardiac arrhythmias, and seizure disorders are the principal considerations when loss of consciousness does occur. This order of diagnostic consideration differs substantially from that recommended for older individuals.

In the general population, a peak incidence of TLOC is observed around the age of 15 years. The overall incidence of syncope coming to medical attention in childhood and adolescence is approximately 1 per 1000 (0.1%). By far the most common cause is a neurally mediated reflex syncope and in particular the vasovagal faint. The peak incidence of vasovagal fainting in the teenage period is thought to be related to the period of rapid growth. At the age of 20 years, about 20% of male subjects have experienced at least one vasovagal syncopal episode. The even higher prevalence in young women may be due to the hormonal changes during the menstrual cycle. By comparison, in the general population in this same age group, epilepsy has a much lower prevalence of about 5 per 1000 (0.5%) and cardiac syncope (i.e. cardiac arrhythmias or structural heart disease) is even less common.

Initial approach to the diagnostic evaluation

A detailed patient and family history is the most crucial part of the initial diagnostic work-up of a young patient with TLOC. The first challenge for the attending physician is to differentiate nonsyncope conditions that cause apparent TLOC (e.g. seizure disorders, drug intoxication) from true syncope (see Chapter 1). Then, the second challenge is to determine among the many young fainters whether a given patient with TLOC falls within the small proportion of patients that are prone to serious and potentially lethal conditions such as arrhythmias and other cardiac causes of syncope and seizures. Most young fainters have relatively innocent causes of TLOC, particularly neurally mediated reflex syncope.

The physical examination should focus on examination of the heart and measurement of blood pressure. Heart rate and blood pressure should be assessed with the patient both supine and after 3 min standing (see also Chapter 7 and Chapter 20, Part 2). A 12-lead surface electrocardiogram (ECG) is recommended to screen for rare forms of cardiac syncope, for example, long QT syndrome, preexcitation (e.g. Wolff–Parkinson–White [WPW] syndrome), heart block (congenital or acquired), or ventricular hypertrophy suggesting hypertrophic cardiomyopathy (HCM).

Common causes of syncope in the young
Neurally mediated reflex syncope (neural reflex syncope)

Neurally mediated reflex syncope disorders comprise a heterogeneous group of functional disturbances that are characterized by episodic reflex vasodilatation and/or bradycardia resulting in transient failure of blood pressure control (Figure 21.1). The pathophysiologic and clinical aspects of these disorders are dealt with in Chapters 3, 4, and 20, Part 1, respectively.

Reflex syncope disorders have an excellent prognosis, but may have serious social repercussions and a dramatic impact on the quality of life. Diagnosing these disorders is therefore of great importance. In most young patients without heart disease, if the history is typical for neurally mediated reflex syncope, and the physical examination and ECG is normal, then a presumptive

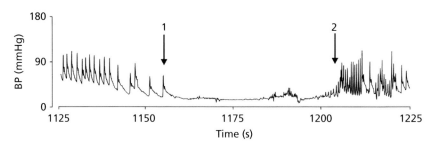

Figure 21.1 Blood pressure recording obtained in a 17-year-old boy with frequent faints due to blood injury phobia when a blood taking provocation was discussed. Just mentioning the procedure induced 50 s of asystole. (Finapres recordings.) Arrows: 1 = last heartbeat before asystole; 2 = first heartbeat after asystole, coinciding with the start of resuscitation. Time (s) taken from onset of ECG recording in this patient. (From van Dijk N, Velzeboer SC, Destree-Vonk A, Linzer M, Wieling W *PACE* 2001; **24**: 122–124 with permission of the editor.)

Table 21.1 Triggers of neurally mediated reflex faints in the young.

Emotional circumstances and pain, venipunctures, immunizations
Prolonged motionless standing, especially in combination with warm
  temperature, confined spaces, crowded rooms ('church syncope')
Fasting, lack of sleep, fatigue, menstruation, illness with fever
Micturition
(Post)exercise (i.e. after termination of long runs or vigorous bursts of
  activity during competitive sports)
Hyperventilation and straining (self-induced syncope)
Stretching
Coughing
Standing up quickly or arising from squatting
Pronounced weight loss
Certain medications, alcohol, and drugs (these need to be distinguished
  from intoxicated states, which can also cause loss of consciousness)

diagnosis of reflex syncope can be made without any other testing. Many young subjects with reflex syncope have a history of syncope in an immediate family member that has not been associated with sudden death and this may be helpful in formulating the differential diagnosis.

The main triggers causing neural reflex syncope in the young are similar to those in older people and are listed in Table 21.1. The more common specific neurally mediated faints are described below.

Vasovagal syncope
In young subjects vasovagal syncope is the most common of the neural reflex disorders (Figure 21.1). Two situations in particular are known to provoke

Table 21.2 Typical
premonitory symptoms
for vasovagal faints in
young subjects.

Lightheadedness
Palpitations
Weakness
Dimming or blurred vision
Nausea, epigastric distress
Feeling warm or cold
Facial pallor
Sweating, dilated pupils

this disorder. First, distressing emotional situations and pain can induce a vasovagal faint. The pathways involved descend from the corticohypo-thalamic centers in the brain to medullary cardiovascular centers. A typical example is an ordinary faint during blood drawing. This condition appears to be more common in young subjects than in adult subjects. Emotional triggers for vasovagal syncope or near-syncope in children and teenagers include having a hair cut, eye examinations, placing a contact lens, dental procedures, or watching television programs about medical matters or animal biology. Second, factors that increase pooling of venous blood below the heart such as long periods of standing motionless in combination with high ambient temperatures are also known to precipitate vasovagal syncope.

Young subjects often experience prodromal symptoms and signs when a spontaneous vasovagal syncope is imminent (Table 21.2). These prodromal symptoms are reported to be more intense than those in elderly subjects, perhaps related to a more intact cerebrovascular supply and a more robust autonomic nervous system responsiveness, and less complete disruption of memory during a vasovagal episode in the young. However, some young subjects have little or no prodromal symptoms and the collapse occurs without apparent warning of any kind.

In young subjects with recurrent episodes of vasovagal syncope, the present-ation can vary markedly encompassing the classical emotionally induced vaso-vagal episodes, posture-induced vasovagal syncope, and occasional vasovagal episodes with no consistent trigger. Apparently benign vasovagal episodes may even occur during normal daily exercises like playing, walking, or cyc-ling. Thus, the clinical presentation may vary widely both within and among young patients.

Other forms of neurally mediated reflex syncope
Situational faints are common in young patients. In this regard the description of these conditions is similar to that provided in Chapter 20, Part 1 for older patients. Carotid sinus syndrome, on the other hand, is not a consideration in

young patients (except in the rare case of a child who may have been subjected to neck surgery and/or radiation therapy to the neck).

Orthostatic syncope: postural orthostatic tachycardia syndrome and autonomic failure)
An orthostatic disorder that has received much attention lately is the so-called postural orthostatic tachycardia syndrome (POTS). It is defined by symptoms of cerebral hypoperfusion (e.g. lightheadedness, fatigue, weakness, blurred vision) and an excessive increase in heart rate in the upright posture (postural tachycardia). Other symptoms of sympathetic activation such as diaphoresis, nausea, and tremulousness may also occur (see also Chapter 4). The prevalence in the general population is not known, but is probably low.

Postural tachycardia is related to age, with lower incidence in older age groups. Thus the normal ranges need to be adjusted for age. We consider an increase in heart rate of >35 bpm or to >120 bpm in upright posture as excessive. The female : male ratio of POTS is about 4 or 5 : 1. Fainting occurs in a minority of these subjects.

The underlying mechanisms for POTS are debated. Partial denervation of the lower limbs as well as central nervous system functional disorders have been suggested as the basis for this disorder. When it is severe in terms of impact on well-being and lifestyle, POTS patients require evaluation at a specialty center in order for the diagnosis to be confirmed and treatment recommended. Mild forms of POTS are reasonably treated in the community. Treatment predominantly focuses on salt and volume repletion, tilt-training, and if necessary the use of vasoconstrictors such as midodrine.

Primary autonomic neuropathy as a cause of orthostatic hypotension and syncope is extremely rare in young subjects. Secondary autonomic neuropathy with symptomatic orthostatic hypotension and (near-) syncope may occur in the setting of chronic diseases like diabetes mellitus and in young patients using vasoactive medications.

Additional distinctive syncopal syndromes observed in the young
Fainting lark Nonreflex-mediated factors that are involved in fainting in young subjects include hyperventilation, where the decrease in $Pa\,CO_2$ may cause constriction of cerebral vessels. Straining, which impedes venous return, may also trigger syncope. These adjunctive factors, in conjunction with prolonged orthostatic stress, have been reported to be involved in epidemic syncope in female teenage fans during rock concerts. They are also incorporated in self-induced fainting. The latter stunt has been used by children, high school students, and military recruits as entertainment for their friends, and by others for more practical purposes such as avoiding imminent exams. The 'fainting lark' is the maneuver most commonly used. It combines the effects of acute arterial hypotension induced by standing up quickly and raised intrathoracic pressure with cerebral vasoconstriction due to hypocapnia. The fainting lark is initiated by the subject first squatting in a full knee bend and then overbreathing. The subject then stands up suddenly and performs a

forced expiration against a closed glottis. Almost instantaneous syncope with little or no warning symptoms occurs. The fainting lark has also been applied as a research tool to study the sequence of events during fainting in young adults (for more details see Chapter 3).

Syncope upon standing up. Abrupt onset of syncope or near-syncope upon standing is another relatively distinctive syncopal syndrome observed in young subjects (although similar symptoms also occur in older individuals) (Figure 21.2). The early onset after postural change, and rapid termination, distinguish this syndrome from orthostatic hypotension and POTS discussed earlier.

Almost all young subjects are familiar with a brief feeling of lightheadedness shortly after standing up quickly, characterized by its time of onset (5–10 s after standing up) and short duration (disappearance of symptoms within 30 s). The complaints occur especially after prolonged supine rest or after arising from the squatted position. In some instances, true syncope may occur upon standing in otherwise healthy teenagers and adolescents. The complaints are caused by a transient fall in systemic blood pressure, which occurs upon active standing, but not so dramatically (or not at all) upon passive head-up tilt (Figure 21.1). The initial transient fall in blood pressure in healthy subjects is ascribed to vasodilatation in the active muscles during standing up. The majority of the patients involved are reported to be tall with an asthenic habitus and poorly developed musculature.

Stretch syncope. Stretch syncope may occur during stretching with the neck hyperextended while standing. It is reported to occur in teenage boys with a familial tendency to faint. It has been attributed to effects of straining (which decreases systemic blood pressure) in combination with decreased cerebral blood flow caused by mechanical compression of the vertebral arteries. The latter element of the pathophysiology seems somewhat unlikely, but cannot be excluded.

Migraine. Migraine-related syncope is another syncopal syndrome thought to occur predominantly in young subjects. There are uncertainties regarding the relation of migraine to syncope. Most cases are probably vasovagal or orthostatic faints (see Chapter 20, Part 5).

It has been reported that syncope associated with migraine may be accompanied with prodromal symptoms that suggest brainstem ischemia due to basilar artery involvement (brainstem migraine). A 'typical' attack starts with bilateral visual symptoms, dysarthria, rotational vertigo, diplopia, nystagmus, ataxia, and TLOC, followed by a headache that is usually bioccipital and throbbing. The headache may not always be present. Patients are often adolescent females with a positive family history. Other symptoms and signs of abnormal vasomotor regulation, in particular Raynaud's phenomenon, are often

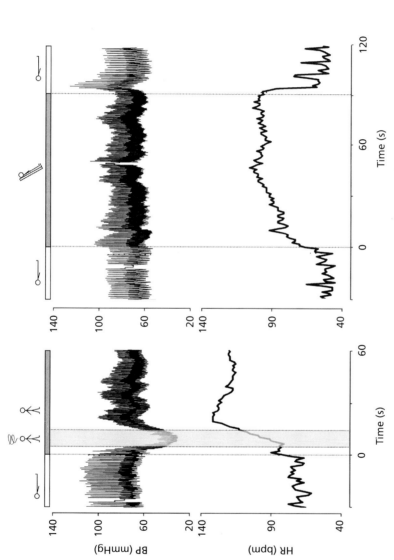

Figure 21.2 Changes in heart rate and blood pressure in a 20-year-old male with an asthenic habitus (197 cm and 73 kg) and a 10-year long history of almost daily near-syncope and occasional syncope upon standing up. Note the marked initial fall in finger blood pressure accompanied by lightheadedness upon active standing, but not upon a passive head-up tilt. (Revised from van Dijk N, Harms MP, Wieling W, *Ned Tijdschr Geneesk* 2000; **144**: 249–254 with permission of the editor.)

present. A role for orthostatic syncope in migraine sufferers has also been reported.

Breath-holding spells. Between the age of 0 and 4 years, the most common cause of syncope is what has been termed breath-holding spells, but they are only occasionally triggered by true breath-holding. In many cases there is a familial history.

There are two types of breath-holding spells.

• Pallid breath-holding spells occur if there is a sudden fright, a fall, or slight trauma. The crying phase is short or absent and often described as a 'silent cry' mimicking a Valsalva maneuver. The loss of consciousness occurs within seconds and is associated with hypotonia, which passes into rigidity with myoclonic jerks. Marked pallor is observed. The condition is most commonly caused by a vagally mediated cardiac inhibition. Some believe that these spells are the equivalent of the vasovagal faint of older individuals (see Chapter 20, Part 5).

• Cyanotic breath-holding spells are usually elicited by unpleasant emotionally charged situations. They usually happen if the child is upset or angry. Crying occurs at the beginning. The event increases in intensity and finally terminates with prolonged expiration and visible cyanosis. Loss of consciousness and hypotonia followed by a few myoclonic jerks often occur. The etiology of cyanotic breath-holding spells is not entirely clear. However, a few scenarios have been hypothesized including hypocapnic cerebral vasoconstriction due to hyperventilation during the crying phase, cerebral hypoxia due to hypoventilation, and reflex closure of the vocal cords inducing a Valsalva-like increase in intrathoracic pressure and intrapulmonary shunting with ventilation–perfusion mismatch. Importantly, syncope in toddlers may also occur unassociated with any event or crying, but is often still labeled as a 'breath-holding' spell.

Less frequent causes of syncope in the young
Cardiac syncope
Cardiac etiology should be considered first in patients who have any of the following:

• congenital or structural heart disease (including postoperative congenital heart disease, long QT syndrome, obstructive cardiomyopathy);

• few, if any, prodromal symptoms suggestive of neurally mediated reflex syncope;

• palpitations or chest pain as prodrome;

• syncope induced by exercise, auditory stimuli, swimming, or diving; or

• a positive family history for unexplained cardiac syncope or sudden death.

Arrhythmias
Arrhythmias tend to be the most common cause of cardiac syncope in young subjects. Table 21.3 summarizes the conditions of greatest concern

Table 21.3 Most important conditions associated with arrhythmias in the young.

Tachycardias

Postoperative congenital heart disease (e.g. ventricular septal defect repair, tetralogy of Fallot)

Hypertrophic obstructive cardiomyopathy (HOCM)

Preexcitation syndromes, especially WPW syndrome and concealed accessory AV connections (common)

Long QT syndrome (rare but potentially life-threatening ventricular tachyarrhythmias, torsades)

Brugada syndrome (rare, but life-threatening ventricular tachyarrhythmias)

Arrhythmogenic right ventricular dysplasia (relatively common, but variable manifestations)

Idiopathic ventricular fibrillation (rare)

Bradycardias

Acquired atrioventricular block (relatively rare, but occurs more frequently with postoperative congenital heart repairs)

Congenital AV block (syncope is now known to be more common than previously thought)

Acquired sinus node dysfunction (again most often seen with postoperative congenital heart repairs)

Familial sinus node disease (rare)

Bradycardia – tachycardia syndrome

Atrial or ventricular arrhythmias after surgical treatment for congenital heart disease (common)

---

predisposing to arrhythmic causes of syncope. Myocardial dysfunction is seldom a direct cause of syncope in young subjects. Exceptions are certain individuals with a cardiomyopathic picture resulting from congenital heart disease or on an idiopathic basis. In such cases, susceptibility to symptomatic arrhythmias is increased.

The syncope that occurs in the congenital long QT syndromes is due to hemodynamic compromise caused by a polymorphous *torsade de pointes* ventricular tachycardia (Figure 21.3). Most patients exhibit their first event in the first two decades of life. Episodes have been associated with fright, being awakened by a loud noise, or extreme emotional stress. Other triggering causes include diving and exercise. In many patients there is a positive family history of sudden death. The various forms of long QT syndromes (LQTS) and related 'ion channelopathies' have been the subject of intensive study in recent years. The reader is referred to detailed reviews of the subject.

Ventricular tachycardia (VT) due to arrhythmogenic right ventricular dysplasia/cardiomyopathy may be associated with syncope. It is often associated with exercise. However, sustained and nonsustained symptomatic VT can

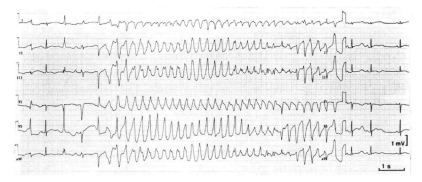

Figure 21.3 Six-lead ECG (leads I, II, III, AVF, V1, and V5) of a 14-year-old girl with syncopal attacks typically triggered by auditory stimuli. The tracings show a 10-s episode of *torsades de pointes*, which terminate spontaneously. Grossly abnormal QT intervals are observed immediately after termination of the arrhythmia. Long QT syndrome (LQTS) type 2 was diagnosed. (Courtesy of AAM Wilde, Professor of Experimental Cardiology, Academic Medical Center, Amsterdam, The Netherlands.)

occur at any time. This and other forms of VT are dealt with in more detail in Chapter 20, Part 3.

In patients with WPW syndrome and other forms of ventricular preexcitation, either paroxysmal supraventricular tachycardia alone or atrial fibrillation with a rapid ventricular response can be the cause of syncope. Many young patients may have paroxysmal supraventricular tachycardia using concealed accessory pathways and exhibit no evidence of preexcitation. The reentry mechanism is identical to that of conventional WPW regular (usually narrow) QRS tachycardia, and both are curable with catheter ablation techniques.

With a hypotensive tachycardia or marked bradycardia, the patient may appear to be pulseless and may have myoclonic jerks and urinary incontinence. Recovery is typically rapid with a sudden return of the pulse, flushing of the face, and usually full orientation of the patient. Certain of these rhythm disturbances may, however, lead to life-threatening consequences.

Primary obstructive cardiac causes of syncope

Obstructive conditions causing syncope in the young are in many respects similar to those seen in older subjects with the exception of atherosclerotic cardiovascular disease, which is rarely encountered in young individuals, and congenital anomalies that are more commonly detected in the young. As is true in older subjects, the basis of the faint may be the hemodynamic limitation imposed by the lesion, but could also be the result of arrhythmias or even neural reflex events. Multiple causes of syncope need to be kept in mind when contemplating therapy strategy. Obstructive conditions of particular importance in young subjects are:
• valvular/supravalvular aortic stenosis;
• hypertrophic cardiomyopathy (HOCM);

- primary pulmonary hypertension;
- tetralogy of Fallot;
- congenital anomalies of the coronary arteries
- postoperative congenital heart disease (especially ventricular septal defect repair); and
- Eisenmenger's syndrome.

Congenital anomalies of the coronary arteries are particularly important conditions to consider when syncope is associated with exercise. Entrapment of a coronary artery between the pulmonary artery and aorta is among the more common of these abnormalities. Angiography is usually needed, and surgical correction is necessary.

Syncope-Mimics

Psychogenic causes (pseudosyncope)

A conversion reaction is a rare cause of apparent TLOC in young subjects. However, it may occur in adolescents, and especially in females.

Consideration should be given to this diagnosis in the instance of a relatively high frequency of syncope recurrences (up to several times a day) and absence of associated physical injury. The duration of the apparent (not real) loss of consciousness is often prolonged. During an episode, it is common for tightly closed eyes or voluntary lid closure with lid flutter to be observed; in contrast during true syncope or epilepsy the eyes are often open and deviated. An unusual posture may be assumed. Some of these patients are found to have suffered from sexual abuse or battering. Malingering with simulated convulsions (pseudoseizures) has also been reported in young subjects as a cause of TLOC. Finally, illicit substance abuse, in particular of alcohol and cocaine, is associated with exotic unexplained episodes of syncope in young subjects. The reader is referred to Chapter 18 for additional discussion of psychogenic 'pseudo-syncope'.

Distinguishing syncope and epilepsy

Myoclonic jerks mimicking a seizure may occur during vasovagal syncope and in other forms of syncope as well. An asystole of about 10 s duration is needed in adults before myoclonic jerks occur. In young persons, the anoxic threshold is reported to be lower than in adults. It is lowest in early childhood. Clinical features known to be helpful for distinguishing myoclonic jerks from the abnormal motor activity associated with 'grand mal' seizures are summarized in Table 21.4.

Subsequent diagnostic work-up

The history and the physical examination guide the attending physicians in choosing the subsequent diagnostic work-up. In the case of a history typical for reflex-mediated syncope (e.g. vasovagal faint, postmicturition syncope, etc.), the absence of abnormalities on physical examination and a normal ECG are

Table 21.4 Distinguishing myoclonic jerks from the abnormal motor activity associated with 'grand mal' (generalized) seizures.

In neurally mediated reflex syncope, myoclonic jerks start after the subject has fallen on the floor, whereas in epilepsy the tonic clonic movements start while standing.

Young subjects having an ordinary faint normally become very pale, while patients having a seizure may be cyanotic.

In epilepsy, the duration of the loss of consciousness is longer (usually >5 min), whereas in reflex syncope loss of consciousness is usually short (often 1 min or less).

Urinary incontinence can happen both in reflex syncope and in epilepsy but seems to be more common in epilepsy.

Loss of bowel control suggests epilepsy.

Tongue biting almost exclusively occurs in epilepsy.

Postictal confusion always happens in epilepsy and is prolonged, whereas it is less intense and shortlasting in reflex syncope. However, prolonged fatigue may occur after reflex syncope and is very characteristic of the vasovagal faint.

The ability to stand upright occurs in epilepsy before complete recovery of mental function, whereas in reflex syncope it usually occurs after complete recovery of mental function (although the patient may remain 'fatigued').

---

usually sufficient to make a diagnosis. Further investigations are not necessary. The work-up for other than reflex-mediated syncopes is case specific.

Ambulatory ECG (AECG) recorders should be used for patients with a history of palpitations associated with syncope. Whether to choose a 24-h, 48-h, or longer-term recorder depends on the anticipated frequency of attacks suggested in the medical history. Implantable loop recorders (ILRs) may be particularly effective in cases of troublesome but infrequent syncope and in younger patients who may not be able to manage an external recording system at school or when very active.

Cardiology consultation including echocardigraphy should be obtained in the case of a heart murmur. Whenever syncope occurs during exertion or emotion an echocardiogram and an exercise test should be performed in addition to the careful history, physical examination, and ECG. Electro-encephalography (EEG) is indicated for patients showing prolonged loss of consciousness, seizure activity, and a significant postictal phase of lethargy and confusion. The EEG is not, however, recommended as a 'screening tool' in the evaluation of most patients who present with TLOC.

Electrophysiologic study has a very minor role in pediatric patients with syncope, especially in the absence of structural heart disease. Testing may be warranted if a tachyarrhythmia is suspected, particularly in the case of operated congenital heart disease, HOCM, arrhythmogenic right ventricular dysplasia/cardiomyopathy (ARVD), and preexcitation syndromes.

In patients with 'atypical' vasovagal syncope or unexplained syncope and a normal cardiac evaluation, tilt-table testing can be helpful. Such testing may not be warranted given a single syncope, but is certainly warranted if a second occurrence develops and in patients with multiple faints. Head-up tilt tests may have a relatively high 'false-positive' rate (15–20% in adults) and should therefore be interpreted with caution for the primary identification of patients with vasovagal syncope. The false-positive rate may be higher in children and adolescents than in adult patients, especially after instrumentation (e.g. placement of venous or arterial cannula): an incidence of near-fainting of 40% was reported during a head-up tilt test after placement of a simple intravenous line in healthy children and teenagers. The false-negative rate in adults has been estimated to be as high as 50%, but this number is uncertain. In young subjects the 'false-negative' rate is probably lower.

Tilt-table testing can be helpful for patients with conversion reactions. In such cases, loss of consciousness may occur with little or no significant decrease in heart rate, blood pressure, or cerebral blood flow. A normal EEG may be observed during monitored episodes. Further, the patient can be observed by the physician and typical markers of vasovagal syndrome are absent.

Therapy

The cause of the syncopal event determines the appropriate therapy. Therapy for other than reflex-mediated syncopes like cardiac arrhythmias and seizures is straightforward and case specific. Since vasovagal syncope is so common in this age group, it is reasonable to discuss its treatment strategy in greater detail (see also Chapter 20, Part 1).

Aborting the acute episode

For acute management of the vasovagal faint (and certain situational faints), recognition of warning symptoms and subsequent resumption of the supine position is usually sufficient. Elevation of the legs may be performed in order to increase venous return to the heart. Traditionally sitting with lowering the head between the knees has been advocated to abort an attack.

Instruction to apply physical counter-maneuvers that can decrease downward pooling of venous blood and thereby increase stroke volume and cardiac output at the earliest recognition of presyncope is helpful in many young patients (see also Chapter 20, Part 2). We have found the combination of leg crossing and muscle tensing easily taught and effective in young patients with reflex syncope (Figure 21.4) (see also Chapter 3). Patients are advised to use leg crossing as a preventive measure to improve orthostatic tolerance under stressful conditions and to combine leg crossing with tensing of leg and abdominal muscles when a faint is imminent (Figure 21.4). Squatting can be used as an emergency measure to prevent loss of consciousness when presyncopal symptoms develop rapidly. A major advantage of applying physical counter-maneuvers is that they can be applied immediately at the start of hypotensive symptoms and the patient can regain self-confidence in stressful situations. In the longer term, tilt-training may be a useful consideration. However, questionable compliance may limit its effectiveness in young individuals.

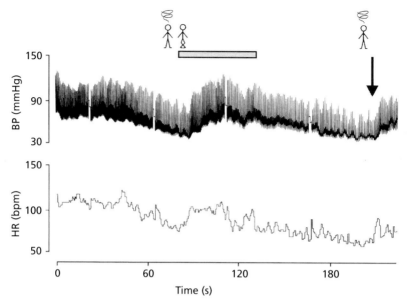

Figure 21.4 Aborting a vasovagal faint by the combination of leg crossing and muscle tensing. In a 15-year-old female subject with recurrent syncope, a typical vasovagal syncope episode was induced during orthostatic stress testing on a tilt-table. Note progressive fall in finger arterial pressure and heart rate. After crossing of the legs and tensing of leg and abdominal muscles, blood pressure and heart rate recover quickly. After uncrossing of the legs a vasovagal reaction is observed (arrow) and the subject has to be returned to supine position. Bar indicates onset of leg crossing and muscle tensing. (From Krediet and Wieling, unpublished.)

Long-term treatment options

In the long term, the most important point in patients with neural reflex syncope is explanation (education) and reassurance regarding the nature of the condition. Patients should be informed that there is minimal risk of sudden death but that physical injury is still of some concern. Initial advice should include early recognition of warning symptoms and avoidance of triggering events. A tilt-table test can be employed for explanation and to teach the patient to recognize early premonitory symptoms in a safe setting. The frequency of syncope events decreases substantially after tilt-table testing. It has been suggested that the clinical encounter, education, and counseling that are associated with this diagnostic procedure have the effect of a positive therapeutic intervention.

A low salt diet should be avoided. Advice for 'superhydration', that is, enough liquid intake to produce colorless urine at a frequency of twice in the morning and twice in the afternoon may help. Two glasses of water with meals is practical advice. During sporting activities and when symptomatic, 'electrolyte' (NaCl)-containing liquids, which expand the extracellular fluid volume, should be advised. These may also be used on everyday to facilitate hydration.

In highly motivated patients with recurrent vasovagal symptoms, the prescription of progressively prolonged periods of enforced upright posture (so-called 'tilt training') is reported to reduce syncope recurrence (see Chapter 20, Part 1). The mechanism underlying its effectiveness is unknown. Compliance with this procedure limits its use in our experience in young subjects.

In young patients with vasovagal reflex syncope due to blood phobia, psychologic deconditioning is the first choice of therapy. In one to five sessions, depending on the seriousness of the phobia, patients are exposed to phobic stimuli and taught to apply body tension. Prognosis after psychologic counseling seems to be very good.

Pharmacologic therapy should be reserved for the rare patient with continued symptoms despite behavior modification. However, undesirable side-effects associated with drugs often outweigh any proposed beneficial effects. Additionally, pharmacologic treatment is less successful for hypotension induced by physical exercise or in warm surroundings. Another unresolved issue is for how long prophylactic therapy with any compound should be advised, since reflex syncope is a self-limited, non-life-threatening condition. Beta-blockers are often used but the overall evidence in their favor is weak (see recently reported POST study). Despite the absence of controlled studies, the mineralocorticoid fludrocortisone is often used early in the management of vasovagal syncope in an attempt to increase blood volume in young subjects. The combination of fludrocortisone with increased salt intake is required for an optimal effect. Fluid retention and hypertension in young subjects are reported to be less problematic than in the elderly. Other medications include alpha-adrenergic agonists like midodrine or pseudoephedrine to increase the peripheral vascular resistance and venous tone.

Even in the instance of cardioinhibitory syncope with an exaggerated asystolic response, pacemaker therapy should be avoided whenever possible. Management with conventional therapy without the need for pacemaker implantation is almost always effective and clearly preferable in young patients. It seems sensible to reserve pacing for rare young subjects who have repeatedly exhibited prolonged asystole during a typical attack and in whom the treatments discussed earlier have not proved effective. In many cases an ILR may need to be implanted to document such episodes. Breath-holding spells generally do not require specific therapy unless connected with long asystole periods associated with potential cerebral injury.

Summary

Syncope is common in children, teenagers, and adolescents. It is usually attributable to neurally mediated reflex syncope, but the differential diagnosis includes other less common but potentially dangerous disorders such as cardiac dysrythmias or ventricular outflow tract obstruction. The most important part of the diagnostic evaluation is taking a good history. An ECG is a helpful screening tool for identifying those who may have structural disease and for unmasking rarer cardiac causes such as preexcitation or long QT syndrome.

The patient's symptoms before and after the syncopal episode and an observer's description of the event will help to determine the cause in the vast majority of patients. If there is doubt about the diagnosis, cardiac causes must be ruled out and if necessary a tilt-table test can be done.

The mainstay of management of young patients with reflex syncope consists of advice and education on the various factors that influence systemic blood pressure in conjunction with chronic expansion of the intravascular volume or reducing the vascular volume into which pooling occurs.

Additional reading

Benrud-Larson LM, Devar MS, Sandroni P, Rummans TA, Haythornthwaite JA, Low PA. Quality of life in patients with postural tachycardia syndrome. *Mayo Clinic Proceedings* 2002; **77**: 531–537.

Krediet CTP, Van Dijk N, Linzer M, Van Lieshout JJ, Wieling W. Management of vaso-vagal syncope: controlling or aborting faints by the combination of leg crossing and muscle tensing. *Circulation* 2002; **106**: 1684–1689.

Massin MM, Bourguignont A, Coremans C, et al. Syncope in pediatric patients presenting to an emergency department. *J Pediatr* 2004; **145**: 223–228.

Priori SG, Barhanin J, Hauer RNW *et al.* Genetic and molecular basis of cardiac arrhythmias: impact on clinical management. Parts I and II. *Circulation* 1999; **99**: 518–528.

Singer W, Shen WK, Opfer-Gehrking TL, Mcphee BR, Hilz MJ, Low PA. Evidence of an intrinsic sinus node abnormality in patients with postural tachycardia syndrome. *Mayo Clinic Proceedings* 2002; **77**: 246–252.

Steinberg LA, Knilans TK. Syncope in children: diagnostic tests have a high cost and low yield, *J Pediatr* 2005; **146**: 355–358.

Van Dijk N, Velzeboer SCJM, Destree-Vonk A, Linzer M, Wieling W. Psychological treatment of malignant vasovagal syncope due to blood phobia. *PACE* 2001; **24**: 122–124.

Wieling W, Ganzeboom KS, Saul JP. Syncope in children and adolescents. *Heart* 2004; **90**: 1094–1100.

CHAPTER 22

Syncope in the older adult (including driving implications)

Rose Anne Kenny and David G. Benditt

Introduction

Syncope is a common problem in older persons. The prevalence of syncope increases with advancing years after the age of 60. The prevalence is particularly high in frail older persons. In one study, 23% of residents in a nursing home had syncope episodes over a 2-year period, and 30% of affected individuals had recurrent syncope.

The assessment, investigation, and management of syncope in older persons are for the most part the same as in younger individuals. However, if frailty or cognitive impairment coexist, then assessment and management will have to be tailored to the individual person's needs.

Goals

The objectives of this chapter are to:
• highlight certain unique features associated with the evaluation of transient loss of consciousness (TLOC) in the older individual; and
• provide insight into diagnostic concerns that tend to be more important in the elderly.

Falls, transient loss of consciousness, and syncope in the elderly: general considerations

Compared with younger individuals, older patients are more susceptible to conditions that may be interpreted (or misinterpreted) to be syncope. Thus 'falls' due to accidents, as well as apparent 'falls' that are in fact associated with true syncope, are prevalent in the elderly and not infrequently cause diagnostic dilemmas. Other forms of TLOC including seizures and minor concussions due to accidents further compound the difficulty of diagnosis in many cases. Finally, even 'true syncope' in older individuals presents several important problems. First, older patients are more likely to be unable to provide a detailed medical history due in part to a greater tendency to retrograde amnesia for premonitory events and also in some cases as a result of failing mental capacity. Second, unlike younger generally healthy patients, the elderly fainter is more likely to have multiple coexisting medical issues, any one of which could account for a faint, thereby complicating the evaluation due to the presence of multiple potential causes of syncope. Third, the older frail individual is at higher risk for significant physical injury, especially bony fractures and subdural hematomas. Lastly, susceptibility to faints in the elderly is more likely to result in loss of an independent lifestyle and lead to being prematurely institutionalized. The latter two issues are of particular importance given the enormous cost burden of health care in older age.

A number of age-related factors influence the increased prevalence and altered presentation of syncope with advancing years:
• age-related physiological changes in baroreflex activity, the renin angiotensin system, and intravascular volume homeostasis;
• some conditions are almost exclusively age-related – carotid sinus syndrome is the best example;
• comorbidity is common, particularly cardiovascular and neurological;
• polypharmacy is frequent – 40% of >65 year olds are taking more than three medications;
• cognitive impairment is common, resulting in lack of recall and details of events;
• Events are less likely to be witnessed – about 60% of syncopal events are unwitnessed in >70 year olds;
• multidisciplinary assessment may be necessary – combined medical, nursing, occupational therapy, and physiotherapy assessment;
• more than one possible cause is more likely, requiring a multifaceted assessment and treatment strategy.

Causes of syncope in the older adult

Most common causes of syncope in older adults are neurally mediated reflex syncope (particularly carotid sinus hypersensitivity), orthostatic hypotension, and cardiac arrhythmias.

Neurally mediated reflex syncope is relatively frequent in older individuals; however, medication related triggers and carotid sinus hypersensitivity are far more common than in younger fainters. Over half the episodes are related to prescription of cardiovascular medications.

Carotid sinus hypersensitivity is an age-related diagnosis. It is rare before the age of 50 years, and the prevalence increases with advancing years and with cardiovascular, cerebrovascular, and neurodegenerative comorbidity. Cardioinhibitory carotid sinus syndrome has been considered in recent reports to be an attributable cause of symptoms in up to 20% of syncope.

The prevalence of orthostatic hypotension in older adults varies from 6% in community-dwelling elderly, to 33% in elderly hospital inpatients. Orthostatic hypotension is an attributable cause of syncope in 20 to 30% of older patients. In symptomatic patients up to 25% have 'age-related' orthostatic

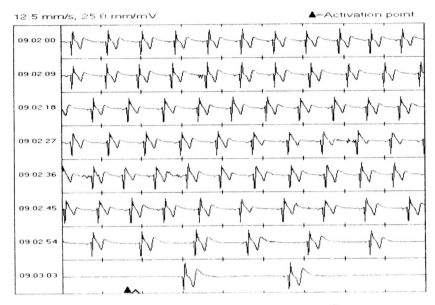

12.5 mm/s, 25.0 mm/mV   ▲=Activation point

Figure 22.1 Ambulatory ECG recording from an ILR (Reveal Plus®, Medtronic Inc., Minneapolis, MN) showing evidence of marked sinus bradycardia in a patient who presented with syncope. The letter 'A' indicates the point in time in which the device was triggered by the heart rate having fallen below a physician programmed predetermined limit. In this instance, the patient was unaware of a problem and did not manually trigger the recording. Nonetheless, the severity of the finding provides a reasonable basis for assuming that the patient's faints were due to bradyarrhythmia.

hypotension, in the remainder orthostatic hypotension is predominantly due to medications. Primary autonomic failure, secondary autonomic failure (e.g., diabetes), and Parkinson's disease are additional causes in this age group. Supine systolic hypertension is often present in older patients with orthostatic hypotension. Hypertension may increase the risk of cerebral ischemia from sudden declines in blood pressure, but it also complicates treatment, given that most agents used for the treatment of orthostatic hypotension will exacerbate supine hypertension (see Chapter 20, Part 2).

Up to 20% of syncope in older patients is due to cardiac arrhythmias. The reader is referred to Chapter 20, Part 3 for more details. In brief, though, older patients with syncope and bundle branch block are now thought to have a relatively high predilection to transient symptomatic high-grade atrioventricular (AV) block and many of them will ultimately prove to need cardiac pacemakers. The use of ILRs for diagnostic assessment can be extremely valuable in this age group as it markedly diminishes the need for the patient to be facile with an external recording apparatus (Figure 22.1).

Diagnostic evaluation

In the elderly patient, an initial evaluation comprising a detailed history, clinical examination, orthostatic blood pressure measurement, and supine and upright carotid sinus massage will provide a diagnosis in over 50% (see Chapter 7). However, about one-third of elderly patients will have more than one possible attributable cause for syncope. Consequently, it is important to be open minded in undertaking the assessment and utilize selected tests to confirm suspected diagnoses when there is any doubt.

History taking

Aspects of history taking in older adults vary in emphasis and clinical details from that obtained from younger adults. Cognitive impairment is present in 5% of 65 year olds and 20% of 80 year olds; cognitive status will influence the accuracy of recall for events. Consequently, older patients who have syncope episodes that are not witnessed may present to the physician as having simply 'fallen' and any evidence of true syncope in the history may have been lost due to retrograde amnesia for the transient loss of consciousness. A further explanation of why older patients present with 'a fall' is loss of balance during cerebral hypoperfusion. Gait and balance instability and slow protective reflexes are common (present in 20 to 50% of community-dwelling elderly) and moderate hemodynamic changes insufficient to cause syncope may result in falls. Up to one-third of syncope or near-syncope events will thus present as 'falls'.

The history should include details of social circumstances, injurious events, impact of events on patient confidence, and ability to remain independent for activities of daily living. The time of day when events occur can also be helpful for diagnosis. Events due to orthostatic hypotension usually occur in the morning. The history should include any association with meals (post-prandial), ingestion of medications, nocturnal micturition, etc. Medications frequently cause or contribute to syncope. Details of the medication history should include duration of treatment, time relationship of this to the onset of events, and times when medications are ingested. It may be helpful to correlate meal times and medication ingestion to 24-h ambulatory blood pressure recordings.

The history should also include details of comorbid diagnoses, in particular associations with physical frailty and locomotor disability (e.g. arthritis, Parkinson's disease, and cerebrovascular disease) and diagnoses that increase the likelihood of cardiovascular syncope (e.g. diabetes, anemia, hypertension, ischemic heart disease, and heart failure).

Physical examination

Elderly patients have a high prevalence of cardiac disease. Consequently careful cardiac and peripheral vascular examination may pay handsome dividends. Evaluation for extra heart sounds and murmurs may suggest the presence of significant structural heart disease. An echocardiogram is then usually warranted to provide quantitative assessment. On the other hand, carotid bruits, although relatively frequent in this population, are almost never the cause of the problem. The physician should not be overly aggressive with neurological tests in such cases, unless evident neurological signs are present or the history is more suggestive of a seizure or drop attack than syncope.

Assessment of the neurological and locomotor systems, including observation of gait and standing balance (eyes open, eyes closed), is recommended as part of the initial evaluation in older patients. If cognitive impairment is suspected this should be formally evaluated. The mini-mental state examination is a 20-item, internationally validated tool adequate for this purpose. Some older persons may require a comprehensive geriatric assessment.

Investigations

In cognitively normal older patients with syncope or unexplained falls, the diagnostic work-up is largely the same as for younger adults. Exceptions include routine supine and upright carotid sinus massage, given the high prevalence of carotid sinus syndrome as a cause of syncope and unexplained falls in the older age group. In up to a third of older patients with carotid sinus syndrome, a diagnostic cardioinhibitory (i.e. demonstration of an induced pause of >3 s duration) response is only present when upright.

Orthostatic hypotension is not always reproducible – particularly so for afternoon measurements in medication-related or age-related orthostatic hypotension. Repeated morning measurements are recommended. If medication-induced or postprandial hypotension is suspected, 24-h ambulatory blood pressure recordings may be helpful. However, the methodology of obtaining ambulatory blood pressure recordings (e.g. repetitive sphygmomanometer measurements) is a limiting factor. In older patients with orthostatic hypotension, diurnal patterns of blood pressure are the mirror image of normal blood pressure behavior, being highest at night and lowest in the mornings (and possibly after meals). Knowledge of diurnal blood pressure behavior can guide treatment and may be particularly helpful in modifying the timing of medications.

The role of insertable loop recorders (ILR) for evaluation of the causes of syncope has been alluded to in several chapters of this book. Very recently, the ISSUE 2 trial results were presented (European Society of Cardiology Scientific Sessions, Stockholm, Sweden, September 2005). These findings indicate that ILR findings are not only of diagnostic value, but can be used effectively to direct therapeutic decisions.

In essence, the ISSUE 2 prospective multicenter observational study assessed the efficacy of specific therapy based on ILR diagnostic observations in patients with recurrent suspected neurally mediated syncope (NMS). Patients with ≥3 clinically severe syncopal episodes in the last 2 years, and without significant electrocardiographic and cardiac abnormalities, were included. Orthostatic hypotension and carotid sinus syncope were excluded. After ILR implantation, patients were followed until the first documented syncope

(Phase I). The ILR documentation of this episode determined the subsequent therapy and commenced Phase II follow-up. Among 392 patients, the 1-year recurrence rate of syncope during Phase I was 33%. Of these, 103 patients had a documented episode and entered Phase II: 53 patients received specific therapy, 47 a pacemaker because of asystole of a median 11.5 s duration and 6 antitachyarrhythmia therapy (catheter ablation – four, implantable defibrillator – one, antiarrhythmic drug) and the remaining 50 patients did not receive specific therapy. The 1-year recurrence rate in 53 patients assigned to a specific therapy was 10% (burden 0.07 ± 0.2 episodes per patient/year) compared with 41% (burden 0.83 ± 1.57 episodes per patient/year) in the patients without specific therapy (80% relative risk reduction for patients, $p = 0.002$, and 92% for burden, $p = 0.002$). The 1-year recurrence rate in patients with pacemakers was 5% (burden 0.05 ± 0.15 episodes per patient/year). Severe trauma secondary to syncope relapse occurred in 2%, mild trauma in 4% of the patients. Consequently, it appears that a strategy based on early diagnostic ILR application, with therapy delayed until documentation of syncope allows a safe, specific and effective therapy is of value in NMS patients of the type included in this study.

Evaluation of the frail elderly

Age *per se* is not a contraindication to assessment and intervention. However, in the more frail patients, the rigor of the assessment will depend on compliance with tests, overall prognosis, and patient and family wishes. Orthostatic blood pressure measurements, carotid sinus massage, and head-up tilt studies are usually well-tolerated tests, even in the frail elderly with cognitive impairment. If patients have difficulty standing unaided, the tilt table can be used to assess orthostatic blood pressure changes.

As a rule, the conventional 12-lead ECG only rarely provides an unequivocal basis for syncope, since the recording is only rarely taken at a time when symptoms are present. However, the 12-lead ECG may provide strong suggestive evidence in cases in which the observed abnormality is severe, such as intermittent AV block or sinus pauses (Figure 22.2). On the other hand, ambulatory ECG recorders can be of great value in the early stages of diagnostic evaluation of the older fainter (Figure 22.1, also see Chapter 12). In particular, implantable loop recorders (ILRs) offer long-term diagnostic monitoring with a minimally invasive procedure. The utility and cost-effectiveness of this approach has been well-demonstrated. MCOT-type systems (e.g. Cardionet®, San Diego, CA) are rapidly evolving and will be of importance for patients who are reluctant to undergo even the relatively minor ILR invasive procedure (see Chapter 12). Finally, the ATP test is being evaluated as a means of unmasking subtle forms of bradycardia in older patients. This test can be easily carried out in the clinic, is very safe, and may obviate the need for continued outpatient monitoring.

In those cases in which any invasive diagnostic procedure and repeated hospital admission are deemed inappropriate or refused by the patient, it may be

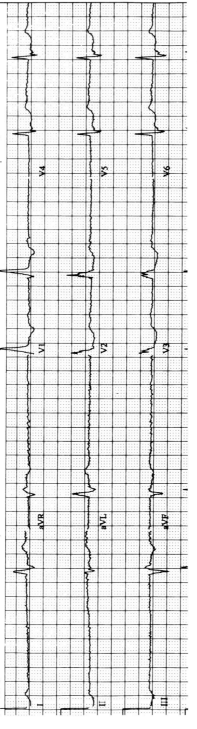

Figure 22.2 12-lead ECG recording in an older patient with syncope, bifascicular conduction system disease, moderately depressed ejection fraction (EF = 45%), and second degree Type 1 AV block. Although the patient was asymptomatic during the recording, in this instance the likelihood of block within the infra-nodal conduction system is very high and is reasonably assumed to account for syncope. A pacemaker was deemed to be indicated.

necessary to treat 'blind' using limited clinical data, that is, by altering possible culprit medication, prescribing antiarrhythmic agents, and/or cardiac pacing. Thus, in the frail elderly, it may be more frequently necessary for physicians to make clinical judgments as to the most likely cause of loss of consciousness than is the case in younger patients.

There is good evidence that modification of cardiovascular risk factors for falls/syncope reduces the incidence of subsequent events. Whether or not treatment of hypotension or arrhythmias decelerates cognitive decline in older patients is not known.

Driving and syncope

The vast majority of road accidents are caused by drowsiness and/or alcohol and perhaps increasingly due to inattention related to driving conveniences such as use of mobile telephones. Younger drivers tend to be more susceptible to driving impairment as a consequence of various forms of intoxication or lack of attention, than are older drivers. Medically related causes of motor vehicle accidents are in fact unusual. Most medical causes of road accidents occur in drivers who are already known to have preexisting disease. Thus older drivers are more likely to be at risk in terms of syncope and also perhaps sleep disorders.

Sudden driver incapacity has been reported with an incidence approximating only 1/1000 of all traffic accidents. Apart from intoxicated states such as those occurring with alcohol or other drugs, the medical condition of a driver tends not to be an important factor in road accidents causing injury to others. The most common causes of road accidents involving presumed TLOC at the wheel are listed in Table 22.1.

An American Heart Association (AHA)/North American Society of Pacing and Electrophysiology (NASPE) medical/scientific statement dealing with personal and public safety issues related to arrhythmias that may affect

Table 22.1 Causes of 2000 road accidents involving collapse at wheel, based on reports by the police to Driver Vehicle Licensing Agency.

Causes	Reported (%)
Epilepsy	38%
Blackouts	21%
Diabetes on insulin	18%
Heart condition	8%
Stroke	7%
Others	7%

consciousness, proposed recommendations on driving after syncope. Recommendations were provided for the following groups of drivers and the reader is referred to that publication for details:

• Drivers of ordinary motorcycles, cars, and other small vehicles with and without a trailer.

• Drivers of vehicles over 5 metric tons or passenger-carrying vehicles exceeding eight seats excluding the driver.

• Drivers of taxis, small ambulances, and other vehicles that form an intermediate category between the ordinary private driver and the vocational driver.

The ESC Syncope Task Force guidelines advise only minimal restrictions for ordinary drivers with heart disease and syncope. Only temporary suspension of driving is needed during the diagnostic evaluation. However, local government regulations should be consulted before making a final recommendation. Depending on the specific rules in each jurisdiction, professional drivers may be required to undergo prolonged restriction from driving (6 months or longer) until an effective treatment is demonstrated. Regulations for commercial drivers (and for airmen) tend to be much stricter, and the physician is advised to consult government regulations for these cases.

Summary

The evaluation of mobile, independent, cognitively normal older adults is similar to that of younger individuals. However, risk factor stratification and the contribution of individual abnormalities to symptom reproduction are more complex in the older individual than in healthier younger individuals. Multiple risk factors are more common in the elderly and the boundaries between falls, accidents, and syncope are often blurred.

Older patients have a median of five risk factors for syncope or falls. Morning orthostatic blood pressure measurements and, supine and upright carotid sinus massage are a more integral part of the initial evaluation in the older patient (unless contraindicated) than is the case in the younger subject. In frailer older adults, the evaluation should be modified according to prognosis. Driving and avocation restrictions must consider local government regulations and should be individualized.

Further reading

Armstrong VL. Lawson J. Kamper AM. Newton J. Kenny RA. The use of an implantable loop recorder in the investigation of unexplained syncope in older people. *Age & Ageing* 2003; **32**: 185–188.

Driving and heart disease. Task Force Report. Prepared on behalf of the ESC Task Force by MC Petch. *Eur Heart J* 1998; **19**: 1165–1177.

Epstein AE, Miles WM, Benditt DG, Camm AJ *et al.* Personal and public safety issues related to arrhythmias that may affect consciousness: implications for regulation and physician recommendations. *Circulation* 1996; **94**: 1147–1166.

Ermis C, Zhu AX, Pham S, *et al.* Comparison of automatic and patient-activated arrhythmia recordings by implantable loop recorders in the evaluation of syncope. *Amer J Cardiol* 2003; **92**: 815–819.

Herner B, Smedby B, Ysander L. Sudden illness as a cause of motor vehicle accidents. *Br J Int Med* 1966; **23**: 37–41.

Kenny RA. Syncope in the elderly: diagnosis, evaluation, and treatment. *J Cardiovasc Electrophysiol* 2003; **14**: S74–77.

Kenny RA, Richardson DA, Steen N, Bexton RS, Shaw FE, Bond J. Carotid sinus syndrome: a modifiable risk factor for nonaccidental falls in older adults (SAFE PACE). *J Am Coll Cardiol* 2001; **38**: 1491–1496.

Kurbaan AS, Bowker TJ, Wijesekera N, Franzen AC, Heaven D, Itty S, Sutton R. Age and hemodynamic responses to tilt testing in those with syncope of unknown origin. *J Am Coll Cardiol* 2003; **41**: 1004–1007.

O'Shea D. Setting up a falls and syncope service for the elderly. *Clinics in Geriatric Medicine* 2002; **18**: 269–278.

Parry SW. Steen IN. Baptist M. Kenny RA. Amnesia for loss of consciousness in carotid sinus syndrome: implications for presentation with falls. *J Am Coll Cardiol.* 2005; **45**: 1840–1843.

Varga E. Worum F. Szabo Z. Varga M. Lorincz I. Motor vehicle accident with complete loss of consciousness due to vasovagal syncope. Forensic Science International. 2002; **130**: 156–159.

Ward C, Kenny RA. Reproducibility of orthostatic hypotension in symptomatic elderly. *Am J Med* 1996; **100**: 418–422.

CHAPTER 23

Conditions that mimic syncope

J. Gert van Dijk

Introduction

Certain medical conditions may cause a real or apparent loss of consciousness that might appear to be syncope but is in fact not a true syncope. In order to understand which conditions may mimic syncope, we must take one step upwards on a hierarchical tree of definitions towards a larger entity – transient loss of consciousness (TLOC) – of which syncope is a subset (Figure 23.1).

Syncope is defined as a transient, self-limited loss of consciousness with a rapid onset, spontaneous and prompt recovery, and *caused by global cerebral hypoperfusion*. That final element of the definition is crucial to understanding not just what syncope is, but also what the differential diagnosis may be. In essence, 'syncope-mimics' are conditions that are also associated with TLOC or seem to be associated with TLOC, *but are not the result of cerebral hypoperfusion*.

Since there are so many different causes of TLOC, it is important to have an overview of the various possibilities. These possibilities have been the subject of other chapters in this book. With this background, practitioners should consider each presentation carefully, beginning with a detailed medical history and eyewitness observations; without these latter two items as a starting point, physicians may resort to a wasteful 'shotgun diagnostic approach', ordering tests for all disorders that may possibly cause TLOC (and as experience teaches, even testing for some that do not).

Goals

The goals of this chapter are to:
- provide a framework for syncope as part of the larger group of conditions causing TLOC;
- discuss nonsyncope disorders associated with real TLOC;
- discuss disorders with apparent TLOC; and
- provide help with disentangling the clues.

A framework

Transient loss of consciousness (TLOC), if taken at face value, may result from many disorders including concussion of the brain, hypoglycemia, intoxication,

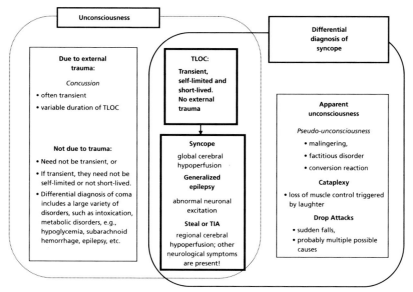

TLOC=transient loss of consciousness (of any etiology)

Figure 23.1 Schematic depicting the clinical relationship among 'unconsciousness', 'transient loss of consciousness (TLOC)', and 'syncope'. Syncope falls within the category of TLOC, but other conditions do as well, so the two terms (TLOC, syncope) are not synonymous. TLOC is defined by four elements (transient, self-limited, short-lived, and no external causative trauma). Although syncope belongs in this group, it is also defined by loss of cerebral perfusion.

subarachnoid hemorrhages, and others that do not really resemble syncope that much; there are too many differences in clinical presentation.

Disorders that do mimic syncope obviously have TLOC in common, but several other features as well:
• A short duration, of usually not more than a few minutes (coma does not belong in the same list as syncope).
• TLOC must be self-limited (conditions requiring resuscitation do not usually cause confusion with syncope).
• TLOC should not be due to external trauma to the head. (This is mainly to exclude a concussion that can easily be differentiated from the other causes of TLOC in the vast majority of cases, but also other conditions (e.g. intracranial bleed) that are caused by some internal process in the patient rather than due to an external cause). Of course, trauma may occur as a consequence of TLOC (e.g. injury due to a TLOC-initiated fall).

Bearing these points in mind, we may define TLOC as a *transient, short-lived, and self-limited loss of consciousness not due to an external traumatic cause*. By its very nature, this means that doctors usually do not see patients during TLOC but only afterwards. Most clues to select the precise cause of TLOC in a given patient will therefore have to be unearthed through careful history-taking.

In some cases, the basis for syncope may be readily apparent. For instance, TLOC in a nervous young girl immediately following ear piercing: this is almost certainly a case of neurally mediated reflex syncope. Note that while an external factor plays a part here, it is only a *trigger*; the *cause* of the unconsciousness is cerebral hypoperfusion, which is of an internal rather than external nature. Another example is TLOC accompanied by first unilateral and then generalized jerking movements in a known epileptic: this should be considered an epileptic seizure, unless there are overwhelming arguments for something else. Then again, what does one do with someone who had a 'spell' or 'attack' in a busy shopping center, in whom 'some jerks' were reported but for whom otherwise no eyewitness account is available? Epilepsy? Syncope? Especially in the elderly it may not even be possible to establish that consciousness was indeed lost; all that is clear is that there was an attack of some sort in which consciousness *seemed to have been* lost.

This chapter will not only deal with nonsyncope disorders causing TLOC but will also go into disorders in which consciousness is only apparently lost (Figure 23.1). However, before doing so, we may consider which entities are encountered by changing some of the items in the list of criteria that define TLOC; altering any one of them changes the list of possible disorders. How about an elderly woman, living alone, who has a bump on the head and little recollection of events? The bump might be due to a syncope-related fall or the unconsciousness might also have been the result of head trauma caused by stumbling. If we cannot be certain whether the head trauma was the cause rather than the result of unconsciousness, we have to consider TLOC as well as a concussion. Another series of disorders come into play when the items 'short-lived' or 'transient' are altered. In such cases, metabolic disorders, intoxication, and other neurological disorders including structural cerebral damage, will have to be considered. Figure 23.1 shows the results of these mental exercises.

Real, nonsyncope TLOC
Epilepsy
Epilepsy is, like syncope, clinically characterized by (usually) transient (usually) short-lived attacks of a (usually) self-limited nature. For some, the word 'seizure' is limited to epileptic attacks, while for others, particularly in the United Kingdom, it may denote attacks from other causes as well (sometimes including syncope!). Here, the word 'seizure' will be used exclusively as a synonym for 'epileptic attack'. From this point on, there may be two important differences from syncope. The first is that the pathophysiology is totally different and the second is that consciousness need not be lost.

Epilepsy is due to aberrant functioning of neural networks. Somehow they escape their normal firing pattern. The result is uncontrolled firing of cortical neurons. What this does to the patient is simply the result of which functions are governed by the misbehaving neurons. Thus, any cortical function may appear as a result of epilepsy. Hence, seizures may take the form of

Table 23.1 Classification of epilepsy (shortened).

Partial seizures (seizures beginning locally)
A Simple partial seizures (consciousness not impaired).
   Attacks may be motor, sensory, psychic, or autonomic in nature.
B Complex partial seizures (with impairment of consciousness).
   In such cases, consciousness may be altered at the start of the attack but this may also
      develop during it.
C Partial seizures with secondary generalization.

Generalized seizures (bilaterally symmetric and without local onset)
A Absence seizures
B Myoclonic seizures
C Clonic seizures*
D Tonic seizures*
E Tonic–clonic seizures*
F Atonic seizures*

Unclassified epileptic seizures
This category is used when there are inadequate or incomplete data to use the other two
   groups.

Forms of epilepsy that are relevant in the differential diagnosis of syncope are noted by
an asterisk (*).

simple movements, but sensations affecting any sense, emotions, thoughts, and complex behavior patterns may also be due to epilepsy. The brain area that functions abnormally often changes in the course of an attack and this is reflected in a changing clinical expression. For instance, the textbook aura in which the patient experiences a strange sensation welling upwards from the abdomen, or senses a strange smell or unprovoked fear, signifies that only a small portion of the cortex is actually out of control. If the abnormal activity spreads to motor areas, movements may be seen which, depending on the spread of abnormal activity over the cortex may first affect one limb or body side or affect all limbs simultaneously. The international classification of epilepsy (Table 23.1) is based on the concept of spreading activity: the two main categories are partial seizures, beginning locally in a part of the cortex, and generalized ones, without an apparent local beginning.

Epilepsy and consciousness
Consciousness can be defined as the awareness of one self and one's surroundings. It has 'arousal' and 'content' aspects. The first can be seen as a continuum between being wide awake and alert on the one hand and a profoundly deep coma on the other hand. The 'content' aspect describes what one is aware of. Obviously, it is not possible to apply 'content' when one is deeply unconscious. While this sounds very philosophical it does have a practical consequence, as neurologists sometimes use loss of consciousness in an equally complex sense.

For most people, unconsciousness is a total loss of alertness, that is, something resembling sleep but from which one cannot be awakened. This meaning of consciousness is restricted to the 'arousal' part of consciousness that resides either in the brainstem or in the integrity of a very large part of the cerebral cortex. Loss of consciousness is then always associated with the ability to control one's posture, that is, to remain upright. Unconsciousness thus leads to falls (if one is initially upright). Generalized epileptic seizures (Table 23.1) of the tonic–clonic variety disrupt the function of the entire cortex and are therefore a prime syncope mimic.

Some disorders affect the 'content' aspect of consciousness. The best examples of such states of altered consciousness are also found in epilepsy, in the form of 'absence' seizures in children and complex partial seizures in adults. Patients during such attacks may blink and stare. They may have 'automatisms', such as chewing or lip movements. During complex partial seizures, patients may carry out fairly complex but aimless acts, such as replacing objects. Patients usually do not respond or respond only vaguely when addressed. They normally remain upright, however, and this feature is enough to cancel them out as syncope mimics. The reason to mention them here is that neurologists sometimes use the phrase 'loss of consciousness' for this state, with the risk of causing confusion with the common meaning of unconsciousness that implies falling down and lying down unresponsively. The formal way of labeling consciousness in these conditions is to call it 'altered' or 'impaired' (but not 'lost').

Types of epilepsy that may mimic syncope
Returning to differential diagnosis, there are a number of forms of epilepsy (Table 23.1) to consider for purposes of differentiating them from syncope. These are subdivided according to the type of movement.

'Myoclonic' refers to bilateral jerks, alone or in short series, usually without impairment of consciousness; this type need not concern us. 'Tonic' here refers to the body and limbs being held in a stiff position, usually with the limbs extended. 'Clonic' refers to coarse, large-scale, and powerful jerking movements of the arms and legs. These are usually synchronized over the body. 'Tonic–clonic' refers to a succession of stiffness and movements. During the tonic phase, the patient may utter a cry and may keel over like a falling log. Thereafter massive synchronous jerking movements occur. These gradually decrease in frequency and severity. This scenario lasts for a period of varying length, but usually only about a minute (estimates of bystanders are usually much longer than the actual duration). Finally, 'atonic' seizures, as the name suggests, are not accompanied by movements of any kind. Nevertheless, control over postural muscles is lost. Patients fall limply to the floor with flaccid muscles. Such attacks often last only long enough to cause a fall and then it may not be clear whether consciousness was lost. Attacks may, however, last for 1 min or longer and are then accompanied by unconsciousness. These attacks can certainly resemble syncope, but luckily for differential diagnosis they are rare and almost exclusively seen in children with learning difficulties or other neurological abnormalities.

It should be understood that both stiffness and jerking movements may definitely occur in syncope. Both have been observed in intentionally provoked syncope (using the so-called 'mess trick'). Most subjects were then seen to fall limply to the floor, but a minority fell rather stiffly to the floor in a manner resembling epilepsy. Jerking movements occurred in no less than 90% of cases; this observation is extremely important as both lay people and most medical and paramedical personnel commonly assume that jerking movements equal epilepsy. Luckily, the movements differed from those seen in epilepsy: in syncope, the movements were smaller and not synchronous over various parts of the body. The difference from the much more massive and synchronous clonic movements can be used to diagnostic advantage. Although most eyewitnesses may not be able to describe the movements they have seen in much detail, they are often able to choose between the two types of movement, if a doctor mimics them. It should be noted that jerking movements probably do not occur in 90% of all syncope attacks: in fainting blood donors, the movements were only seen in as few as 12% of patients. The extreme and very sudden cessation of blood flow in the mess trick may account for the difference.

There are additional aspects that may help to ascribe jerks to either syncope or epilepsy. In syncope, jerks follow the fall, and never precede it, as may occur in epilepsy. If the jerks are unilateral at any moment during the attack, epilepsy is more likely than syncope. And finally, if the jerks start before consciousness is lost epilepsy is quite likely (Tables 23.2–23.6 list a series of diagnostic clues).

Triggers in syncope and epilepsy
Epileptic attacks are usually not provoked by evident triggers. However, certain types of epilepsy, such as absences and complex partial seizures, tend not to appear during times of high activity. In contrast, many types of syncope are related to specific circumstances or triggers. For instance, the triggers that evoke the abnormal reflex in classic vasovagal syncope are well known. These may include pain, fear, or anxiety. Only syncope due to arrhythmia regularly occurs under various circumstances without any recognizable common ground; in fact, lack of this during evaluation should alert the physician to think of arrhythmia (provided syncope is likelier than epilepsy on other grounds).

'Reflex epilepsy' is often triggered by specific stimuli. The most common type is visually induced epilepsy: repeated visual stimuli may provoke an attack. A classical example is the sun flickering through the trees but video games may now be more relevant. Nonspecific startling sounds may also cause epilepsy. Finally, there is a wide array of other triggers that may induce epilepsy; this includes music (often restricted to a specific song), mental activity (again often restricted to a highly specific activity, such as arithmetic),

Table 23.2 History in TLOC: events prior to the attack.

Posture	
Lying	Reflex syncope and autonomic failure less likely, otherwise all possible causes are possible
Standing	Reflex syncope and autonomic failure (in that case occurrence related to duration of standing)
Activity	
Standing up	Autonomic failure (in that case occurrence related to duration of standing)
Micturition, defecation	Reflex syncope
Protracted coughing	Reflex syncope
Swallowing	Reflex syncope including carotid sinus hypersensitivity
Predisposing factors	
After a meal	Autonomic failure, particularly in the elderly
Head movements, pressure on the neck, shaving	Carotid sinus hypersensitivity
Fear, pain, stress	Reflex syncope (classic vasovagal variant)
During physical exercise	Cardiac: structural cardiopulmonary disease
Directly after cessation of physical exercise	Autonomic failure
During exercise of the arms	Steal syndrome
Palpitations	Cardiac arrhythmia
Startling (e.g. alarm clock)	Prolonged QT syndrome
Seeing flashing light	Epilepsy with photosensitivity
Sleep deprivation	Epilepsy
None; attacks appear to occur randomly	Epilepsy or cardiac: arrhythmia
Laughter	Cataplexy
Heat	Reflex syncope, autonomic failure

Note: These items have been gathered from several sources, and were ordered according to the course of events in an attack, ending with antecedent disorders. For most of the items not enough information is available to evaluate their utility in terms of sensitivity and specificity.

Table 23.3 History in TLOC: events at the onset of the attack.

Nausea, sweating, pallor	Autonomic activation: reflex syncope
Pain in shoulders, neck (coat-hanger pattern)	Ischemia of local muscles: autonomic failure
Rising sensation from abdomen, unpleasant smell or taste, or other phenomena specific to subject but recurring over attacks	Epileptic aura

Table 23.4 History in TLOC: events during the attack.

Fall	
Keeling over, stiff	Tonic phase epilepsy, rarely syncope
Flaccid collapse	Syncope (all variants)
*Movements**	
Beginning before the fall	Epilepsy
Beginning after the fall	Epilepsy, syncope
Symmetric, synchronous	Epilepsy
Asymmetric, asynchronous	Syncope, may be epilepsy
Beginning at onset of unconsciousness	Epilepsy
Beginning after onset of unconsciousness	Syncope
Lasting less than about 15 s	Syncope more likely than epilepsy
Lasting for 30 s to minutes	Epilepsy
Restricted to one limb or one side	Epilepsy
Other aspects	
Automatisms (chewing, smacking, blinking)	Epilepsy
Cyanotic face	Epilepsy
Eyes open	Epilepsy as likely as syncope
Tongue bitten	Epilepsy
Head consistently turned to one side	Epilepsy
Incontinence	Epilepsy as likely as syncope

*The word clonic is in everyday use restricted to epilepsy, while the word myoclonus is used for the movements in syncope as well as for certain types of epilepsy and to describe postanoxic movements (perhaps these share the same pathophysiology with syncopal myoclonus). The word 'convulsions' is best reserved for epilepsy. 'Myoclonic jerks' has little connotation with a specific cause and is preferable to avoid jumping to conclusions.

Table 23.5 History in TLOC: events after the attack.

Nausea, sweating, pallor	Autonomic activation: syncope
Clearheaded immediately on regaining consciousness	Syncope, may occur in epilepsy
Confused during minutes after regaining consciousness	Epilepsy
Aching muscles (not to be confused with local bruises)	Epilepsy
Palpitations	Cardiac: arrhythmia
Chest pain	Cardiac: ischemia

hot water baths, eating, reading, etc. Usually, it takes repeated occurrences of such events for patients and doctors to become aware of the association. Most triggers that can evoke reflex epilepsy do not evoke any type of syncope and should therefore not cause much diagnostic confusion. One exception may be important: startling auditory stimuli may both cause epilepsy and syncope in the prolonged QT syndrome; both conditions are very rare, though.

Table 23.6 History in TLOC: antecedent disorders.

Recent start or change of medication	Autonomic failure, may be arrhythmia
History of heart disease	Cardiac: arrhythmia or structural cardiac disease
Parkinsonism	Autonomic failure (primary type)
History of epilepsy	Epilepsy
Psychiatric history	May be psychogenic, but remember to check for autonomic failure due to medication!
Occurrence of sudden death in family members	Arrhythmia, specifically prolonged QT syndrome
Metabolic disorders (e.g. diabetes)	Real, noncirculatory TLOC or autonomic failure (secondary)
Use of medication (antihypertensives, antiangina, antidepressives, phenothiazines, antiarrhythmics, diuretics)	Autonomic failure due to medication or hypovolemia; arrhythmia

Steal syndrome

'Steal' refers to the condition in which a stenosis or occlusion of an artery causes such a low blood pressure beyond the stenosis that blood flow is diverted from another artery to flow into the low-pressure region. This presupposes that there are preexisting connections between the 'donor' artery and the poststenotic 'acceptor' artery. The best-known example is a stenosis of the subclavian artery, in which the poststenotic artery receives an additional blood supply through the ipsilateral vertebral artery. Blood in that artery then flows down instead of upwards. Blood flows into that vertebral artery through the basilar artery, itself supplied through either the other vertebral artery or, through Willis' circle primarily supplied by the carotid system.

Do 'steal syndromes' cause syncope? This is certainly possible, as the vertebrobasilar system may be hard pressed to keep both the arm and the brainstem and occipital lobes supplied with blood. Indeed, symptoms attributed to vertebrobasilar steal include vertigo, diplopia, blurred vision, and cranial nerve dysfunction, but also 'syncope' or 'drop attacks' may occur. Strictly speaking, TLOC resulting from steal should not be labeled as 'syncope', as it is not due to a *global* but to a *regional* cerebral hypoperfusion. If there are several signs or symptoms implicating the brainstem, the diagnosis is not difficult. It is unfortunately unknown how often an isolated TLOC without any brainstem signs or symptoms results from a steal phenomenon. The following considerations may help.

A blood pressure difference between the arms or complaints of claudication of one arm may point towards the presence of a steal phenomenon. However the presence of 'steal' does not mean that any transient ischemic attacks (TIAs) or TLOC may be ascribed to it. In fact, slightly more than half (54%) of the patients with a proven steal phenomenon have no clinical symptoms at all.

Of the patients who do, only about one-half have symptoms restricted to the vertebrobasilar region; the rest have carotid or combined symptoms. Pathologic and longitudinal studies have shown that infarctions of the vertebrobasilar artery apparently do not, or hardly ever, occur in this condition, meaning that it may be seen as a rather benign condition. It has gradually become clear that TIAs in a patient with steal only occur if there is atherosclerosis in other extracranial arteries as well. Physicians should therefore be wary of ascribing any TIA, let alone isolated TLOC, to a documented steal phenomenon. This holds true especially if the TIA involves the carotid territory.

In short, the chances that TLOC without any brainstem signs are due to subclavian steal are probably very small. Having said that, complaints may be ascribed to steal with more likelihood if they are clearly associated with exercise of one arm; under such circumstances the increased demands of the arm may decrease brainstem flow to below critical levels. Note that this concerns the left arm much more often than the right.

Apparent TLOC

Whether this category can mimic syncope largely depends on the quality of the account of the events, as given by the patient or an eyewitness. Two factors are particularly important for history-taking: true loss of consciousness is absolutely incompatible with actively staying upright and must be associated with amnesia for the event. Here, we will discuss disorders in which loss of consciousness is not present although it may appear to be so, as well as some conditions commonly but incorrectly thought to be accompanied by loss of consciousness. We will discuss cataplexy, psychiatric causes, hyperventilation, TIAs, and drop attacks.

Cataplexy

The symptom cataplexy occurs for all practical purposes only in the context of the disease narcolepsy. Although cataplexy is not widely known orrecognized, it is not particularly rare. Cataplexy refers to loss of muscle tone due to emotions, particularly laughter. In contrast to vasovagal syncope, pain, fear and anxiety are not strong triggers. Startle may provoke cataplexy, but over a series of attacks it is never the only trigger, or the most common one. According to most textbooks, patients suddenly slump to the ground with complete paralysis. Partial attacks are, however, more common. These can be restricted to dropping of the jaw and sagging or nodding of the head. Attacks may develop slowly enough to allow the patient to stagger and break the fall before he or she comes to lie on the floor. In effect, such attacks look rather 'unreal' and 'psychogenic', which they are not. Complete attacks look like syncope in that the patient is unable to respond at all, although he or she is completely conscious and aware of what is going on. The presence of consciousness can in fact only be assessed later through the absence of amnesia. Although narcolepsy may start with cataplexy, this is rare. Faced with laughter-related attacks, physicians should ask for the presence of excessive daytime sleepiness, narcolepsy's main symptom. When in doubt, refer to a neurologist: the condition is well treatable.

Psychiatry and syncope

Although the term 'psychogenic syncope' may be found in the literature, authors probably mean 'psychogenic pseudo-syncope' (see also Chapter 18). Otherwise there would have to be a way to shut down cerebral perfusion through a mental process (none exists). In a broader sense, 'psychogenic' should be treated with much caution when dealing with epidemiologic or individual studies on real or apparent TLOC. Often, the diagnosis of 'psychogenic' relies on exclusion of other causes rather than on a positive ground or on a careful psychiatric examination. Estimates of how often attacks are 'psychogenic' should therefore be viewed with caution. On this somewhat shaky basis, we may discuss several entities touching on psychiatry.

Pseudo-unconsciousness is not a common term. Here, it denotes that patients act as if they are unconsciousness while they are not. This is not uncommon in emergency rooms. In the *DSM-IV*, the standard psychiatric diagnostic manual, a distinction is made between three entities:

1 In 'conversion disorder' patients show unexplained somatic symptoms at a time when psychologic factors are also apparent. In the past, it was thought this action was due to represented suppressed problems, was not under voluntary control, and that patients were unaware of the psychogenic origin of the complaint; the *DSM-IV* now shies away from any explanation (see also Chapter 18),

2 a 'factitious disorder' means that patients intentionally pretend to be ill in order to assume the sick role,

3 in 'malingering' they do the same as in factitious disorder, but to gain some other advantage, such as avoiding some task or duty.

These three forms look alike from a somatic point of view, so we will focus on how to distinguish them from true unconsciousness.

Usually, a state of pseudo-unconsciousness will probably have lasted too long for it to be confused with syncope, so the differential diagnosis is one of coma rather than of syncope. Still, similar states may occur during consultation or tilt-table testing, so it is important to know a few tell-tale features that help differentiate them from true unconsciousness. First of all, there should be no gross abnormalities during a neurologic examination, except for a lack of responsiveness. Although such patients lie relaxed with their eyes shut their muscle tone differs from that of truly unconscious subjects, resulting in a nonflaccid posture of the limbs, recognizable to trained eyes. There may be a tendency to sudden and active closure of the eyes when these are opened passively. When a lifted limb is let go it may hesitate shortly in midair before it starts to fall. Likewise, the patient's hand held above the face and let go will not drop onto the face but will just miss it. There may be reflexive gaze movements or the eyes may be turned upwards, downwards, or consistently away from the observer. Such patients may show an incredible ability to suppress any response to pain, so this has little value for the diagnosis. A slightly more invasive test concerns ice-water irrigation of the ears, producing an eye deviation in comatose subjects but a lively nystagmus in awake ones. Note that 'tricks' as described here should not be used to hold a patient in contempt as a fraud, but simply to restore communication, allowing the problem to be addressed. Remarks made to others in the patient's hearing range that such states 'usually pass quickly' may be more helpful than a confrontational approach.

During a tilt-table test, apparent unconsciousness with intact blood pressure and heart rate may indicate a feigned or conversive response. However, there are other ways to lose consciousness than through abnormalities of the systemic circulation, so this is not enough to establish pseudo-unconsciousness. This requires features as outlined earlier or, even better, the documentation that there are no functional cerebral disturbances on an electroencephalogram (EEG): if the EEG does not change while consciousness is apparently being lost, true unconsciousness is ruled out.

Psychogenic attacks such as described earlier can mimic syncope, but there is another type that mimics epilepsy. The difference probably depends on the absence or presence of convulsive movements, giving rise to 'pseudo-syncope' as well 'pseudo-seizures'. Pseudo-seizures are sometimes labeled as 'non epileptic attack disorder' (NEAD) in epileptology papers. To the mind of the author, this is an unfortunate term, as it states what it is not (epilepsy) instead of what it is (psychogenic). Taken literally, syncope falls under the NEAD heading, which is about as useful as labeling epilepsy as a 'nonsyncopal attack disorder'.

Hyperventilation

Hyperventilation is not the same as the 'hyperventilation syndrome', and the 'hyperventilation syndrome' does not occur at all in the *DSM-IV*. 'Hyperventilation' simply refers to breathing more than metabolic needs warrant. This leads to a series of physiologic events, including hypocapnia, constriction of cerebral vessels, and reduced cerebral blood flow. As such, the act of hyperventilation could certainly contribute to syncope or theoretically even cause it. Lightheadedness and tingling fingers or toes may with good reason be seen as physiologic manifestations of breathing too much and do not necessarily indicate psychologic factors. This does not hold for a large variety of other complaints, such as anxiety, fear, or various other somatic-sounding phenomena, that may occur together under stressful circumstances and that are often bundled together as the 'hyperventilation syndrome'.

Within the term 'hyperventilation syndrome' is the assumption that hyperventilation is evoked by stress, and that the resulting overbreathing and hypocapnia cause the complaints. However, a series of intriguing studies have called this concept into question. Experiments in which hyperventilating subjects were supplied with extra CO_2 to make them normocapnic suggest that many complaints were in fact not linked to hypocapnia. The matter has not however been completely resolved, however. Overbreathing can at least contribute to the complaints, even if it is not at their root. The particular set of complaints may be found in the *DSM-IV* under 'panic disorder'.

Can hyperventilation cause syncope? As noted earlier, the resulting reduction of cerebral perfusion might contribute to syncope, but it is at present unknown whether or not hyperventilation on its own can cause syncope. An argument against this is that one of the first effects of impaired consciousness would probably be that voluntary control over ventilation is lost. Autonomic circuits, taking over, would immediately end hyperventilation and thereby restore consciousness. Theoretically, syncope could still ensue if this resumption of normal control would lag significantly behind the constriction of cerebral vessels. A perhaps likelier association between hyperventilation and syncope is that the anxiety in a panic attack evokes both hyperventilation as a stress response, as well as a vasovagal reflex syncope. The only exceptions are those with clear and documented autonomic failure: hyperventilation can cause hypotension in such cases, aggravating orthostatic hypotension.

In patients without autonomic failure, it seems prudent to consider hyperventilation as a physiologic phenomenon that might at most increase the chances of syncope due to other processes, but does not cause it on its own. Also, keep in mind that the term 'hyperventilation syndrome' may be a misnomer because that particular constellation of complaints does not necessarily require the act of hyperventilation.

Syncope in psychiatric patients

Nonpsychiatrists may tend to label complaints of patients with a psychiatric history as 'psychogenic'. As we have seen, the three psychiatric disorders resembling syncope are conversion, factitious disorders, and malingering. There is no reason to suppose that these occur overly often in major psychiatric diseases such as depression, schizophrenia, and bipolar disorder, any more than they would in many somatic diseases. Note that true syncope may, however, occur with increased frequency in these disorders, due to medication causing orthostatic hypotension, (i.e. secondary autonomic failure) or cardiac arrhythmias. Main culprits are phenothiazines, tricyclic antidepressives, and monoamine oxidase inhibitors. Rather than turning to the 'blind-alley' approach of labeling attacks in such patients as 'psychogenic', a careful history should determine whether the attacks fit the pattern of syncope in autonomic failure. If so, a revision of medication may be called for.

Transient ischemic attacks

As a rule, TIAs do not cause attacks of TLOC. The majority of TIAs affect the territory of one carotid artery. When this happens, a large variety of neurologic functions may be lost, but consciousness is not foremost among them. As has been said, loss of consciousness points to a severe loss of function of the brainstem or a very large portion of the cortex. In patients with a massive stroke of one hemisphere and additional damage, consciousness may indeed be lowered, so we may theoretically expect that this can also occur in a TIA. This is not a common presentation however, and the accompanying impressive loss of hemispheric function with hemiparesis as the most obvious feature rules out any chance that this can be mistaken for syncope, in which only consciousness is lost, and no other neurologic function.

The same reasoning applies for vertebrobasilar TIAs. Here, consciousness may be supposed to be affected more often than in a carotid TIA, but it is not likely that loss of consciousness would be the only feature of such TIAs. Ataxia, dysarthria, paresis, hemianopia, and a variety of other signs predominate in vertebrobasilar TIAs. This knowledge should affect the choice of any additional investigations in patients with TLOC without accompanying neurologic deficits: ultrasound studies of cerebral vessels are not indicated.

Drop attacks
The term 'drop attack' is one of the vaguest and least helpful in medical terminology. A conservative approach to deal with it would be to reserve it for a specific clinical phenomenon without attributing any specific cause to it. The phenomenon would then be a very short-lasting attack in which a patient suddenly falls without any warning and without any other feature whatsoever. The attacks last for too short a time for patients to be certain whether there was any loss of consciousness. Commonly, they remember landing on the floor so any loss of conscience would have to be extremely short, if it existed at all. Apart from possible injuries and being startled, patients have nothing else to tell about the attacks. When used in this sense, a variety of disorders come into play as possible causes of this phenomenon. Unfortunately, many researchers use the term as a substitute for a particular cause. Several will be discussed.

First, the term 'drop attacks' was coined in 1974 to describe a syndrome in which the individual 'dropped' without loss of consciousness. The attacks occurred in middle-aged people and more often in women. Patients often bruised their knees. There were no other features and patients did not develop other signs or symptoms. This may be the best use of the term, also known in French as 'blue knee disease'. Second, the term is also used to describe 'astatic' or 'atonic' epileptic seizures. In such cases, the attacks may last longer than described above. They are accompanied by specific EEG abnormalities. These attacks occur in the context of myoclonic attacks in young children. Third, the term 'drop attacks' was used to describe episodes of falling in patients with Ménière's disease. Short-lived disturbances of the vestibular system may have caused sudden disequilibrium, described as being 'pushed' by patients. Finally, some authors appear to use 'drop attacks' simply as a substitute for unexplained falling. In this sense, the term has no advantage over 'falling' itself, which at least carries no connotation of any specific cause.

Disentangling the clues: considerations for various specialists

For medical specialists, it is daunting, if not impossible, to step over the borders of one's speciality and consider a differential diagnosis mixing neurological, cardiac, psychiatric, and internal medicine disorders. In truth, however, this conundrum does not occur that often, suggesting that the initial assignment to a speciality-based category usually works well. When errors are made, the patient will usually have moved on to a specialist, who now has to move up one step in the hierarchy of disorders, that is, from epilepsy or syncope to TLOC.

The best approach is to see whether anything was missed in the history of the TLOC episodes. A thorough step-by-step history of as many attacks as possible needs to be taken from both patients and any eyewitnesses. To help with this, pointers from various sources have been compiled (Tables 23.2–23.6). More specific advice may be directed by neurologists and cardiologists, who often see each others' patients. Note that both have a similar problem: in episodic cardiac rhythm disturbances as well as in epilepsy, interictal abnormalities need not be present on the ECG or the EEG. The problem is not unlike fishing: you can only be certain that there are fish when one is caught; until then, the presence of fish cannot be excluded. To avoid misunderstanding test results, the presence or absence of any clinical attacks during long-term ECG or EEG recordings should always be mentioned in the reports.

What if you are a neurologist?

The most obvious mistake in this case was that a patient with syncope was referred as having epilepsy. The initial judgment was probably to blame for the mistake, in which myoclonic jerks were interpreted as epileptic clonic movements. Note that the difference can indeed be difficult to distinguish, and that an eyewitness may understandably be hard pressed to give a detailed description of a very impressive and apparently life-threatening event. When a neurologist suspects syncope, a division into the main categories must be made. Reflex syncope and autonomic failure in the form of orthostatic hypotension may be treated by neurologists and do not necessarily require cardiologic expertise. However the one form that must never be missed is syncope due to cardiac disease, in view of the high associated mortality. Neurologists should therefore know how to differentiate between the main categories (Table 23.2). The difficulty increases if there was only one event and if the EEG does not show clear epileptiform abnormalities. An erroneous diagnosis of epilepsy may profoundly affect quality of life: consider the loss of driving a car, the burden of being labeled an 'epileptic', and side-effects that include drowsiness, weight gain, and even malformed children. Withholding antiepileptic medication can therefore be warranted until more evidence in favor of epilepsy is gained. If there are epileptiform abnormalities on the EEG, one should keep in mind that there is a chance of about 1% that the EEG is falsely abnormal, and that there are several normal EEG phenomena that may be mistaken as 'epileptiform'. In case of repeated attacks history-taking should focus on a trigger pattern and on features such as postictal confusion that may help differentiate between types of TLOC. The absence of any recognizable trigger pattern is compatible with epilepsy but should also raise suspicions of rhythm disturbances.

What if you are a cardiologist?
Here, the reverse situation applies: as it is gradually becoming better known that syncope may be associated with myoclonic jerks, there is now a chance that epilepsy may be mistaken for syncope. Table 23.2 may be helpful in selecting a proper cause. In the case of a single attack, the history should determine what to do. If there are features suggesting epilepsy, such as prolonged confusion, referral is warranted. In the case of repeated attacks a pattern should be sought. If none is found, epilepsy is possible and should be investigated.

What if you are an emergency room physician?
As doctors in emergency rooms are among the first to see a patient with TLOC, they are less likely than others further up the chain to suffer from others' faulty diagnoses. A possible danger is relying too much on overly quick associations made by passers-by or paramedical personnel. The real challenge for the emergency room physician is not to reach a faulty diagnosis oneself, and in this respect the greatest danger is to jump too quickly to a specific syndrome instead of starting at the root, that is, TLOC. It is probably wise to consider diagnostic actions from three angles:
1 always expect the common (reflex syncope, epilepsy),
2 be wary of the dangerous (cardiac syncope), and
3 consider whether any tests need to be carried out now or after referral.

What if you are a general practitioner?
General practitioners face the same problem as emergency room physicians, with two differences: they do not have a hospital's array of tests at their immediate disposal and see more patients in whom no further action is necessary. The task of correctly picking out the dangerous conditions is therefore less easy, while the danger of letting them go undetected is greater. More than any other physician, general practitioners must therefore be skilled in taking a detailed TLOC history.

What if you are a pediatrician?
The array of disorders causing TLOC in children differs from that in adults. Cardiac causes are rare and the types of epilepsy affecting children differ from those in adults. Some forms of epilepsy, such as absence epilepsy or Rolandic attacks, hardly ever affect adults. The terminology of syncope is even more confusing in children than in adults. There are two types of breath-holding spells, 'pallid' and 'cyanotic'. 'Pallid breath-holding spells', also called 'reflex anoxic seizures', are the same form of reflex syncope that is called vasovagal

syncope in adolescents and adults. The nature of cyanotic breath-holding spells
is not quite clear; hyperventilation or a Valsalva maneuver may be to blame.

In small children, common triggers for reflex syncope are a fall or bumping
the head. The resulting unconsciousness does not ensue immediately, proving
that it was not due to brain trauma but to emotion caused by the attack. As in
adults, the presence of a trigger is very important in deciding between epilepsy
and syncope.

Summary

'Syncope' does not have the same meaning as TLOC. In this chapter several key points were addressed. In undetermined attacks, thinking or talking
about 'unexplained syncope' limits thinking to syncope, while 'TLOC' does
not. Further, all that shakes is not epilepsy. While syncope is commonly
triggered, epilepsy is usually not. Beware of medication-induced orthostatic
hypotension in subjects with a psychiatric history. 'Psychogenic syncope' is
an impossibility, but 'psychogenic pseudosyncope' certainly occurs. The complaints in the 'hyperventilation syndrome' do not necessarily require the act
of hyperventilation. If loss of consciousness is not accompanied by signs or
symptoms suggesting dysfunction of the brainstem or a hemisphere, then a
TIA or steal syndrome is highly unlikely.

Additional reading

Benbadis SR. The problem of psychogenic symptoms: is the psychiatric community in
denial? *Epilepsy Behav* 2005; **6**: 9–14.
Commission on classification and terminology of the international league against
epilepsy. Proposal for revised classification of epilepsies and epileptic syndromes.
Epilepsia 1989; **30**: 389–399.
DSM-IV. Diagnostic and statistical manual of mental disorders. American Psychiatric
Association. Washington 1994.
Hornsveld HK, Garssen B, Dop MJ, van Spiegel PI, de Haes JC. Double-blind placebo-
controlled study of the hyperventilation provocation test and the validity of the
hyperventilation syndrome. *Lancet* 1996; **348**: 1584–1588.
Lempert T, Bauer M, Schmidt D. Syncope: a videometric analysis of 56 episodes of
transient cerebral hypoxia. *Ann Neurol* 1994; **36**: 233–237.
Taylor CL, Selman WR, Ratcheson RA. Steal affecting the central nervous system.
Neurosurg 2002; **50**: 679–689.
Thijs RD, Benditt DG, Mathias CJ, Schondorf R, Sutton R, Wieling W, van Dijk JG.
Unconscious confusion – a literature search for definitions of syncope and related
disorders. *Clin Auton Res* 2005; **15**: 35–39.

Section five:
Selected references since 1990

Key selected references

(primarily published since 1990 and organized by principal topic)

Guidelines/task force statements/consensus statements

Brignole M, Alboni P, Benditt DG *et al.* Guidelines on management (diagnosis and treatment) of syncope – Update 2004. *Europace* 2004; **6**: 467–537.

Department of Health. *Improving services for people with epilepsy.* Department of Health Action Plan in response to the National Clinical Audit of Epilepsy-related Death. London: Department of Health, 2003. Available from: URL: http://www.dh.gov.uk.

Bernstein AD, Daubert JC, Fletcher R *et al.* The revised NASPE/BPEG generic code for antibradycardia, adaptive-rate, and multisite pacing. *PACE* 2002; **25**: 260–264.

Flink R, Pedersen B, Guekht AB *et al.* Guidelines for the use of EEG methodology in the diagnosis of epilepsy. International League Against Epilepsy: commission report. Commission on European Affairs: Subcommission on European Guidelines. *Acta Neurol Scand* 2002; **106**: 1–7.

Gregoratos G, Abrams J, Epstein AE *et al.* ACC/AHA/NASPE 2002 guideline update for implantation of cardiac pacemakers and antiarrhythmia devices: summary article. *Circulation* 2002; **106**: 2145–2161.

Priori SG, Aliot E, Blomstrom-Ludqvist C *et al.* Task Force on Sudden Cardiac Death. European Society of Cardiology. Summary of recommmendations. *Europace* 2002; **4**: 3–18.

Guideline for the prevention of falls in older persons. American Geriatrics Society, British Geriatrics Society, and American Academy of Orthopaedic Surgeons Panel on Falls Prevention. *J Am Geriatr Soc* 2001; **49**: 664–672.

Haverkamp W, Breithardt G, Camm AJ *et al.* The potential for QT prolongation and proarrhythmia by non-antiarrhythmic drugs: clinical and regulatory implications. Report on a Policy Conference of the European Society of Cardiology. *Eur Heart J* 2000; **21**: 1216–1231.

Crawford MH, Bernstein SJ, Deedwania PC *et al.* ACC/AHA Guidelines for Ambulatory Electrocardiography. *J Am Coll Cardiol* 1999; **34**: 912–948 (Executive summary and recommendations. *Circulation* 1999; **100**: 886–893).

Gilman S, Low PA, Quinn N *et al.* Consensus statement on the diagnosis of multiple system atrophy. *J Neurol Sci* 1999; 163; 94–98.

Petch MC. Driving and heart disease. Task Force Report. Prepared on behalf of the ESC Task Force. *Eur Heart J* 1998; **19**: 1165–1177.

Linzer M, Yang E, Estes M *et al.* Clinical Guideline. Diagnosing syncope. Part 1: Value of history, clinical examination, and electrocardiography. *Ann Intern Med* 1997; **126**: 989–996.

Linzer M, Yang E, Estes M *et al.* Clinical Guideline. Diagnosing syncope. Part 2: Unexplained syncope. *Ann Intern Med* 1997; **127**: 76–86.

Royal College of Physicians. *Adults with poorly controlled epilepsy: Clinical guidelines for treatment & Practical tools for aiding epilepsy management.* July 1997. ISBN 1 86016 062 X. Code 15113 002.

Benditt DG, Ferguson DW, Grubb BP *et al.* Tilt table testing for assessing syncope. ACC expert consensus document. *J Am Coll Cardiol* 1996; **28**: 263–275.

Epstein AE, Miles WM, Benditt DG *et al.* Personal and public safety issues related to arrhythmias that may affect consciousness: implications for regulation and physician recommendations. *Circulation* 1996; **94**: 1147–1166.

The Consensus Committee of the American Autonomic Society and the American Academy of Neurology. Consensus statement on the definition of orthostatic hypotension, pure autonomic failure, and multiple system atrophy. *Neurology* 1996; **46**: 1470.

DSM IV. *Diagnostic and statistical manual of mental disorders.* American Psychiatric Association. Washington 1994.

Breithardt G, Cain ME, El-Sherif N *et al.* Standards for analysis of ventricular late potentials using high resolution or signal-averaged electrocardiography. A statement by a Task Force Committee between the European Society of Cardiology, the American Heart Association and the American College of Cardiology. *Eur Heart J* 1991; **12**: 473–480.

Commission on classification and terminology of the international league against epilepsy. Proposal for revised classification of epilepsies and epileptic syndromes. *Epilepsia* 1989; **30**: 389–399.

Pathophysiology of syncope

Grubb BP. Neurocardiogenic syncope and related disorders of orthostatic intolerance. *Circulation* 2005; **111**: 2997–3006.

Giese AE, Li V, McKnite S, Sakaguchi S, Ermis C, Samniah N, Benditt DG. Impact of age and blood pressure on the lower arterial pressure limit for maintenance of consciousness during passive upright posture in healthy vasovagal fainters: preliminary observations. *Europace* 2004; **6**: 457–462.

Gisolf J, van Lieshout JJ, van Heusden K, Pott F, Stok WJ, Karemaker JM. Human cerebral venous outflow pathway depends on posture and central venous pressure. *J Physiol* 2004; **560**: 317–327.

Gisolf J, Westerhof BE, Van Dijk N, Wesseling KH, Wieling W, Karemaker JM. Sublingual nitroglycerin used in routine tilt testing provokes a cardiac output-mediated vasovagal response. *J Am Coll Cardiol* 2004; **44**: 588–593.

Gisolf J, Wilders R, Immink RV, van Lieshout JJ, Karemaker JM. Tidal volume, cardiac output and functional residual capacity determine end-tidal CO(2) transient during standing up in humans. *J Physiol* 2004; **554**: 579–590.

Mathias CJ. Disorders of the autonomic nervous system. In WG Bradley, RB Daroff, GM Fenichel, Jancovich J, (eds). *Neurology in Clinical Practice.* 3rd edn. Butterworth-Heinemann, Boston, 2004: 2403–2240.

Mathias CJ. Role of autonomic evaluation in the diagnosis and management of syncope. *Clinical Autonomic Research* 2004, **14**: S1, 45–54.

Mathias CJ. Autonomic diseases – clinical features and laboratory evaluation. *J Neurol Neurosurg Psychiatry* 2003; **74**: 31–41.

Mathias CJ. Autonomic diseases – management. *J Neurol Neurosurg Psychiatry* 2003; **74**: 42–47.

Van Lieshout JJ, Wieling W, Karemaker JM, Secher NH. Syncope, cerebral blood velocity and oxygenation. *J Appl Physiol* 2003; **94**: 833–848.

Goldstein DS, Robertson D, Esler M, Straus SE, Eisenhofer G. Dysautonomias: Clinical disorders of the autonomic nervous system. *Ann Int Med* 2002; **137**: 753–763.

Mathias CJ, Bannister R (eds). *Autonomic Failure: A Textbook of Clinical Disorders of the Autonomic Nervous System.* 4th ed, Oxford University Press, Oxford, 2002.

Mathias CJ. To stand on one's own legs. *Clin Med* 2002; **2**: 237–245.

Mukai S, Lipsitz LA. Orthostatic hypotension. *Clin Geriatr Med* 2002; **18**: 253–268.

Wieling W, Halliwill JR, Karemaker JM. Orthostatic intolerance after space flight (Editorial). *J Physiol* 2002; **538**: 1.

Mathias CJ, Deguchi K, Schatz I. Observations on recurrent syncope and presyncope in 641 patients. *Lancet* 2001; **357**: 348–353.

Omboni S, Smit AA, van Lieshout JJ *et al.* Mechanisms underlying the impairment in orthostatic intolerance after nocturnal recumbency in patients with autonomic failure. *Clin Sci* 2001; **101**: 609–618.

Harms MPM, Collier W, Wieling W, Lenders JWM, Secher NH, van Lieshout JJ. Cerebral blood flow velocity and oxygenation in patients with neurogenic orthostatic hypotension during orthostic stress. *Stroke* 2000; **31**: 1608–1614.

Schondorf R, Wieling W. Vasoconstrictor reserve in neurally mediated syncope. *Clin Auton Res* 2000; **10**: 53–56.

Hainsworth R. Syncope and fainting: classification and pathophysiological basis. In: Mathias CJ, Bannister R, eds. *Autonomic Failure. A textbook of clinical disorders of the autonomic nervous system.* 4th edn. Oxford University Press, Oxford, 1999: 428–436.

Robertson RM, Medina E, Shah N, Furlan R, Mosqueda-Garcia R. Neurally mediated syncope: pathophysiology and implications for treatment. *Am J Med Sci* 1999; **317**: 102–109.

Smit AAJ, Halliwill JR, Low PA, Wieling W. Topical Review. Pathophysiological basis of orthostatic hypotension in autonomic failure. *J Physiol* 1999; **519**: 1–10.

Wieling W, van Lieshout JJ, ten Harkel ADJ. Dynanmics of circulatory adjustments to head up tilt and tilt back in healthy and sympathetically denervated subjects. *Clin Sci* 1998; **94**: 347–352.

Blanc JJ, L'Heveder G, Mansourati J *et al.* Assessment of newly recognized association: carotid sinus hypersensitivity and denervation of sternocleidomastoid muscles. *Circulation* 1997; **95**: 2548–2551.

Tea SH, Mansourati J, L'Heveder G, Mabin D, Blanc JJ. New insights into the pathophysiology of carotid sinus syndrome. *Circulation* 1996; **93**: 1411–1416.

El-Sayed H, Hainsworth R. Relationship between plasma volume, carotid baroreceptor sensitivity and orthostatic tolerance. *Clin Sci* 1995; **88**: 463–470.

Hainsworth R, El Bedawi KM. Orthostatic tolerance in patients with unexplained syncope. *Clin Auton Res* 1994; **4**: 239–244.

Lempert T, Bauer M, Schmidt D. Syncope: A videometric analysis of 56 episodes of transient cerebral hypoxia. *Ann Neurol* 1994; **36**: 233–237.

Alboni P, Menozzi C, Brignole M *et al.* An abnormal neural reflex plays a role in causing syncope in sinus bradycardia. *J Am Coll Cardiol* 1993; **22**: 1130–1134.

Brignole M, Gianfranchi L, Menozzi C *et al.* Role of autonomic reflexes in syncope associated with paroxysmal atrial fibrillation. *J Am Coll Cardiol* 1993; **22**: 1123–1129.

Rowell LB. *Human Cardiovascular Control.* Oxford University Press, New York, 1993. 117–136.

Leitch JW, Klein GJ, Yee R *et al.* Syncope associated with supraventricular tachycardia: An expression of tachycardia or vasomotor response. *Circulation* 1992; **85**: 1064–1071.

Minaker KL, Meneilly GS, Young JB *et al.* Blood pressures, pulse and neurohumeral responses to nitroprusside induced hypotension in normotensive men. *J Gerontol Med Sci* 1991; **46**: M151–154.

Van Lieshout JJ, Wieling W, Karemaker JM, Eckberg D. The vasovagal response. *Clin Sci* 1991; **81**: 575–586.

Wahba MMAE, Morley CA, Al-Shamma YMH, Hainsworth R. Cardiovascular reflex responses in patients with unexplained syncope. *Clin Sci* 1989; **77**: 547–553.

Hainsworth R, Al-Shamma, Yns H. Cardiovascular responses to upright tilting in healthy subjects. *Clin Sci* 1988; **74**; 17–22.

Shannon RP, Wei JY, Rosa RM *et al.* The effect of age and sodium depletion on cardiovascular response to orthostasis. *Hypertension* 1986; **8**: 438–443.

Lipsitz LA. Nyquist P, Wei JY, Rowe JW. Postprandial reduction in blood pressure in the elderly. *N Engl J Med* 1983; **309**: 81–83.

Jansen R, Penterman BJM, Van Lier HJT, Hoefnagels WHL. Blood pressure reduction after oral glucose loading and its relation to age, blood pressure and insulin. *Am J Cardiol* 1982; **60**: 1087–1091.

Wollner L, McCarthy ST, Soper NDW, Macy DJ. Failure of cerebral autoregulation as a cause of brain dysfunction in the elderly. *Br Med J* 1979; **1**: 1117–1118.

Gribbin B, Pickering TG, Sleight P, Peto R. Effect of age and high blood pressure on baroreflex sensitivity in man. Circ Res 1971; **29**: 424–431.

Johnson AM. Aortic stenosis, sudden death, and the left ventricular baroreceptors. *Br Heart J* 1971; **33**: 1–5.

Sharpey-Schafer EP, Hayter CJ, Barlow ED. Mechanism of acute hypotension from fear and nausea. *Br Med J* 1958; **2**: 878–880.

Scheinberg P, Blackburn I, Rich M *et al.* Effects of aging on cerebral circulation and metabolism. *Arch Neurol Psych* 1953; **70**: 77–85.

Barcroft H, Edholm OG. On the vasodilatation in human skeletal muscle during posthaemorrhagic fainting. *J Physiol* [London] 1945; **104**: 161–175.

Barcroft H, Edholm OG, McMichael J, Sharpey-Shafer EP. Posthaemorrhagic fainting. *Lancet* 1944; **i**: 489–491.

Rossen R, Kabat H, Anderson JP. Acute arrest of cerebral circulation in man. *Arch Neurol Psychiatr* 1943; **50**: 510-528.

Epidemiology

Morag RM, Murdock LF, Khan ZA, Heller MJ, Brenner BE. Do patients with a negative Emergency Department evaluation for syncope require hospital admission? *J Emerg Med* 2004; **27**: 339–343.

Shen WK, Decker WW, Smars PA *et al.* Syncope Evaluation in the Emergency Department Study (SEEDS): a multidisciplinary approach to syncope management. *Circulation* 2004; **110**: 3636–3645.

Sun BC. Emond JA, Camargo CA Jr. Characteristics and admission patterns of patients presenting with syncope to U.S. emergency departments, 1992–2000. *Academic Emerg Med* 2004; **11**: 1029–1034.

Ganzeboom KS, Colman N, Reitsma JB, Shen WK, Wieling W. Prevalence and triggers of syncope in medical students. *Am J Cardiol* 2003; **91**: 1006–1008.

Scuffham P, Chaplin S, Legood RJ. Incidence and costs of unintentional falls in older people in the United Kingdom. *Epidemiol Community Health* 2003; **57**: 740–744.

Blanc J-J, L'Her C, Touiza A *et al.* Prospective evaluation and outcome of patients admitted for syncope over a 1 year period. *Eur Heart J* 2002; **23**: 815–820.

Soteriades ES, Evans JC, Larson MG *et al.* Incidence and prognosis of syncope. *N Engl J Med* 2002; **347**: 878–885.

Sarasin FP, Louis-Simonet M, Carballo D *et al.* Prospective evaluation of patients with syncope: a population-based study. *Am J Med* 2001; **111**: 177–184.

Ammirati F, Colivicchi F, Santini M *et al.* Diagnosing syncope in clinical practice. Implementation of a simplified diagnostic algorithm in a multicentre prospective trial – the OESIL 2 study (Observatorio Epidemiologico della Sincope nel Lazio. *Eur Heart J* 2000; **21**: 935–940.

Lewis DA, Dhala A. Syncope in the pediatric patient. The cardiologist's perspective. *Pediatr Clin North Am* 1999; **46**: 205–219.

Morichetti A, Astorino G. Epidemiological and clinical findings in 697 syncope events. *Minerva Medica* 1998; **89**: 211–220.

Feruglio GA, Perraro F. Rilievi epidemiologici sulla sincope nella popolazione generale e come causa di ricovero. *G Ital Cardiol* 1987; **17**: 11–13.

Ben-Chetrit E, Flugeiman M, Eliakim M. Syncope: a retrospective study of 101 hospitalized patients. *Isr J Med Sci Med* 1985; **21**: 950–953.

Lipsitz LA, Pluchino FC, Wei JY, Rowe JW. Syncope in an elderly institutionalized population: prevalence, incidence and associated risk. *Q J Med* 1985; **55**: 45–54.

Savage DD, Corwin L, McGee DL *et al.* Epidemiologic features of isolated syncope: The Framingham Study. *Stroke* 1985; **16**: 626–629.

Martin GJ, Adams SL, Martin HG *et al.* Prospective evaluation of syncope. *Ann Emerg Med* 1984; **13**: 499–504.

Day SC, Cook EF, Funkenstein H, Goldman L. Evaluation and outcome of emergency room patients with transient loss of consciousness. *Am J Med* 1982; **73**: 15–23.

Silverstein MD, Singer DE, Mulley A *et al.* Patients with syncope admitted to medical intensive care units. *JAMA* 1982; **248**: 1185–1189.

Murdoch BD. Loss of consciousness in healthy South African men: incidence, causes and relationship to EEG abnormality. *SA Med J* 1980; **57**: 771–774.

Lamb L, Green HC, Combs JJ, Cheesman SA, Hammond J. Incidence of loss of consciousness in 1980 Air Force personnel. *Aerospace Med* 1960; **12**: 973–988.

Dermkasian G, Lamb LE. Syncope in a population of healthy young adults. *JAMA* 1958; **168**: 1200–1207.

Economics/social costs

Sun BC, Emond JA, Camargo CA Jr. Direct medical costs of syncope-related hospitalizations in the United States. *Am J Cardiol* 2005; **95**: 668–671.

Winker R. Orthostatic intolerance-prevalence, diagnostic management and its significance for occupational medicine. *Wiener Klinische Wochenschrift* 2004; **116**: 40–46.

Kenny RA, O'Shea D, Walker HF. Impact of a dedicated syncope and falls facility for older adults on emergency beds. *Age Ageing* 2002; **31**: 272–275.

Ammirati F, Colivicchi F, Santini M. Diagnosing syncope in the clinical practice.Implementation of a simplified diagnostic algorithm in a multicentre prospective trial – the OESIL 2 study (Osservatorio Epidemiologico della Sincope nel Lazio). *Eur Heart J* 2000; **21**: 935–940.

Nyman J, Krahn A, Bland P, Criffiths S, Manda V. The costs of recurrent syncope of unknown origin in elderly patients. *PACE* 1999; **22**: 1386–1394.

Sutton R, Petersen ME. The economics of treating vasovagal syncope. *PACE* 1997; **20**: 849–850.

Kapoor W, Karpf M, Maher Y *et al.* Syncope of unknown origin: the need for a more cost-effective approach to its diagnostic evaluation. *JAMA* 1982; **247**: 2687–2691.

Risk stratification

Brugada P, Brugada R, Brugada J. Patients with asymptomatic Brugada electrocardiogram should undergo pharmacological and electrophysiological testing. *Circulation* 2005; **112**: 279–292.

Van Dijk N, Colman N, Dambrink JHA, Wieling W. Pilots with vasovagal sincope: Fit to fly? *Aviat, Space, Environ Med* 2003; **74**: 571–574.

Sheldon R, Rose S, Ritchie D *et al.* Historical criteria that distinguish syncope from seizures. *J Am Coll Cardiol* 2002; **40**: 142–148.

Rose MS, Koshman ML, Spreng S, Sheldon R. The relationship between health related quality of life and frequency of spells in patients with syncope. *J Clin Epidemiol* 2000; **35**: 1209–1216.

Oh JH, Hanusa BH, Kapoor WN. Do symptoms predict cardiac arrhythmias and mortality in patients with syncope? *Arch Intern Med* 1999; **159**: 375–380.

Martin TP, Hanusa BH, Kapoor WN. Risk stratification of patients with syncope. *Ann Emerg Med* 1997; **29**: 459–466.

Kapoor WN, Hanusa B. Is syncope a risk factor for poor outcomes? Comparison of patients with and without syncope. *Am J Med* 1996; **100**: 646–655.

Sheldon R, Rose S, Flanagan P, Koshman ML, Killam S. Risk factors for syncope recurrence after a positive tilt-table test in patients with syncope. *Circulation* 1996; **93**: 973–981.

Middlekauff H, Stevenson W, Stevenson L, Saxon L. Syncope in advanced heart failure: high risk of sudden death regardless of origin of syncope. *J Am Coll Cardiol* 1993; **21**: 110–116.

Kapoor W. Evaluation and outcome of patients with syncope. *Medicine* 1990; **69**: 169–175.

Nienaber CA, Hiller S, Spielmann RP, Geiger M, Kuck KH. Syncope in hypertrophic cardiomyopathy: multivariate analysis of prognostic determinants. *J Am Coll Cardiol* 1990; **15**: 948–955.

Raviele A, Proclemer A, Gasparini G *et al.* Long-term follow-up of patients with unexplained syncope and negative electrophysiologic study. *Eur Heart J* 1989; **10**: 127–132.

Kapoor W, Peterson J, Wieand HS, Karpf M. Diagnostic and prognostic implications of recurrences in patients with syncope. *Am J Med* 1987; **83**: 700–708.

Kapoor W, Karpf M, Wieand S, Peterson J, Levey G. A prospective evaluation and follow-up of patients with syncope. *New Engl J Med* 1983; **309**: 197–204.

Initial evaluation

Sheldon R. Tilt testing for syncope: a reappraisal. *Curr Opin Cardiol* 2005; **20**: 38–41.

Brignole M, Alboni P, Benditt D *et al.* Guidelines on management (diagnosis and treatment) of syncope – Update 2004. *Europace J* 2004; **6**: 467–537.

Colman N, Nahm K, van Dijk JG, Reitsma JB, Wieling W, Kaufmann H. Diagnostic value of history taking in reflex syncope. *Clin Auton Res* 2004 Oct; **1**: 37–44.

Benditt DG, Brignole M. Syncope: is a diagnosis a diagnosis? *J Am Coll Cardiol* 2003; **41**: 791–794.

Donateo P, Brignole M, Alboni P *et al.* A standardised conventional evaluation of the mechanism of syncope in patients with bundle-branch block. *Europace* 2002; **4**: 357–360.

Sheldon R, Rose S, Ritchie D *et al.* Historical criteria that distinguish syncope from seizures. *J Am Coll Cardiol* 2002; **40**: 142–148.

Alboni P, Brignole M, Menozzi C *et al.* The diagnostic value of history in patients with syncope with or without heart disease. *J Am Coll Cardiol* 2001; **37**: 1921–1928.

Farwell D, Sulke N. How do we diagnose syncope? *J Cardiovasc Electrophysiol* 2001; **13**: S9–S13.

Kapoor WH. Syncope. *N Engl J Med* 2000; **343**: 1856–1862.

Linzer M, Yang EH, Estes III M *et al.* Diagnosing syncope. Part 1: Value of history, physical examination, and electrocardiography. *Ann Intern Med* 1997; **126**: 989–996.

Calkins H, Shyr Y, Frumin H, Schork A, Morady F. The value of clinical history in the differentiation of syncope due to ventricular tachycardia, atrioventricular block and neurocardiogenic syncope. *Am J Med* 1995; **98**: 365–373.

Hoefnagels WAJ, Padberg GW, Overweg J *et al.* Transient loss of consciousness: the value of the history for distinguishing seizure from syncope. *J Neurol* 1991; **238**: 39–43.

Syncope evaluation/management unit

Bourdeaux L, Matthews L, Richards NL, SanAgustin G, Thomas P, Veltigian S. Comparative study of case management program for patients with syncope. *J Nurs Care Qual* 2005; **20**: 140–144.

Maisel WH. Specialized syncope evaluation [comment]. *Circulation* 2004; **110**: 3621–3623.

Shen WK, Decker WW, Smars PA *et al.* Syncope Evaluation in the Emergency Department Study (SEEDS): a multidisciplinary approach to syncope management. *Circulation* 2004; **110**: 3636–3645.

Brignole M, Disertori M, Menozzi C *et al.* Evaluation of Guidelines in Syncope Study group. Management of syncope referred urgently to general hospitals with and without syncope units. *Europace* 2003; **5**: 293–298.

Shaw FE, Bond J, Richardson DA *et al.* Multifactorial intervention after a fall in older people with cognitive impairment and dementia presenting to the accident and emergency department. *Br Med J* 2003; **326**: 73–77.

Croci F, Brignole M, Alboni P *et al.* The application of a standardised strategy of evaluation in patients referred to three syncope units. *Europace* 2002; **4**: 351–356.

Kenny RA, O'Shea D, Walker HF. Impact of a dedicated syncope and falls facility for older adults on emergency beds. *Age Ageing* 2002; **31**: 272–275.

Diagnostic testing

Ambulatory electrocardiography/implantable ECG recorders

Joshi AK, Kowey PR, Prystowsky EN *et al.* First experience with a mobile cardiac outpatient telemetry (MCOT) system for the diagnosis and management of cardiac arrhythmia. *Am J Cardiol* 2005; **95**: 878–881.

Krahn AD, Klein GJ, Yee R, Skanes AC. The use of monitoring strategies in patients with unexplained sincope – Role of the external and implantable loop recorder. *Clin Auton Res* 2004; **14**: 55–61.

Ross PE. Managing care through the air. *IEEE Spectrum* Dec 2004; 26–31.

Armstrong VL, Lawson J, Kamper AM, Newton J, Kenny RA. The use of an implantable loop recorder in the investigation of unexplained syncope in older people. *Age & Ageing* 2003; **32**: 185–188.

Ermis C, Zhu AX, Pham S *et al.* Comparison of automatic and patient-activated arrhythmia recordings by implantable loop recorders in the evaluation of syncope. *Amer J Cardiol* 2003; **92**: 815–819.

Menozzi C, Brignole M, Garcia-Civera R *et al.* Mechanism of syncope in patients with heart disease and negative electrophysiologic test. *Circulation* 2002; **105**: 2741–2745.

Brignole M, Menozzi C, Moya A *et al.* Mechanism of syncope in patients with bundle branch block and negative electrophysiologic test. *Circulation* 2001; **104**: 2045–2050.

Krahn A, Klein GJ, Yee R, Skanes AC. Randomized assessment of syncope trial. Conventional diagnostic testing versus a prolonged monitoring strategy. *Circulation* 2001; **104**: 46–51.

Moya A, Brignole M, Menozzi C *et al.* and ISSUE Investigators. Mechanism of syncope in patients with isolated syncope and in patients with tilt-positive syncope. *Circulation* 2001; **104**: 1261–1267.

Kurbaan AS, Erickson M, Petersen ME, Franzen AC, Stack Z, Williams T, Sutton R. Respiratory changes in vasovagal syncope. *J Cardiovasc Electrophysiol* 2000; **11**: 607–611.

Seidl K, Ramekan M, Breuning S *et al.* Diagnostic assessment of recurrent unexplained syncope with a new subcutaneously implantable loop recorder. *Europace* 2000; **2**: 256–262.

Krahn AD, Klein GJ, Yee R, Takle-Newhouse T, Norris C. Use of an extended monitoring strategy in patients with problematic syncope. Reveal Investigators. *Circulation* 1999; 26: **99**: 406–410.

Krahn A, Klein GJ, Yee R, Norris C. Final results from a pilot study with an implantable loop recorder to determine the etiology of syncope in patients with negative noninvasive and invasive testing. *Am J Cardiol* 1998; **82**: 117–119.

Linzer M, Pritchett ELC, Pontinen M, McCarthy E, Divine GW. Incremental diagnostic yield of loop electrocardiographic recorders in unexplained syncope. *Am J Cardiol* 1990; **66**: 214–219.

Bass EB, Curtiss EJ, Arena VC *et al.* The duration of Holter monitoring in patients with syncope: is 24 hours enough? *Arch Intern Med* 1990; **150**: 1073–1078.

Gibson TC, Heitzman MR. Diagnostic efficacy of 24-hour electrocardiographic monitoring for syncope. *Am J Cardiol* 1984; **53**: 1013–1017.

Tilt-table testing – clinical application, protocols, limitations

Mathias CJ. Role of autonomic evaluation in the diagnosis and management of syncope. *Clin Auton Res* 2004; **14**; 45–54.

Foglia-Manzillo G, Romano M, Corrado G *et al.* Reproducibility of asystole during head-up tilt testing in patients with neurally-mediated syncope. *Europace* 2002; **4**: 365–368.

Moya A, Brignole M, Menozzi C *et al.* and ISSUE Investigators. Mechanism of syncope in patients with isolated syncope and in patients with tilt-positive syncope. *Circulation* 2001; **104**: 1261–1267.

Brignole M, Menozzi C, Del Rosso A *et al.* New classification of hemodynamics of vasovagal syncope: beyond the VASIS classification. Analysis of the presyncopal phase of the tilt test without and with nitroglycerin challenge. Vasovagal Syncope International Study. *Europace* 2000; **2**: 66–76.

Raviele A, Giada F, Brignole M *et al.* Diagnostic accuracy of sublingual nitroglycerin test and low-dose isoproterenol test in patients with unexplained syncope. A comparative study. *Am J Cardiol* 2000; **85**: 1194–1198.

Theodorakis G, Markianos M, Zarvalis E *et al.* Provocation of neurocardiogenic syncope by clomipramine administration during the head-up tilt test in vasovagal syncope. *J Am Coll Cardiol* 2000; **36**: 174–178.

Bartoletti A, Gaggioli G, Bottoni N *et al.* Head-up tilt testing potentiated with oral nitroglycerin. A randomized trial of the contribution of a drug-free phase and a nitroglycerin phase in the diagnosis of neurally meaidted syncope. *Europace* 1999; **1**: 183–186.

Foglia Manzillo G, Giada F, Beretta S, Corrado G, Santarone M, Raviele A. Reproducibility of head-up tilt testing potentiated with sublingual nitroglycerin in patients with unexplained syncope. *Am J Cardiol* 1999; **84**: 284–288.

Ammirati F, Colivicchi F, Biffi A, Magris B, Pandozi C, Santini M. Head-up tilt testing potentiated with low-dose sublingual isosorbide dinitratte: A simplified time-saving approach for the evaluation of unexplained syncope. *Am Heart J* 1998; **135**: 671–676.

Del Rosso A, Bartoli P, Bartoletti A *et al.* Shortened head-up tilt testing potentiated with sublingual nitroglycerin in patients with unexplained syncope. *Am Heart J* 1998; **135**: 564–570.

Imholz BPM, Wieling W, Montfrans GA van, Wesseling KH. Fifty-years-experience with finger arterial pressure monitoring: Assessment of the technology. *Cardiovasc Res* 1998; **38**: 605–616.

Natale A, Sra J, Akhtar M *et al.* Use of sublingual nitroglycerin in patients with unexplained syncope. *Am Heart J* 1998; **135**: 564–570.

Voice RA, Lurie KG, Sakaguchi S, Rector TS, Benditt DG. Comparison of tilt angles and provocative agents (edrophonium and isoproterenol) to improve head-upright tilt-table testing. *Am J Cardiol* 1998; **81**: 346–351.

Gaggioli G, Bottoni N, Mureddu R *et al.* Effects of chronic vasodilator therapy to enhance susceptibility to vasovagal syncope during upright tilt testing. *Am J Cardiol* 1997; **80**: 1092–1094.

Fitzpatrick AP, Lee RJ, Epstein LM, Lesh MD, Eisenberg S, Sheinman MM. Effect of patient characteristics on the yield of prolonged baseline head-up tilt testing and the additional yield of drug provocation. *Heart* 1996; **76**: 406–411.

Kapoor WN, Fortunato M, Hanusa SH, Schulberg HC. Psychiatric illnesses in patients with syncope. *Am J Med* 1995; **99**: 505–512.

Morillo CA, Klein GJ, Zandri S, Yee R. Diagnostic accuracy of a low-dose isoproterenol head-up tilt protocol. *Am Heart J* 1995; **129**: 901–906.

Moya A, Permanyer-Miralda G, Sagrista-Sauleda J *et al.* Limitations of head-up tilt test for evaluating the efficacy of therapeutic interventions in patients with vasovagal syncope: results of a controlled study of etilefrine versus placebo. *J Am Coll Cardiol* 1995; **25**: 65–69.

Natale A, Aktar M, Jazayeri M *et al.* Provocation of hypotension during head-up tilt testing in subjects with no history of syncope or presyncope. *Circulation* 1995; **92**: 54–58.

Raviele SA, Menozzi C, Brignole M *et al.* Value of head-up tilt testing potentiated with sublingual nitriglycerin to assess the origin of unexplained syncope. *Am J Cardiol* 1995; **76**: 267–272.

Kapoor WN, Smith M, Miller NL. Upright tilt testing in evaluating syncope: a comprehensive literature review. *Am J Med* 1994; **97**: 78–88.

McIntosh SJ, Lawson J, Kenny RA. Intravenous cannulation alters the specificity of head-up tilt testing for vasovagal syncope in elderly patients. *Age Ageing* 1994; **63**: 58–65.

Raviele A, Gasparini G, Di Pede F *et al.* Nitroglycerin infusion during upright tilt: a new test for the diagnosis of vasovagal syncope. *Am Heart J* 1994; **127**: 103–111.

Tonnesen G, Haft J, Fulton J, Rubenstein D. The value of tilt testing with isoproterenol in determining therapy in adults with syncope and presyncope of unexplained origin. *Arch Intern Med* 1994; **154**: 1613–1617.

Blanc JJ, Mansourati J, Maheu B, Boughaleb D, Genet L. Reproducibility of a positive passive upright tilt test at a seven-day interval in patients with syncope. *Am J Cardiol* 1993 15; **72**: 469–471.

Brooks R, Ruskin JN, Powell AC *et al.* Prospective evaluation of day-to-day reproducibility of upright tilt-table testing in unexplained syncope. *Am J Cardiol* 1993; **71**: 1289–1292.

De Buitler M, Grogan EW Jr, Picone MF, Casteen JA. Immediate reproducibility of the tilt table test in adults with unexplained syncope. *Am J Cardiol* 1993; **71**: 304–307.

Grubb BP, Wolfe D, Tenesy Armos P, Hahn H, Elliot L. Reproducibility of head upright tilt-table test in patients with syncope. *PACE* 1992; **15**: 1477–1481.

Kapoor WN, Brant N. Evaluation of syncope by upright tilt testing with isoproterenol. A nonspecific test. *Ann Intern Med* 1992; **116**: 358–363.

Sheldon R, Killam S. Methodology of isoproterenol-tilt table testing in patients with syncope. *J Am Coll Cardiol* 1992; **19**: 773–779.

Sheldon R, Splawinski J, Killam S. Reproducibility of isoproterenol tilt-table tests in patients with syncope. *Am J Cardiol* 1992; **69**: 1300–1305.

Fitzpatrick AP, Theodorakis G, Vardas P, Sutton R. Methodology of head-up tilt testing in patients with unexplained syncope. *J Am Coll Cardiol* 1991; **17**: 125–130.

Almquist A, Goldenberg IF, Milstein S *et al.* Provocation of bradycardia and hypotension by isoproterenol and upright posture in patients with unexplained syncope. *N Engl J Med* 1989; **320**: 346–351.

Waxman MB, Yao L, Cameron DA, Wald RW, Roseman J. Isoproterenol induction of vasodepressor-type reaction in vasodepressor-prone persons. *Am J Cardiol* 1989; **63**: 58–65.

Kenny RA, Ingram A, Bayliss J, Sutton R Head-up tilt: a useful test for investigating unexplained syncope. *Lancet* 1986; **1**: 1352–1355.

Electrophysiological testing

Weerasooriya R, Jais P, Hocini M, *et al.* Effect of catheter ablation on quality of life of patients with paroxysmal atrial fibrillation. *Heart Rhythm* 2005; **2**: 619–623.

Seidl K, Drogemuller A, Rameken M, Schneider S, Zahn R, Senges J, Two year follow-up in 643 patients with non-invasively unexplained syncope and therapy guided by electrophysiologic study. *Zeit Kardiol* 2003; **92**: 852–861.

Menozzi C, Brignole M, Garcia-Civera R *et al.* Mechanism of syncope in patients with heart disease and negative electrophysiologic test. *Circulation* 2002; **105**: 2741–2745.

Brignole M, Menozzi C, Moya A *et al.* The mechanism of syncope in patients with bundle branch block and negative electrophysiologic test. *Circulation* 2001, **104**: 2045–2050.

Fei L, Trohman RG. Advances in cardiac electrophysiology and pacing. *Crit Care Clin* 2001; **17**: 337–364.

Link M, Kim KM, Homoud M, Estes III M, Wang P. Long-term outcome of patients with syncope associated with coronary artery disease and a non-diagnostic electro-physiological evaluation. *Am J Cardiol* 1999; **83**: 1334–1337.

Olshansky B, Hahn EA, Hartz VL, Prater SP, Mason JW. Clinical significance of syncope in the electrophysiologic study versus electrocardiographic monitoring (ESVEM) trial. *Am Heart J* 1999; **137**: 878–886.

Englund A, Bergfeldt L, Rosenqvist M. Pharmacological stress testing of the His-Purkinje system in patients with bifascicular block. *PACE* 1998; **21**: 1979–1987.

Menozzi C, Brignole M, Alboni P *et al.* The natural course of untreated sick sinus syn-drome and identification of the variables predictive of unfavourable outcome. *Am J Cardiol* 1998; **82**: 1205–1209.

Bergfeldt L, Vallin H, Rosenqvist M, Insulander P, Åström H, Nordlander R. Sinus node recovery time assessment revisited: role of pharmacological blockade of the autonomic nervous system. *J Cardiovasc Electrophysiol* 1996; **7**: 95–101.

Petrac D, Radic B, Birtic K, Gjurovic J. Prospective evaluation of infrahis second-degree AV block induced by atrial pacing in the presence of chronic bundle branch block and syncope. *PACE* 1996, **19**: 679–687.

Brignole M, Menozzi C, Bottoni N *et al.* Mechanisms of syncope caused by transient bradycardia and the diagnostic value of electrophysiologic testing and cardiovascular reflexivity maneuvers. *Am J Cardiol* 1995; **76**: 273–278.

Englund A, Bergfeldt L, Rehnqvist N, Åström H, Rosenqvist M. Diagnostic value of programmed ventricular stimulation in patients with bifascicular block: a prospective study of patients with and without syncope. *J Am Coll Cardiol* 1995; **26**: 1508–1515.

Bergfeldt L, Edvardsson N, Rosenqvist M, Vallin H, Edhag O. Atrioventricular block pro-gression in patients with bifascicular block assessed by repeated electrocardiography and a bradycardia-detecting pacemaker. *Am J Cardiol* 1994; **74**: 1129–1132.

Gaggioli G, Bottoni N, Brignole M *et al.* Progression to second or third-degree atri-oventricular block in patients electrostimulated for bundle branch block: a long-term study. *G Ital Cardiol* 1994: **24**: 409–416.

Lacroix D, Dubuc M, Kus T, Savard P, Shenasa M, Nadeau R. Evaluation of arrhythmic causes of syncope: correlation between Holter monitoring, electrophysiologic testing, and body surface potential mapping. *Am Heart J* 1991; **122**: 1346–1352.

Moazez F, Peter T, Simonson J, Mandel W, Vaughn C, Gang E. Syncope of unknown origin: clinical, noninvasive, and electrophysiologic determinants of arrhythmia induction and symptom recurrence during long-term follow-up. *Am Heart J* 1991; **121**: 81–88.

Sra J, Anderson A, Sheikh S *et al.* Unexplained syncope evaluated by electrophysiologic studies and head-up tilt testing. *Ann Intern Med* 1991; **114**: 1013–1019.

Fujimura O, Yee R, Klein G, Sharma A, Boahene A. The diagnostic sensitivity of electrophysiologic testing in patients with syncope caused by transient bradycardia. *N Engl J Med* 1989; **321**: 1703–1707.

Kaul U, Dev V, Narula J, Malhotra A, Talwar K, Bhatia M. Evaluation of patients with bundle branch block and "unexplained" syncope: a study based on comprehensive electrophysiologic testing and ajmaline stress. *PACE* 1988; **11**: 289–297.

Twidale N, Heddle W, Tonkin A. Procainamide administration during electrophysiologic study – Utility as a provocative test for intermittent atrioventricular block. *PACE* 1988; **11**: 1388–1397.

Hammill SC, Holmes DR, Wood DL *et al.* Electrophysiologic testing in the upright position: Improved evaluation of patients with rhythm disturbances using a tilt table. *J Am Coll Cardiol* 1984; **4**: 65–71.

Morady F, Higgins J, Peters R *et al.* Electrophysiologic testing in bundle branch block and unexplained syncope. *Am J Cardiol* 1984; **54**: 587–591.

McAnulty JH, Rahimtoola SH, Murphy E *et al.* Natural history of "high risk" bundle branch block. Final report of a prospective study. *N Engl J Med* 1982; **307**: 137–143.

Scheinman MM, Peters RW, Sauvé MJ *et al.* Value of the H-Q interval in patients with bundle branch block and the role of prophylactic permanent pacing. *Am J Cardiol* 1982; **50**: 1316–1322.

Dhingra RC, Palileo E, Strasberg B *et al.* Significance of the HV interval in 517 patients with chronic bifascicular block. *Circulation* 1981; **64**; 1265–1271

ATP/adenosine test

Flammang D, Benditt D, Pelleg A. Apport du test à l'adénosine-5′-triphosphate (ATP) dans l'évaluation diagnostique et l'approche thérapeutique des syncopes d'origine indéterminée (vasovagale ou neurocardiogénique). The adenosine-5′-triphosphate (ATP) test: a diagnostic tool in the management of syncope of unknown origin. Basic and clinical aspects. *Ann Cardiol et d'Angeiol* 2005; **54**: 144–150.

Flammang D, Pelleg A, Benditt DG. The adenosine triphospate (ATP) test for evaluation of syncope of unknown origin. *J Cardiovas Electrophysiol* 2005 (In Press)

Cheung JW, Stein KM, Markowitz SM *et al.* Significance of adenosine-induced atrioventricular block in patients with unexplained syncope. *Heart Rhythm* 2004; **1**: 664–668.

Donateo P, Brignole M, Menozzi C *et al.* Mechanism of syncope in patients with positive adenosine tests. *J Am Coll Cardiol* 2003; **41**:93–98.

Brignole M, Gaggioli G, Menozzi C *et al.* Clinical features of Adenosine sensitive syncope and tilt-induced vasovagal syncope. *Heart* 2000; **83**: 24–28.

Flammang D, Erickson M, Mc Carville S, Church T, Hamani D, Donal E. Contribution of head-up tilt testing and ATP testing in assessing the mechanisms of vasovagal syndrome. Preliminary results and potential therapeutic implications. *Circulation* 1999; **99**: 2427–2433.

Mittal S, Stein K, Markowitz S *et al.* Induction of neurally mediated syncope with Adenosine. *Circulation* 1999; **99**: 1318–1324.

Flammang D, Chassing A, Donal E, Hamani D, Erickson M, Mc Carville S. Reproducibility of the adenosine 5'triphosphate test in vasovagal syndrome. *J Cardiovasc Electrophysiol* 1998; **9**: 1161–1166.

Brignole M, Gaggioli G, Menozzi C *et al.* Adenosine-induced atrioventricular block in patients with unexplained syncope. The diagnostic value of ATP test. *Circulation* 1997; **96**: 3921–3927.

Flammang D, Church T, Waynberger M, Chassing A, Antiel M. Can Adenosine 5'triphosphate be used to select treatment in severe vasovagal syndrome? *Circulation* 1997; **96**: 1201–1208.

Shen WK, Hammil S, Munger T *et al.* Adenosine: potential modulator for vasovagal syncope. *J Am Coll Cardiol* 1996; **28**: 146–154.

Signal-averaged ECG and related recordings

Steinberg JS, Prystowsky E, Freedman RA *et al.* Use of the signal-averaged electrocardiogram for predicting inducible ventricular tachycardia in patients with unexplained syncope: relation to clinical variables in a multivariate analysis. *J Am Coll Cardiol* 1994; **23**: 99–106.

Winters SL, Steward D, Gomes JA. Signal averaging of the surface QRS complex predicts inducibility of ventricular tachycardia in patients with syncope of unknown origin: a prospective study. *J Am Coll Cardiol* 1987; **10**: 775–781.

Gang ES, Peter T, Rosenthal ME, Mandel WJ, Lass Z. Detection of late potentials on the surface electrocardiogram in unexplained syncope. *Am J Cardiol* 1986; **58**: 1014–1020.

Kuchar DL, Thorburn CW, Sammel NL. Signal averaged electrocardiogram for evaluation of recurrent syncope. *Am J Cardiol* 1986; **58**: 949–953.

Echocardiogaphy

Panther R, Mahmood S, Gal R. Echocardiography in the diagnostic evaluation of syncope. *J Am Soc Echocardiogr* 1998; **11**: 294–298.

Recchia D, Barzilai B. Echocardiography in the evaluation of patients with syncope. *J Gen Intern Med* 1995; **10**: 649–655.

Alam M, Silverman N. Apical left ventricular lipoma presenting as syncope. *Am Heart J* 1993; **125**: 1788–1790.

Bogaert AM, De Scheerder I, Colardyn F. Successful treatment of aortic rupture presenting as a syncope: the role of echocardiography in diagnosis. *Int J Cardiol* 1987; **16**: 212–214.

Grigg LE, Downey W, Tatoulis J, Hunt D. Benign congenital intracardiac thyroid and polycistic tumor causing right ventricular outflow tract obstruction and conduction disturbance. *J Am Coll Cardiol* 1987; **9**: 227–227.

Hoegholm A, Clementsen P, Mortensen SA. Syncope due to right atrial thromboembolism: diagnostic importance of two-dimensional echocardiography. *Acta Cardiol* 1987; **42**: 469–473.

Peters MN, Hall RJ, Cooley DA, Leachman RD, Garcia E. The clinical syndrome of atrial myxoma. *JAMA* 1974; **230**: 695–701.

Clinical trial techniques

Brignole M. Randomized clinical trials of neurally mediated syncope. *J Cardiovasc Electrophys* 2003; **14**: S64–69.

Gajek J, Zysko D, Halawa B. Controversies in the conduction and evaluation of clinical trials results for the treatment in vasovagal syncope. *Polski Merkuriusz Lekarski* 2003; **14**: 464–467.

Sheldon R, Connolly S. Vasovagal Pacemaker Study II. Second Vasovagal Pacemaker Study (VPS II): rationale, design, results, and implications for practice and future clinical trials. *Card Electrophysiol Rev* 2003; **7**: 411–415.

Steering Committee of the ISSUE 2 study. International Study on Syncope of Uncertain Etiology 2: the management of patients with suspected or certain neurally mediated syncope after the initial evaluation rationale and study design. *Europace* 2003; **5**: 317–321.

Raviele A, Giada F, Sutton R *et al.* The vasovagal Syncope and pacing (Synpace) trial: rationale and study design. *Europace* 2001; **3**: 336–341.

Sheldon R, Rose R. Components of clinical trials for vasovagal syncope. *Europace* 2001; **3**: 233–240.

Ammirati F, Colivicchi F, Santini M. Diagnosing syncope in clinical practice: implementation of a simplified diagnostic algorithm in a multicentre prospective trial. *Eur Heart J* 2000; **21**: 935–940.

Specific conditions

Neurally mediated reflex syncope
Vasovagal syncope

Colman N, Nahm K, van Dijk JG, Reitsma JB, Wieling W, Kaufmann H. Diagnostic value of history taking in reflex syncope. *Clin Auton Res* 2004; **14**: 37–44.

Alboni P, Dinelli M, Gruppillo P *et al.* Haemodynamic changes early in prodromal symptoms of vasovagal syncope. *Europace* 2002; **4**: 311–316.

Brignole M, Menozzi C, Del Rosso A *et al.* New classification of haemodynamics of vasovagal syncope: beyond the VASIS classification. Analysis of the pre-syncopal phase of the tilt test without and with nitroglycerin challenge. *Europace* 2000; **2**: 66–76.

Sutton R, Brignole M, Menozzi C *et al.* Dual-chamber pacing in treatment of neurally-mediated tilt-positive cardioinhibitory syncope. Pacemaker versus no therapy: a multicentre randomized study. *Circulation* 2000; **102**: 294–299.

Raviele A, Brignole M, Sutton R *et al.* Effect of etilefrine in preventing syncopal recurrence in patients with vasovagal syncope: a double-blind, randomized, placebo-controlled trial. The Vasovagal Syncope International Study. *Circulation* 1999; **99**: 1452–1457.

Leitch J, Klein G, Yee R, Murdick C, Teo WS. Neurally-mediated syncope and atrial fibrillation. *N Engl J Med* 1991; **324**: 495–496 (letter) dysfunction of the sinus node. *PACE* 1995; **18**: 1075–107.

Menozzi C, Brignole M, Lolli G *et al.* Follow-up of asystolic episodes in patients with cardioinhibitory, neurally mediated syncope and VVI pacemaker. *Am J Cardiol* 1993; **72**: 1152–1155.

Kapoor WN. Evaluation and management of the patient with syncope. *JAMA* 1992; **268**: 2553–2560.

Sutton R, Petersen M, Brignole M, Raviele A, Menozzi C, Giani P. Proposed classific-ation for tilt induced vasovagal syncope. *Eur J Cardiac Pacing Electrophysiol* 1992; **3**: 180–183.

Carotid sinus syndrome

Richardson DA, Bexton R, Shaw FE *et al.* How reproducible is the cardioinhibitory response to carotid sinus massage in fallers. *Europace* 2002; **4**: 361–364.

Kenny RA, Richardson DA, Steen N *et al.* Carotid sinus syndrome: a modifiable risk factor for non-accidental falls in older adults (SAFE PACE). *J Am Coll Cardiol* 2001; **38**: 1491–1496.

Parry SW, Richardson D, O'Shea D, Sen B, Kenny RA. Diagnosis of carotid sinus hyper-sensitivity in older adults: carotid sinus massage in the upright position is essential. *Heart* 2000; **83**: 22–23.

Davies AG, Kenny RA. Neurological complications following carotid sinus massage. *Am J Cardiol* 1998; **81**: 1256–1257.

Gaggioli G, Brignole M, Menozzi C *et al.* Reappraisal of the vasodepressor reflex in carotid sinus syndrome. *Am J Cardiol* 1995; **75**: 518–521.

Munro N, Mc Intosh S, Lawson J *et al.* The incidence of complications after carotid sinus massage in older patients with syncope. *J Am Geriatr Soc* 1994; **42**: 1248–1251.

Brignole M, Menozzi C. Carotid sinus syndrome: diagnosis natural history and treatment. *Eur J Cardiac Pacing Electrophysiol* 1992; **4**: 247–254.

Brignole M, Menozzi C, Lolli G, Bottoni N, Gaggioli G. Long-term outcome of paced and non paced patients with severe carotid sinus syndrome. *Am J Cardiol* 1992; **69**: 1039–1043.

Brignole M, Menozzi C, Gianfranchi L, Oddone D, Lolli G, Bertulla A. Carotid sinus mas-sage, eyeball compression and head-up tilt test in patients with syncope of uncertain origin and in healthy control subjects. *Am Heart J* 1991; **122**: 1644–1651.

Brignole M, Menozzi C, Gianfranchi L, Oddone D, Lolli G, Bertulla A. Neurally medi-ated syncope detected by carotid sinus massage and head-up tilt test in sick sinus syndrome. *Am J Cardiol* 1991; **68**: 1032–1036.

Brignole M, Menozzi C, Lolli G, Oddone D, Gianfranchi L, Bertulla A. Validation of a method for choice of pacing mode in carotid sinus syndrome with or without sinus bradycardia. *PACE* 1991; **14**: 196–203.

Brignole M, Gigli G, Altomonte F *et al.* The cardioinhibitory reflex evoked by carotid sinus stimulation in normals and in patients with cardiovascular disorders. *G Ital Cardiol* 1985; **15**: 514–519.

Miscellaneous

Calkins H, Seifert M, Morady F. Clinical presentation and long-term follow-up of athletes with exercise-induced vasodepressor syncope. *Am Heart J* 1995; **129**: 1159–1164.

Ferrante I, Artico M, Nadacci B *et al.* Glossopharyngeal neuralgia with cardiac syncope. *Neurosurgery* 1995; **36**: 58–63.

Sakaguchi S, Shultz JJ, Remole SC *et al.* Syncope associated with exercise, a manifest-ation of neurally mediated syncope. *Am J Cardiol* 1995; **75**: 476–481.

Morgan-Hughes NJ, Kenny RA, Scott CD, Dark JH, McComb JM. Vasodepressor reac-tions after orthotopic cardiac transplantation: relationship to reinnervation status. *Clin Auton Res* 1994; **4**: 125–129.

Fitzpatrick AP, Banner N, Cheng A, Yacoub M, Sutton R. Vasovagal syncope may occur after orthotopic heart transplantation. *J Am Coll Cardiol* 1993; **21**: 1132–1137.

Johnston RT, Redding V. Glossopharyngeal neuralgia associated with cardiac syncope: long term treatment with permanent pacing and carbamazepine. *Br Heart J* 1990; **36**: 58–63.

Scherrer U, Vissing S, Morgan BJ, Hanson P, Victor RG. Vasovagal syncope after infusion of a vasodilator in a heart-transplant recipient. *New Engl J Med* 1990; **322**: 602–604.

Rushton JG, Stevens JC, Miller RH. Glossopharyngeal (vagoglossopharyngeal) neuralgia. A study of 217 cases. *Arch Neurol* 1981; **38**: 201–205.

Orthostatic syncope

Jordan J. Acute effects of water on blood pressure – What do we know. *Clin Auton Res* 2002; **12**: 250–255.

Mukai S, Lipsitz LA. Orthostatic hypotension. *Clin Geriatr Med* 2002; **18**: 253–268.

Schatz IJ. Orthostatic hypotension predicts mortality. Lessons from the Honolulu heart program. *Clin Auton Res* 2002; **12**: 223–224.

Grubb BP, Kanjwal Y, Kosinski DJ. The postural orthostatic tachycardia syndrome; Current concepts in pathophysiology dignosis and management. *J Intervent Cardiac Electrophysiol* 2001; **5**: 9–16.

Omboni S, Smit AA, van Lieshout JJ, Settels JJ, Langewouters GJ, Wieling W. Mechanisms underlying the impairment in orthostatic intolerance after nocturnal recumbency in patients with autonomic failure. *Clin Sci* 2001; **101**: 609–18.

Wieling W, Harms MPM, Kortz RAM, Linzer M. Initial orthostatic hypotension as a cause of recurrent syncope: a case report. *Clin Auton Res* 2001; **11**: 269–270.

Smit AAJ, Halliwill JR, Low PA, Wieling W. Topical Review. Pathophysiological bais of orthostatic hypotension in autonomic failure. *J Physiol* 1999; **519**: 1–10.

Cardiac arrhythmias as primary cause
(see also Electrophysiologic Testing)

Long QT syndromes/Brugada syndrome

Gaita F, Giustetto C, Bianchi F *et al.* Short QT syndrome: pharmacological treatment. *J Am Coll Cardiol.* 2004; **43**: 1494–1499.

Gaita F, Giustetto C, Bianchi F *et al.* Short QT syndrome. A familial cause of sudden death. *Circulation* 2003; **108**: 965.

Alings M, Wilde A. "Brugada" syndrome. Clinical data and suggested pathophysiological mechanism. *Circulation* 1999; **99**: 666–673.

Brugada J, Brugada P, Brugada R. The syndrome of right bundle branch block ST segment elevation in V1 to V3 and sudden death – the Brugada syndrome. *Europace* 1999; **1**: 156–166.

Brugada J, Brugada P. Further characterization of the syndrome of right bundle branch block, ST segment elevation and sudden cardiac death. *J Cardiovasc Electrophysiol* 1997; **8**: 325–331.

Schwartz PJ, Zaza A, Locati EH, Moss AJ. Stress and sudden death: the case of the long QT syndrome. *Circulation* 1991; **83**: 71–80.

Syncope with myocardial ischemia

Silvetti MS, Grutter G, Di Ciommo V, Drago F. Paroxysmal atrioventricular block in young patients. *Ped Cardiol* 2004; **25**: 506–512.

Ascheim DD, Markowitz SM, Lai H, Engelstein ED, Stein KM, Lerman BB. Vasodepressor syncope due to subclinical myocardial ischemia. *J Cardiovasc Electrophysiol* 1997; **8**: 215–221.

Kovac JD, Murgatroyd FD, Skehan JD. Recurrent syncope due to complete atrioventricular block, a rare presenting symptom of otherwise silent coronary artery disease: successful treatment by PTCA. *Cathet Cardiovasc Diagn* 1997; **42**: 216–218.

Watanabe K, Inomata T, Miyakita Y *et al.* Electrophysiologic study and ergonovine provocation of coronary spasm in unexplained syncope. *Jpn Heart J* 1993; **34**: 171–182.

Havranek EP, Dunbar DN. Exertional syncope caused by left main coronary artery spasm. *Am Heart J* 1992; **123**: 792–794.

Hattori R, Murohara Y, Yui Y, Takatsu Y, Kawai C. Diffuse triple-vessel coronary artery spasm complicated by idioventricular rhythm and syncope. *Chest* 1987; **92**: 183–185.

Syncope with exercise (Neural-reflex, primary cardiac arrhythmias)

Colivicchi F, Ammirati F, Santini M. Epidemiology and prognostic implications of syncope in young competing athletes. *Eur Heart J* 2004; **25**: 1749–1753.

Fox WC. Lockette W. Unexpected syncope and death during intense physical training: evolving role of molecular genetics. *Aviat Space & Environ Med* 2003; **74**: 1223–1230.

Maron BJ. Hypertrophic cardiomyopathy. *Circulation* 2002; **106**: 2419–2421.

Kosinski D, Grubb BP, Kip K, Hahn H. Exercise-induced neurocardiogenic syncope. *Am Heart J* 1996; **132**: 451–452.

Thomson HL, Atherton JJ, Khafagi FA, Frenneaux MP. Failure of reflex venoconstriction during exercise in patients with vasovagal syncope. *Circulation* 1996; **93**: 953–959.

Calkins H, Seifert M, Morady F. Clinical presentation and long-term follow-up of athletes with exercise-induced vasodepressor syncope. *Am Heart J* 1995; **129**: 1159–1164.

Sakaguchi S, Shultz JJ, Remole SC, Adler SW, Lurie KG, Benditt DG. Syncope associated with exercise, a manifestation of neurally mediated syncope. *Am J Cardiol* 1995; **75**: 476–481.

Smith GPD, Mathias CJ. Postural hypotension enhanced by exercise in patients with chronic autonomic failure. *Q J Med* 1995; **88**: 251–256.

Byrne JM, Marais HJ, Cheek GA. Exercise-induced complete heart block in a patient with chronic bifascicular block. *J Electrocardiol* 1994; **27**: 339–342.

Osswald S, Brooks R, O'Nunain SS *et al.* Asystole after exercise in healthy persons. *Ann Intern Med* 1994; **120**: 1008–1011.

Sneddon JF, Scalia G, Ward DE, McKenna WJ, Camm AJ, Frenneaux MP. Exercise induced vasodepressor syncope. *Br Heart J* 1994; **71**: 554–557.

Arad M, Solomon A, Roth A, Atsmon J, Rabinowitz B. Postexercise syncope: evidence for increased activity of the sympathetic nervous system. *Cardiology* 1993; **83**: 121–123.

Leitch JW, Klein GJ, Yee R *et al.* Syncope associated with supraventricular tachycardia: An expression of tachycardia or vasomotor response. *Circulation* 1992; **85**: 1064–1071.

Greci ED, Ramsdale DR. Exertional syncope in aortic stenosis: evidence to support inappropriate left ventricular baroreceptor response. *Am Heart J* 1991; **121**: 603–606.

Pavlovic S, Kocovic D, Djordjevic M *et al.* The etiology of syncope in pacemaker patients. *PACE* 1991; **14**: 2086–2091.

Huycke EC, Card HG, Sobol SM, Nguyen NX, Sung RJ. Postexertional cardiac asystole in a young man without organic heart disease. *Ann Intern Med* 1987; **106**: 844–845.

Yerg JE 2d, Seals DR, Hagberg JM, Ehsani AA. Syncope secondary to ventricular asystole in an endurance athlete. *Clin Cardiol* 1986; **9**: 220–222.

Ausubel K, Furman S. The pacemaker syndrome. *Ann Intern Med* 1985; **103**: 420.

Barra M, Brignole M, Menozzi C, Sartore B, De Marchi E, Bertulla A. Exercise induced intermittent atrio-ventricular block. Three cases report. *G Ital Cardiol* 1985; **15**: 1051–1055.

Woeifel AK, Simpson RJ, Gettes LS, Foster JR. Exercise-induced distal atrio-ventricular block. *J Am Coll Cardiol* 1983; **2**: 578–582.

Neurological disorders

Wasson S, Bedi A, Singh A. Determining functional significance of subclavian artery stenosis using exercise thallium-201 stress imaging. *South Med J* 2005; **98**: 559–560,

Devuyst G, Bogousslavsky J, Meuli R, Moncayo J, de Freitas G, van Melle G. Stroke or transient ischemic attacks with basilar artery stenosis or occlusion: clinical patterns and outcome. *Arch Neurol* 2002; **59**: 567–573.

Shechter A, Stewart WF, Silberstein SD, Lipton RB. Migraine and autonomic nervous system function. A population-based, case-control study. *Neurology* 2002; **58**: 422–427.

Mathias CJ, Polinsky RJ. Separating the primary autonomic failure syndromes, multiple system atrophy, and pure autonomic failure from Parkinson's disease. In: Stern GM, ed. *Parkinson's disease: Advances in Neurology*, vol 80. Lippincott, Philadelphia, 1999: 353–361

Tonkin AL, Frewin DB. Drugs, toxins and chemicals that alter autonomic function. In: Mathias CJ, Bannister R, eds. *Autonomic failure*. 4th edn. Oxford university Press, Oxford, 1999: 527–533.

Wenning GK, Tison F, Shlomo YB, Daniel SE, Quinn NP. Multiple system atrophy: a review of 203 pathologically proven cases. *Mov Dis* 1997; **12**: 133–147.

Gosselin C, Walker PM. Subclavian steal syndrome. Existence, cinical features, diagnosis, management. *Seminars in Vasc Surg* 1996; **9**: 93–97.

Bannister R, Mathias C. Introduction and classification of autonomic disorders. In: Mathias CJ, Bannister R, eds. *Autonomic failure*. 4th edn. Oxford University Press, Oxford, 1999: xvii–xxii.

Davidson E, Rotenbeg Z, Fuchs J, Weinberger I, Agmon J. Transient ischemic attack-related syncope. *Clin Cardiol* 1991; **14**: 141–144.

Hoefnagels WA, Padberg GW, Overweg J, Roos RA, van Dijk JG, Karnphuisen HA. Syncope or seizure? The diagnostic value of the EEG and hyperventilation test in transient loss of consciousness. *J Neurol Neurosurg Psychiatry* 1991; **54**: 953–956.

Davis TL, Freemon FR. Electroencephalography should not be routine in the evaluation of syncope in adults. *Arch Intern Med* 1990; **150**: 2027–2029.

Van Donselaar CA, Geerts AT, Schimsheimer RJ. Usefullness of an aura for classification of a first generalised seizure. *Epilepsia* 1990; **31**: 529–535.

Becker AE, Becker MJ, Edwards JE. Congenital anatomic potentials for subclavian steal. *Chest* 1971; **60**: 4.

Syncope in childhood and adolescents

Steinberg LA, Knilans TK. Syncope in children: diagnostic tests have a high cost and low yield. *J Pediatr* 2005; **146**: 355–358.

Massin MM, Bourguignont A, Coremans C *et al.* Syncope in pediatric patients presenting to an emergency department. *J Pediatr* 2004; **145**: 223–228.

Stewart JM. Chronic orthostatic intolerance and the postural tachycardia syndrome (POTS). *J Pediatr* 2004; **145**: 725–730.

Wieling W, Ganzeboom KS, Saul JP. Reflex sincope in children and adolescente. *Heart* 2004; **90**: 1094–1100.

Levine MM. Neurally mediated syncope in children: results of tilt testing, treatment, and long-term follow-up. *Pediatr Cardiol* 1999; **20**: 331–335.

Lewis DA, Dhala A. Syncope in the pediatric patient. The cardiologist's perspective. *Pediatr Clin North Am* 1999; **46**: 205–219.

McLeod KA, Wilson N, Hewitt J *et al.* Cardiac pacing for severe childhood neurally mediated syncope with reflex anoxic seizures. *Heart* 1999; **82**: 721–725.

Saul JP. Syncope: etiology, management, and when to refer. *J SC Med Assoc* 1999; **95**: 385–387.

Tanaka H, Yamaguchi H, Matashima R, Tamai H. Instantaneous orthostatic hypotension in children and adolescents: a new entity of orthostatic intolerance. *Pediatric Res* 1999; **46**: 691–697.

Deal BJ, Strieper M, Scagliotti D *et al.* The medical therapy of cardioinhibitory syncope in pediatric patients. *Pacing Clin Electrophysiol* 1997; **20**: 1759–1761.

De Jong-de Vos van Steenwijk CCE, Wieling W, Harms MPM, Wesseling KH. Variability of near-fainting esponses in healthy 6–16-year-old subjects. *Clin Sci* 1997; **93**: 205–211.

Driscoll DJ, Jacobsen SJ, Porter CJ, Wollan PC. Syncope in children and adolescents. *J Am Coll Cardiol* 1997; **29**: 1039–1045.

Lenk M, Alehan , Ozme S, Celiker A, Ozer S. The role of serotonin re-uptake inhibitors in preventing recurrent unexplained childhood syncope – a preliminary report. *Eur J Pediat* 1997; **156**: 747–750.

Lewis DA, Zlotocha J, Henke L, Dhala A. Specificity of head-up tilt testing in adolescents: effect of various degrees of tilt challenge in normal control subjects. *J Am Coll Cardiol* 1997; **30**: 1057–1060.

McHarg ML, Shinnar S, Rascoff H, Walsh CA. Syncope in childhood. *Pediatr Cardiol* 1997; **18**: 367–371.

Daliento L, Turrini P, Nava A *et al.* Arrhythmogenic right ventricular cardiomyopathy in young versus adult patients: similarities and differences. *J Am Coll Cardiol* 1995; **25**: 655–664.

De Jong-de Vos van Steenwijk CCE, Wieling W, Harms MP, Wesseling KH. Incidence and hemodynamics of near-fainting in healthy 6–16 year old subjects. *JACC* 1995; **25**: 1615–1621.

Michaelsson M, Jonzon A, Riesenfeld T. Isolated congenital complete atrioventricular block in adult life. *Circulation* 1995; **92**: 442–449.

Lucet V, Grau F, Denjoy I *et al.* Long term course of catecholaminergic polymorphic ventricular tachycardia in children. Apropos of 20 cases with an 8 year-follow-up. *Arch Pediatr* 1994; **1**: 26–32.

O'Marcaigh AS, MacLellan-Tobert SG, Porter CJ. Tilt-table testing and oral metoprolol therapy in young patients with unexplained syncope. *Pediatrics* 1994; **93**: 278–283.

Garson A Jr, Dick M, Fournier A *et al.* The long QT syndrome in children. An international study of 287 patients. *Circulation* 1993; **87**: 1866–1872.

Strieper MJ, Campbell RM J. Efficacy of alpha-adrenergic agonist therapy for prevention of pediatric neurocardiogenic syncope. *Am Coll Cardiol* 1993; **22**: 594–597.

Grubb BP, Temesy-Armos P, Moore J, Wolfe D, Hahn H, Elliott L. The use of head-upright tilt table testing in the evaluation and management of syncope in children and adolescents. *Pacing Clin Electrophysiol* 1992; **15**: 742–748.

Konig D, Linzer M, Pontinen M, Divine GW. Syncope in young adults: evidence for a combined medical and psychiatric approach. *J Intern Med* 1992; **232**: 169–176.

Dambrink JHA, Imholz BPM, Karemaker JM, Wieling W. Postural and transient hypotension in two healthy teenagers. *Clin Auton Res* 1991; **1**: 281–287.

Dambrink JHA, Imholz BPM, Karemaker JM, Wieling W. Circulatory adaptation to orthostatic stress in healthy 10–14 year old children investigated in a general practice. *Clin Sci* 1991; **81**: 51–58.

Perry JC, Garson A Jr. The child with recurrent syncope: autonomic function testing and beta-adrenergic hypersensitivity. *J Am Coll Cardiol* 1991; **17**: 1168–1171.

Camfield PR, Camfield CS. Syncope in childhood: a case control clinical study of the familial tendency to faint. *Can J Neurol Sci* 1990; **17**: 306–308.

Chandar JS, Wolff GS, Garson A Jr *et al.* Ventricular arrhythmias in postoperative tetralogy of Fallot. *Am J Cardiol* 1990; **65**: 655–661.

Paul T, Guccione P, Garson A Jr. Relation of syncope in young patients with Wolff–Parkinson–White syndrome to rapid ventricular response during atrial fibrillation. *Am J Cardiol* 1990; **65**: 318–321.

Pratt J, Fleisher G. Syncope in children and adolescents. *Pediatr Emerg Care* 1989; **5**: 80–82.

Lombroso CT, Lerman P. Breathholding spells (cyanotic and pallid infant syncope). *Pediatrics* 1967; **39**: 563–581.

Syncope in older adults and the elderly

Parry SW. Steen IN. Baptist M. Kenny RA. Amnesia for loss of consciousness in carotid sinus syndrome: implications for presentation with falls. *J Amer Coll Cardiol* 2005; **45**: 1840–1843.

Kenny RA. Syncope in the elderly: diagnosis, evaluation, and treatment. *J Cardiovasc Electrophysiol* 2003; **14**: S74–77.

Kurbaan AS, Bowker TJ, Wijesekera N, Franzen AC, Heaven D, Itty S, Sutton R. Age and hemodynamic responses to tilt testing in those with syncope of unknown origin. *J Am Coll Cardiol* 2003; **41**: 1004–1007.

O'Shea D. Setting up a falls and syncope service for the elderly. *Clin Geriatr Med* 2002; **18**: 269–278.

Varga E, Worum F, Szabo Z, Varga M, Lorincz I. Motor vehicle accident with complete loss of consciousness due to vasovagal syncope. *Forensic Sci Int* 2002; **130**: 156–159.

Zubcevic S, Gavranovic M, Katica V, Brajkovic D, Catibusic F. Frequency of misdiagnosis of epilepsy in a group of 79 children with diagnosis of intractable epilepsy. *Epilepsia* 2001. Proceedings of International League Against Epilepsy, 2001.

Allcock LM, O'Shea D. Diagnostic yield and development of a neurocardiovascular investigation unit for older adults in a district hospital. *J Gerontol A Biol Med Sci* 2000; **55**: M458–462.

Zaidi A, Clough P, Cooper P, Scheepers B, Fitzpatrick AP. Misdiagnosis of epilepsy: many seizure-like attacks have a cardiovascular cause. *J Am Coll Cardiol.* 2000; **36**: 181–184.

Ballard C, Shaw F, McKeith I, Kenny RA. Prevalence, assessment and associations of falls in dementia with Lewy Bodies and Alzheimers disease dementia. *Dementia* 1999; **10**: 97–103.

Smith D, Defalla BA, Chadwick DW. The misdiagnosis of epilepsy and the management of refractory epilepsy in a specialist clinic. *Q J Med* 1999; **92**: 15–23.

Ward C, McIntosh SJ, Kenny RA. Carotid sinus hypersensitivity – a modifiable risk factor for fractured neck of femur. *Age Ageing* 1999; **28**: 127–133.

Ballard C, Shaw F, McKeith, Kenny RA. High prevalence of neurocardiovascular instability in Alzheimer's disease and dementia with Lewy bodies; potential treatment implications. *Neurology* 1998; **51**: 1760–1762.

Masaki KH, Schatz IJ, Burchfiel CM *et al.* Orthostatic hypotension predicts mortality in elderly men: the Honolulu Heart program. *Circulation* 1998; **98**: 2290–2295.

Shaw FE, Kenny RA. Overlap between syncope and falls in the elderly. *Postgrad Med J* 1997; **73**: 635–639.

Shaw FE, Kenny RA. Can falls in patients with dementia be prevented. *Age Ageing* 1997; **27**: 1–7.

Hussain RM, McIntosh SJ, Lawson J, Kenny RA. Fludrocortisone in the treatment of hypotensive disorders in the elderly. *Heart* 1996; **76**: 507–509.

Ward C, Kenny RA. Reproducibility of Orthostatic Hypotension in symptomatic elderly. *Am J Med* 1996; **100**: 418–411.

Cummings SR, Nevitt MC, Browner WS *et al.* Risk factors for hip fracture in white women. Study of osteoporotic fractures research group. *New Engl J Med* 1995; **332**: 767–773.

Tinetti ME, Mendes de Leon CF, Doncette JT, Baker DI. Fear of falling and fall related efficacy. *J Gerontol* 1994; **49**: 140–147.

Tonkin A, Wing L. Effects of age and isolated systolic hypertension on cardiovascular reflexes. *Hypertension* 1994; **12**: 1083–1088.

McIntosh SJ, da Costa D, Kenny RA. Outcome of an integrated approach to the investigation of dizziness, falls and syncope in elderly patients referred to a syncope clinic. *Age Ageing* 1993; **22**: 53–58.

McIntosh SJ, Lawson J, Kenny RA. Clinical characteristics of vasodepressor, cardioinhibitory and mixed carotid sinus syndrome in the elderly. *Am J Med* 1993; **95**: 203–208.

Brignole M, Oddone D, Cogorno S *et al.* Long term outcome in symptomatic carotid sinus hypersensitivity. *Am Heart J* 1992; **123**: 687–692.

Wieling W, Veerman DP, Dambrink JHA, Imholz BPM. Disparities in circulatory adjustment to standing between young and elderly subjects explained by pulse contour analysis. *Clin Sci* 1992; **83**: 149–155.

Kenny RA, Traynor G. Carotid Sinus Syndrome – Clinical characteristics in elderly patients. *Age Ageing* 1991; **20**: 449–454.

Tonkin A, Wing LMH, Morris MJ, Kapoor V. Afferent baroreflex dysfunction and age-related orthostatic hypotension. *Clin Sci* 1991; **81**: 531–538.

Nevitt MC, Cummings SR, Kidd S. Risk factors for recurrent non syncopal falls. A prospective study. *J Am Med Ass* 1989; **261**: 2663–2667.

Robbins AS, Rubenstien LZ, Josephson KT. Predictors of falls among elderly people. Results of 2 population-based studies. *Arch Intern Med* 1989; **149**: 1628–1631.

Strasberg B, Sagie A, Herdman *et al.* Carotid sinus hypersensitivity in the carotid sinus syndrome. *Prog Cardiovasc Disease* 1989; **31**: 379–391.

Cummings SR, Nevitt MC, Kidd S. Forgetting Falls: the limited accuracy of recall of falls in the elderly. *J Am Geriatr Soc* 1988; **36**: 613–616.

Mader SL, Josephson KR, Rubenstein LZ. Low prevalence of postural hypotension among community dwelling elderly. *JAMA* 1987; **258**: 1511–1514.

Kapoor W, Snustad D, Petersen J *et al.* Syncope in the Elderly. *Am J Med* 1986 **80**: 419–428.

Lipsitz LA, Fullerton KJ. Postprandial blood pressure reduction in healthy elderly. *J Am Ger Soc* 1986; **34**: 267–270.

Murphy AL, Rowbotham BJ, Boyle RS *et al.* Carotid sinus hypersensitivity in elderly nursing home patients. *Aust N Z J Med* 1986; **16**: 24–27.

Tinnetti ME, Williams TF, Mayewski R. Fall risk index for elderly patients based on number of chronic disabilities. *Am J Med* 1986; **80**: 429–451.

Lipsitz LA, Storch HA, Winaker KL, Rowe JW. Intra-individual variability in postural blood pressure in the elderly. *Clin Sci* 1985; **69**: 337–341.

Palmer KT. Studies into postural hypotension in elderly patients. *N Z Med J* 1983; **96**: 43–45.

Strangaard S. Autoregulation of cerebral blood flow in hypertensive patients: the modifying influence of prolonged antihypertensive treatment on the tolerance of acute drug induced hypotension. *Circulation* 1976; **53**: 720–729.

Conditions mimicking syncope

Benbadis SR. The problem of psychogenic symptoms: is the psychiatric community in denial? *Epilepsy Behav* 2005; **6**: 7–14.

Savitz SI, Caplan LR. Vertebrobasilar disease. *N Engl J Med* 2005; **352**: 2618–2626.

Thijs RD, Benditt DG, Mathias CJ, Schondorf R, Sutton R, Wieling W, van Dijk JG. Unconscious confusion – a literature search for definitions of syncope and related disorders. *Clin Auton Res* 2005; **15**: 35–39.

Bergfeldt L. Differential diagnosis of cardiogenic syncope and seizure disorders. *Heart* 2003; **89**: 353–358.

Kouakam C, Lacroix D, Klug D, Baux P, Marquie C, Kacet S. Prevalence and prognostic significance of psychiatric disorders in patients evaluated for recurrent unexplained syncope. *Am J Cardiol* 2002; **89**: 530–535.

Zaidi A, Clough P, Cooper P, Scheepers B, Fitzpatrick AP. Misdiagnosis of epilepsy: Many seizure-like episodes have a cardiovascular cause. *J Am Coll Cardiol* 2000; **36**: 181–184.

Dey AB, Stout NR, Kenny RA. Cardiovascular syncope is the most common cause of drop attacks in the elderly. *Pacing Clin Electrophysiol* 1997; **20**: 818–819.

Kapoor W, Fortunato M, Hanusa BH, Schulberg HC. Psychiatric illnesses in patients with syncope. *Am J Med* 1995; **99**: 505–551.

Grubb BP, Gerard G, Wolfe DA, Samoil D, Davenport CW, Homan RW. Syncope and seizure of psychogenic origin: identification with head-upright tilt table testing. *Clin Cardiol* 1992; **15**: 839–842.

Linzer M, Pontinen M, Gold DT, Divine GW, Felder A, Brooks WB. Impairment of physical and psychosocial function in recurrent syncope. *J Clin Epidemiol* 1991; **44**: 1037–1043.

Linzer M, Felder A, Hackel A, Perry AJ, Varia I, Melville ML. Psychiatric syncope: a new look at an old disease. *Psychosomatics* 1990; **31**: 181–188.

Markush RE, Karp HR, Heyman A, O'Fallon WM. Epidemiologic study of migraine symptoms in young women. *Neurol* 1975; **25**: 430–435.

Personal and public safety issues

Bhatia A, Dhala A, Blanck Z, Deshpande S, Akhtar M, Sra AJ. Driving safety among patients with neurocardiogenic (vasovagal) syncope. *Pacing Clin Electrophysiol* 1999; **22**: 1576–1580.

Sutton R. Vasovagal syncope: prevalence and presentation. An algorithm of management in the aviation environment. *Eur Heart J* (Supp) 1999: D109–113.

Prepared on behalf of the Task Force by MC Petch. Task Force Report. Driving and heart disease. *Eur Heart J* 1998; **19**: 1165–1177.

Trappe HJ, Wenzlaff P, Grellman G. Should patients with implantable cardioverter-defibrillators be allowed to drive? Observations in 291 patients from a single center over an 11-year period. *J Intervent Cardiac Electrophys* 1998; **2**: 193–201.

Epstein AE, Miles WM, Benditt DG, Camm AJ *et al.* Personal and public safety issues related to arrhythmias that may affect consciousness: implications for regulation and physician recommendations. *Circulation* 1996; **94**: 1147–1166.

Herner B, Smedby B, Ysander L. Sudden illness as a cause of motor vehicle accidents. *Br J Int Med* 1966; **23**: 37–41.

Treatment options

Neurally mediated reflex syncope
Carotid sinus syndrome

Brignole M, Menozzi C, Gaggioli G *et al.* Effects of vasodilator therapy in patients with carotid sinus hypersensitivity. *Am Heart J* 1998; **136**: 264–268.

Grubb BP, Samoil D, Kosinski D, Temesy-Armos P, Akpunonu B. The use of serotonin reuptake inhibitors for the treatment of carotid sinus hypersensitivity syndrome unresponsive to dual chamber pacing. *PACE* 1994; **17**: 1434–1436.

Deschamps D, Richard A, Citron B, Chaperon A, Binon JP, Ponsonaille J. Hypersensibilite sino-carotidienne. Evolution a moyen et a long terme des patients traites par stimulation ventriculaire. *Arch Mal Coeur* 1990; **83**: 63–67.

Brignole M, Sartore B, Barra M, Menozzi C, Lolli G. Ventricular and dual chamber pacing for treatment of carotid sinus syndrome. *PACE* 1989; **12**: 582–590.

Brignole M, Sartore B, Barra M, Menozzi C, Lolli G. Is DDD superior to VVI pacing in mixed carotid sinus syndrome? An acute and medium-term study. *PACE* 1988; **11**: 1902–1910.

Sugrue DD, Gersh BJ, Holmes DR, Wood DL, Osborn MJ, Hammill SC. Symptomatic "isolated" carotid sinus hypersensitivity: Natural history and results of treatment with anticholinergic drugs or pacemaker. *J Am Coll Cardiol* 1986; **7**: 158–162.

Almquist A, Gornick CC, Benson DW Jr *et al.* Carotid sinus hypersensitivity: Evaluation of the vasodepressor component. *Circulation* 1985; **67**: 927–936.

Madigan NP, Flaker GC, Curtis JJ, Reid J, Mueller KJ, Murphy TJ. Carotid sinus hypersensitivity: Beneficial effects of dual-chamber pacing. *Am J Cardiol* 1984; **53**: 1034–1040.

Vasovagal syncope

Physical maneuvers/Fluid/Volume

Abe H, Kohshi K, Nakashima Y. Home orthostatic self-training in neurocardiogenic syncope. *Pacing Clin Electrophysiol* 2005; **28**: S246–248.

van Dijk N, de Bruin IG, Gisolf J *et al.* Hemodynamic effects of leg crossing and skeletal muscle tensing during free standing in patients with vasovagal syncope. *J Appl Physiol* 2005; **98**: 584–590.

Abe H, Kondo S, Kohshi K *et al.* Usefulness of orthostatic self-training for the prevention of neurocardiogenic syncope. *PACE* 2002; **25**: 1454–1458.

Kerdiet CTP, van Dijk N, Linzer M, van Lieshout JJ, Wieling W. Management of vaso-vagal syncope: Controlling or aborting faints by leg crossing and muscle tensing. *Circulation* 2002; **106**: 1684–1689.

Di Girolamo E, Di Iorio C, Leonzio L, Sabatini P, Barsotti A. Usefulness of a tilt training program for the prevention of refractory neurocardiogenic syncope in adolescents. A controlled study. *Circulation* 1999; **100**: 1798–1801.

Ector H, Reybrouck T, Heidbuchel H, Gewillig M, Van de Werf F. Tilt training: a new treatment for recurrent neurocardiogenic syncope or severe orthostatic intolerance. *PACE* 1998; **21**: 193–196.

Younoszai AK, Franklin WH, Chan DP, Cassidy SC, Allen HD. Oral fluid therapy. A promising treatment for vasodepressor syncope. *Arch Pediatr Adolesc Med* 1998; **152**: 165–168.

Pharmacologic treatment

Moore A, Watts M, Sheehy T, Hartnett A, Clinch D, Lyons D. Treatment of vasode-pressor carotid sinus syndrome with midodrine: a randomized, controlled pilot study. *J Am Geriatr Soc* 2005; **53**: 114–118.

Madrid A, Ortega I, Rebollo GJ *et al.* Lack of efficacy of atenolol for the prevention of neurally-mediated syncope in highly symptomatic population: a prospective double-blind, randomized and placebo-controlled study. *J Am Coll Cardiol* 2001; **37**: 554–557.

Perez-Lugones A, Schweikert R, Pavia S *et al.* Usefulness of midodrine in patients with severely symptomatic neurocardiogenic syncope: A randomized control study. *J Cardiovasc Electrophysiol* 2001; **12**: 935–938.

Di Girolamo E, Di iorio C, Sabatini O, Leonzio L, Barbone C, Barsotti A. Effects of paroxetine hydrochloride, a selective serotonin reuptake inhibitor, on refractory vasovagal syncope: a randomized, double-blind, placebo-controlled study. *J Am Coll Cardiol.* 1999; **33**: 1227–1230.

Raviele A, Brignole M, Sutton R *et al.* Effect of etilefrine in preventing syncopal recurrence in patients with vasovagal syncope: a double-blind, randomized, placebo-controlled trial. The Vasovagal Syncope International Study. *Circulation* 1999; **99**: 1452–1457.

Di Girolamo E, Di Iorio C, Sabatini P, Leonzio L, Barsotti A. Effects of different treatments vs no treatment on neurocardiogenic syncope. *Cardiologia* 1998; **43**: 833–837.

Iskos D, Dutton J, Scheinman MM, Lurie KG. Usefulness of pindolol in neurocardiogenic syncope. *Am J Cardiol* 1998; **82**: 1121–1124.

Ward CR, Gray JC, Gilroy JJ, Kenny RA. Midodrine: a role in the management of neurocardiogenic syncope. *Heart* 1998; **79**: 45–49.

Biffi M, Boriani G, Sabbatani P *et al.* Malignant vasovagal syncope: a randomised trial of metoprolol and clonidine. *Heart* 1997; **77**: 268–272.

Sra J, Maglio C, Biehl M, Dhala A *et al.* Efficacy of midodrine hydrochloride in neurocardiogenic syncope refractory to standard therapy. *J Cardiovasc Electrophysiol* 1997; **8**: 42–46.

Jhamb DK, Singh B, Sharda B *et al.* Comparative study of the efficacy of metoprolol and verapamil in patients with syncope and positive head-up tilt test response. *Am Heart J* 1996; **132**: 608–611.

Sheldon R, Rose S, Flanagan P, Koshman L, Killam S. Effects of beta blockers on the time to first syncope recurrence in patients after a positive isoproterenol tilt table test. *Am J Cardiol* 1996; **78**: 536–539.

Cohen MB, Snow JS, Grasso V *et al.* Efficacy of pindolol for treatment of vasovagal syncope. *Am Heart J* 1995; **130**: 786–790.

Mahanonda N, Bhuripanyo K, Kangkagate C *et al.* Randomized double-blind, placebo-controlled trial of oral atenolol in patients with unexplained syncope and positive upright tilt table test results. *Am Heart J* 1995; **130**: 1250–1253.

Kelly PA, Mann DE, Adler SW, Fuenzalida CE, Reiter MJ. Low dose disopyramide often fails to prevent neurogenic syncope during head-up tilt testing. *PACE* 1994; **17**: 573–576.

Grubb BP, Wolfe D, Samoil D, Temesy-Armos P, Hahn H, Elliott L. Usefulness of fluoxetine hydrochloride for prevention of resistant upright tilt induced syncope. *PACE* 1993; **16**: 458–464.

Muller G, Deal B, Strasburger JF, Benson DW Jr. Usefulness of metoprolol for unexplained syncope and positive response to tilt testing in young persons. *Am J Cardiol* 1993; **71**: 592–595.

Brignole M, Menozzi C, Gianfranchi L *et al.* A controlled trial of acute and long-term medical therapy in tilt-induced neurally mediated syncope. *Am J Cardiol* 1992; **70**: 339–342.

Fitzpatrick AP, Ahmed R, Williams S *et al.* A randomized trial of medical therapy in malignant vasovagal syndrome or neurally-mediated bradycardia/hypotension syndrome. *Eur J Cardiac Pacing Electrophysiol* 1991; **1**: 191–202.

Milstein S, Buetikofer J, Dunnigan A, Benditt DG, Gornick C, Reyes WJ. Usefulness of disopyramide for prevention of upright tilt-induced hypotension-bradycardia. *Am J Cardiol* 1990; **65**: 1339–1344.

Pacemaker treatment

Kinay O, Yazici M, Nazli C *et al.* Tilt training for recurrent neurocardiogenic syncope: effectiveness, patient compliance, and scheduling the frequency of training sessions. *Jap Heart J* 2004; **45**: 833–843.

Link MS, Hellkamp AS, Estes NA 3rd *et al.* MOST Study Investigators. High incidence of pacemaker syndrome in patients with sinus node dysfunction treated with ventricular-based pacing in the Mode Selection Trial (MOST). *J Am Coll Cardiol* 2004; **43**: 2066–2071.

Occhetta E, Bortnik M, Audoglio R, Vassanelli C. INVASY Study Investigators. Closed loop stimulation in prevention of vasovagal syncope. Inotropy Controlled Pacing in Vasovagal Syncope (INVASY): a multicentre randomized, single blind, controlled study. *Europace* 2004; **6**: 538–547.

Raviele A, Giada F, Menozzi C *et al.* Vasovagal Syncope and Pacing Trial Investigators. A randomized, double-blind, placebo-controlled study of permanent cardiac pacing for the treatment of recurrent tilt-induced vasovagal syncope. The vasovagal syncope and pacing trial (SYNPACE). *Eur Heart J* 2004; **25**: 1741–1748.

Wagshal AB, Weinstein JM, Weinstein O *et al.* Do the recently modified pacemaker guidelines for neurocardiogenic syncope also apply to young patients? Analysis based on five-year follow-up of Israeli soldiers with syncope and a positive tilt test. *Cardiology* 2004; **102**: 200–205.

Ammirati F, Colivicchi F, Santini M *et al.* Permanent cardiac pacing versus medical treatment for the prevention of recurrent vasovagal syncope. A multicenter, randomized, controlled trial. *Circulation* 2001; **104**: 52–56.

Raviele A, Giada F, Sutton R *et al.* The vasovagal syncope and pacing (Synpace) trial: rationale and study design. *Europace* 2001; **3**: 336–341.

Sutton R, Brignole M, Menozzi C *et al.* Dual-chamber pacing in treatment of neurally-mediated tilt-positive cardioinhibitory syncope.Pacemaker versus no therapy: a multicentre randomized study. *Circulation* 2000; **102**: 294–299.

Benditt DG. Cardiac pacing for prevention of vasovagal syncope (editorial). *J Am Coll Cardiol* 1999; **33**: 21–23.

Benditt DG, Sutton R, Gammage M *et al.* Rate-Drop Response Investigators Group. Rate-drop response cardiac pacing for vasovagal syncope. *J Intervent Cardiac Electrophys* 1999; **3**: 27–33.

Connolly SJ, Sheldon R, Roberts RS, Gent M. Vasovagal pacemaker study investigators. The North American vasovagal pacemaker study (VPS): A randomized trial of permanent cardiac pacing for the prevention of vasovagal syncope. *J Am Coll Cardiol* 1999; **33**: 16–20.

Benditt DG, Petersen M, Lurie KG, Grubb BL, Sutton R. Cardiac pacing for prevention of recurrent vasovagal syncope. *Ann Int Med* 1995; **122**: 204–209.

El-Bedawi KM, Wahbha MAE, Hainsworth R. Cardiac pacing does not improve orthostatic tolerance in patients with vasovagal syncope. *Clin Auton Res* 1995: **88**: 463–470.

Petersen MEV, Chamberlain-Webber R, Fizpatrick AP, Ingram A, Williams T, Sutton R. Permanent pacing for cardio-inhibitory malignant vasovagal syndrome. *Br Heart J* 1994; **71**: 274–281.

Samoil D, Grubb BP, Brewster P, Moore J, Temesy-Armos P. Comparison of single and dual chamber pacing techniques in prevention of upright tilt induced vasovagal syncope. *Eur J Cardiac Pacing Electrophysiol* 1993; **1**: 36–41.

Sra J, Jazayeri MR, Avitall B, Dhala A, Deshpande S, Blanck Z, Akhtar M. Comparison of cardiac pacing with drug therapy in the treatment of neurocardiogenic (vasovagal) syncope with bradycardia or asystole. *N Engl J Med* 1993; **328**: 1085–1090.

Fitzpatrick A, Theodorakis G, Ahmed R, Williams T, Sutton R. Dual chamber pacing aborts vasovagal syncope induced by head-up 60 degree tilt. *PACE* 1991; **14**: 13–19.

Miscellaneous treatment options

Pachon JC, Pachon EI, Pachon JC *et al.* "Cardioneuroablation" – new treatment for neurocardiogenic syncope, functional AV block and sinus dysfunction using catheter RF-ablation. *Europace* 2005; **7**: 1–13.

Van Dijk N, Velzeboer S, Destree-Vonk A, Linzer M, Wieling W. Psychological treatment of malignant vasovagal syncope due to bloodphobia. *PACE* 2001; **24**: 122–124.

Khurana R, Lynch J, Craig F. A novel psychological treatment for vasovagal syncope. *Clin Auton Res* 1997; **7**: 191–197.

Orthostatic syncope

Mathias CJ, Young TM. Water drinking in the management of orthostatic intolerance due to orthostatic hypotension, vasovagal syncope and the postural tachycardia syndrome. *Eur J Neurol* 2004; **11**: 613–619.

Kanjwal Y, Kosinski D, Grubb BP. The postural orthostatic tachycardia syndrome: definitions, diagnosis, and management. *Pacing Clin Electrophysiol* 2003; **26**: 1747–1757.

Wieling W, van Lieshout JJ, Hainsworth R. Extracellular fluid volume expansion in patients with posturally related syncope. *Clin Auton Res* 2002; **12**: 243–249.

Van Lieshout JJ, Ten Harkel ADJ, Wieling W. Physiological basis of treatment of orthostatic hypotension by sleeping head-up tilt and fludrocortisone medication. *Clin Auton Res* 2000; **10**: 35–42.

Mathias CJ, Kimber JR. Treatment of postural hypotension. *J Neurol Neurosurg Psychiat* 1998; **65**: 285–289.

Mtinangi BL, Hainsworth R. Early effects of oral salt on plama volume, orthostatic tolerance, and baroreceptor sensitivity in patients with syncope. *Clin Auton Res* 1998; **8**: 231–235.

Mtinangi B, Hainsworth R. Increased orthostatic tolerance following moderate exercise training in patients with unexplained syncope. *Heart* 1998; **80**: 596–600.

Low PA, Gilden JL, Freeman R, Sheng K-N, McElligott MA. Efficacy of midrodrine vs placebo in neurogenic orthostatic hypotension. *JAMA* 1997; **13**: 1046–1051.

Smit AAJ, Hardjowijono MA, Wieling W. Are portable folding chairs useful to combat orthostatic hypotension? *Ann Neurol* 1997; **42**: 975–978.

Tanaka H, Yamaguchi H, Tamai H. Treatment of orthostatic intolerance with inflatable abdominal band. *Lancet* 1997; **349**: 175.

El-Sayed H, Hainsworth R. Salt supplement increases plasma volume and orthostaic tolerance in patients with unexplained syncope. *Heart* 1996; **75**: 114–115.

Kardos A, Avramov K, Dongo A, Gingl Z, Kardos L, Rudas L. Management of severe orthostatic hypotension by head-up tilt posture and administration of fludrocortisone. *Orvosi Hetilap* 1996; **43**: 2407–2411.

Gilden JL. Midodrine in neurogenic orthostatic hypotension. *Int Angiol* 1993; **12**: 125–131.

Jankovic J, Gilden JL, Hiner BC, Brown DC, Rubin M. Neurogenic orthostatic hypotension: A double-blind placebo-controlled study with midodrine. *Am J Med* 1993; **95**: 38–48.

Wieling W, Van Lieshout JJ, Van Leeuwen AM. Physical maneuvers that reduce postural hypotension in autonomic failure. *Clin Auton Res* 1993; **3**: 57–65.

Ten Harkel ADJ, van Lieshout JJ, Wieling W. Treatment of orthostatic hypotension with sleeping in the head-up position, alone and in combination with fludrocortisone. *J Int Med* 1992; **232**: 139–145.

Van Lieshout JJ, Ten Harkel ADJ, Wieling W. Combating orthostatic dizziness in autonomic failure by physical maneuvers. *Lancet* 1992; **339**: 897–898.

McTavish D, Goa KL. Midodrine. A review of its pharmacological properties and therapeutic use in orthostatic hypotension and secondary hypotensive disorders. *Drugs* 1989; **38**: 757–777.

Maclean AR, Allen EV. Orthostatic hypotension and orthostatic tachycardia; treatment with the 'head-up' bed. *J Am Med Assoc* 1940; **115**: 2162–2167.

Cardiac arrhythmias as primary cause
Cardiac pacemakers

Trim GM, Krahn AD, Klein GJ, Skanes AC, Yee R. Pacing for vasovagal syncope after the second Vasovagal Pacemaker Study (VPS II): a matter of judgement. *Card Electrophysiol Rev* 2003; **7**: 416–420.

Lamas G, Orav EJ, Stambler B *et al.* Quality of life and clinical outcome in elderly patients treated with ventricular pacing as compared with dual-chamber pacing. *N Engl J Med* 1998; **338**: 1097–1104.

Alboni P, Menozzi C, Brignole M *et al.* Effects of permanent pacemaker and oral theophylline in sick sinus syndrome. The THEOPACE study: a randomized controlled trial. *Circulation* 1997; **96**: 260–266.

Andersen HR, Nielsen JC, Thomsen PE *et al.* Long-term follow-up of patients from a randomised trial of atrial versus ventricular pacing for sick-sinus syndrome. *Lancet* 1997; **350**: 1210–1216.

Andersen HR, Thuesen L, Bagger JP *et al.* Prospective randomised trial of atrial versus ventricular pacing in sick-sinus syndrome. *Lancet* 1994; **344**: 1523–1528.

Sgarbossa EB, Pinski SL, Jaeger FJ, Trohman RG, Maloney JD. Incidence and predictors of syncope in paced patients with sick sinus syndrome. *PACE* 1992; **15**: 2055–2060.

Lamas GA, Dawley D, Splaine K *et al.* Documented symptomatic bradycardia and symptom relief in patients receiving permanent pacemakers: an evaluation of the joint ACC/AHA pacing guidelines. *PACE* 1988; **11**: 1098.

Rosenqvist M, Brandt J, Schuller H. Long-term pacing in sick sinus node disease: effects of stimulation mode on cardiovascular morbidity and mortality. *Am Heart J* 1988; **116**: 16–22.

Implantable defibrllators

Lerecouvrex M, Ait Said M, Paziaud O *et al.* Automobile driving and implantable defibrillators. *Arch des Mal du Coeur et des Vaiss* 2005; **98**: 288–293.

Akiyama T, Powell JL, Mitchell LB, Ehlert FA, Baessler C. Antiarrhythmics versus Implantable Defibrillators Investigators. Resumption of driving after life-threatening ventricular tachyarrhythmia. *New Engl J Med* 2001; **345**: 391–397.

Steinberg JS, Beckman K, Greene HL *et al.* Follow-up of patients with unexplained syncope and inducible ventricular tachyarrhythmias: analysis of the AVID registry and an AVID substudy. Antiarrhythmics Versus Implantable Defibrillators. *J Cardiovasc Electrophysiol* 2001; **12**: 996–1001.

Fonarow G, Feliciano Z, Boyle N *et al.* Improved survival in patients with nonischemic advanced heart failure and syncope treated with an implantable cardioverter-defibrillator. *Am J Cardiol* 2000; **85**: 981–985.

Pires L, May L, Ravi S *et al.* Comparison of event rates and survival in patients with unexplained syncope without documented ventricular tachyarrhythmias versus patients with documented sustained ventricular tachyarrhythmias both treated with implantable cardioverter-defibrillator. *Am J Cardiol* 2000; **85**: 725–728.

Andrews N, Fogel R, Pelargonio G, Evans J, Prystowsky E. Implantable defibrillator event rates in patients with unexplained syncope and inducible sustained ventricular tachyarrhythmias. *J Am Coll Cardiol* 1999; **34**: 2023–2030.

Knight B, Goyal R, Pelosi F *et al.* Outcome of patients with nonischemic dilated cardiomyopathy and unexplained syncope treated with an implantable defibrillator. *J Am Coll Cardiol* 1999; **33**: 1964–1970.

Mittal S, Iwai S, Stein K *et al.* Long-term outcome of patients with unexplained syncope treated with an electrophysiologic-guided approach in the implantable cardioverter-defibrillator era. *J Am Coll Cardiol* 1999; **34**: 1082–1089.

Link MS, Costeas XF, Griffith JL *et al.* High incidence of appropriate implantable cardioverter-defibrillator therapy in patients with syncope of unknown etiology and inducible ventricular tachycardia. *J Am Coll Cardiol* 1997; **29**: 370–375.

Militianu A, Salacata A, Seibert K *et al.* Implantable cardioverter defibrillator utilization among device recipients presenting exclusively with syncope or near-syncope. *J Cardiovasc Electrophysiol* 1997; **8**: 1087–1097.

Index

Note: page numbers in *italics* refer to figures, those in **bold** refer to tables.